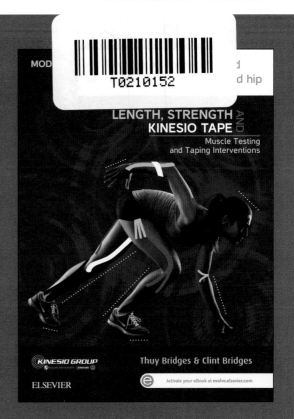

LENGTH, STRENGTH AND KINESIO TAPE

Muscle Testing and Taping Interventions

LENGTH, STRENGTH AND KINESIO TAPE

Muscle Testing and Taping Interventions

Thuy Bridges & Clint Bridges

ELSEVIER

ELSEVIER

Elsevier Australia. ACN 001 002 357
(a division of Reed International Books Australia Pty Ltd)
Tower 1, 475 Victoria Avenue, Chatswood, NSW 2067

Notice

This publication has been carefully reviewed and checked to ensure that the content is as accurate and current as possible at time of publication. We would recommend, however, that the reader verify any procedures, treatments, drug dosages or legal content described in this book. Neither the author, the contributors, nor the publisher assume any liability for injury and/or damage to persons or property arising from any error in or omission from this publication.

National Library of Australia Cataloguing-in-Publication entry

---

Bridges, Thuy, author.
    Length, strength and Kinesio tape : muscle testing and taping interventions / Thuy Bridges,
        Clint Bridges.
    9780729541930 (paperback)
    Includes index.
    Applied kinesiology.
        Musculoskeletal system--Wounds and injuries--Treatment.
        Muscle strength--Testing.
    Bridges, Clint, author.
612.76

Senior Content Strategist: Melinda McEvoy
Senior Content Development Specialists: Natalie Hunt/Elizabeth Coady
Senior Project Manager: Anitha Rajarathnam
Cover and Internals Design by Lisa Petroff
Edited by Laura Davies/Forsyth Publishing Services
Proofread by Melissa Faulkner
Index by Robert Swanson
Typeset by Midland Typesetters Pty Ltd, Australia
Printed by CTPS

DISCLAIMER

The authors of this book and videos do not dispense medical advice nor prescribe the use of the Kinesio Taping® Method as a form of treatment for medical problems or without the advice of a physician. The intent of the authors is only to offer information of a general nature to help you cooperate with your doctor in your mutual quest for good health. In the event you use any of the information in this book for yourself, you are prescribing for yourself. KTAI™ and the authors assume no responsibility for your actions.

The Kinesio® name and visual marks are protected under the copyright laws of the United States and other countries. Permissions granted within the context of this manual and videos do not extend to other uses.

Table of contents

Foreword

Kinesio Taping has been growing in popularity as a method to address many conditions that are often seen by doctors, therapists and trainers across the world.

This popularity, combined with ready access to the internet, has at times diluted the skill of assessments that are fundamental to official Kinesio Taping education.

Practitioners who want to be told what to do and how to tape as a recipe for particular musculoskeletal problems may lose the skill of assessing the fundamentals of movement. This manual brings practitioners back to the joy of basic muscle anatomy to create movement and the relevance of testing for more valuable interventions and to further probe into what creates pain and dysfunction for clients.

Testing for indicated interventions is vitally important to the success of Kinesio Taping, and any other method of treatment, for that matter. For many patients and clients, a common 'recipe' may appear satisfactory; however, for a comprehensive management of a person, it is not enough. The Kinesio Taping Method considers the person as a whole, and this book helps to determine the part of the puzzle that muscles may play in the presenting people and their conditions. The values of 'Ku, Do, Rae' are respectfully introduced to practitioners new to the concept of treating the person as a whole.

Thuy Bridges is one of the longest serving international instructors of the Kinesio Taping Method. Her skill has been to break down what can often come across as the 'art' of Kinesio Taping into the analysis and management of the basics of movement.

Length, Strength and Kinesio Tape is an excellent adjunct to the official Kinesio Taping education process. The artwork on the subjects is a masterpiece of beauty in the context of movement. It serves as a reminder of anatomy during movement and whilst the focus of the text is on the education of practitioners, this art could appear in any esteemed art school.

Practitioners trained properly in the Kinesio Taping Method will recognise the importance of testing to validate treatment interventions and also to reassess outcomes. The assessments and the prioritising of interventions minimises the risk of ineffective applications when dealing with muscular length and strength deficits. This book breaks down the skill and art of Kinesio Taping to the basic muscular mechanics for movement.

The table presented at the end of each chapter ensures that practitioners aim to be thorough with their assessment. The table is a useful reminder for practitioners on how to assess for muscles that they may not commonly treat and offers practitioners assessment skills that are linked with intervention tools. As with any skill, practitioners will start with the science of the taping process and this will eventually become an art with continued practice and reflection on what has been achieved.

It is with pride and satisfaction that I recommend *Length, Strength and Kinesio Tape* as a resource for the skilled practice of Kinesio Taping.

Dr Kenzo Kase

About the authors

Thuy Bridges, BAppSc(Phty)

Senior Physiotherapist and Director, PhysioWISE

Thuy's philosophy has always been 'There's more to fixing people than a university degree'. To be able to treat the whole person rather than an isolated limb or muscle, Thuy founded PhysioWISE Physiotherapy clinics in 2002, where she continues to practise integrating innovative methods with the tried and true ones.

Since gaining her degree in physiotherapy from the University of Sydney, Thuy has travelled the world learning advanced techniques such as Trigenics, Mulligans, Anatomy Trains, Fascial Manipulation, Muscle Energy, Dry Needling, Visceral Manipulation, Functional Movement Screening, Craniosacral techniques, Connect Therapy and of course Kinesio Taping®.

Finding and treating not only the symptomatic but also the diagnostic 'drivers' is key in genuine rehabilitation from acute and chronic conditions. This philosophy and her extensive clinical work led to the development of The Bridges Protocol which provides a diagnosis and specific intervention for otherwise 'non-specific' low-back and pelvic girdle pain. This protocol has been so effective in the PhysioWISE clinics (and for practitioners who have been exposed to it through Thuy's courses), the concepts are now being extended into other areas of the body.

Thuy is a certified practitioner and instructor in Kinesio Taping, tai chi, pilates, yoga; an Associate Instructor for Anatomy Trains, and continues to attend courses at every opportunity. Her personal goal has been to learn at least one brand new technique every year (in addition to upskilling on previously learnt techniques)—an achievement that has been maintained for more than 15 years.

Thuy was introduced to the Kinesio Taping® Method when Dr Kenzo Kase taught his first courses in Australia in 2004. Realising there was more to it than the 'latest fad' that many were writing it off as at the time, Thuy progressed through the advanced courses. Soon afterwards she started her journey as an Accredited Kinesio Taping Instructor. After teaching Kinesio Taping courses across Australasia, she wrote her own Advanced Kinesio Taping manual which was subsequently used as the basis for the Clinical Reasoning KT3 Kinesio Taping Courses taught throughout Australia, New Zealand, Scandinavia and South Africa.

When Thuy has down time from her clinical work, writing and teaching courses, collaborating on research, lecturing at universities, and working at international sporting events, she spends it with her family on adventures in Australia and abroad.

Clint Bridges

Practice Manager, PhysioWISE

Clint's early career in Engineering and Project Management led to a change in direction when he and Thuy started PhysioWISE in 2002 and he took over the Practice Management/IT/Everything-Except-Treatments role. After Thuy had been teaching courses for a few years, Clint became the Education Director for Kinesio Australia which included managing not just Thuy's courses and presentations, but those for other instructors and practitioners as well as coordinating conferences, events, lectures and all things relating to the education of Kinesio in Australia. Over the years, he has attended and assisted on around 50 full Kinesio Taping courses and has managed to pick up a thing or two which helped in his role of compiling, consistency checking, editing and reviewing the content, photos and videos for this book and the associated instructional videos.

Clint's contribution to this book is reflective of the ongoing collaboration with Thuy and other advanced practitioners in bringing high-quality education to therapists in Australia and around the world.

Reviewers

Carlos Bello, Musculoskeletal Physiotherapist APA

Physiotherapist, Physical Spinal and Physiotherapy Clinic, Dynamic Pain Care, Boronia;

Big Hands Australia, Chirnside Park

Victoria, Australia

Phil Doley, BAppSc (Physio), Cert (ortho) APAM

Principal Physiotherapist, Victor Harbor Physiotherapy

Victor Harbor, South Australia, Australia

Patricia Filby, BPhty

Senior Physiotherapist, Royal Hobart Hospital

Hobart, Tasmania, Australia

Emrys Goldsworthy, MSportsCoach, BHSc (MST)

Musculoskeletal Therapist

Red Hill Musculoskeletal Clinic, Red Hill;

Athletica Physical Health, St. Lucia

Queensland, Australia

Kate Moss, BSC Health and Sport Science (Hons), MPhty, Specialist Certificate in Paediatric Orthopaedic Physiotherapy

Sydney, New South Wales, Australia

Nicole Reinke, BSc(Hons), GradCert (Ed), Med, PhD

Lecturer in Pathophysiology, School of Health and Sport Sciences

University of the Sunshine Coast

Sippy Downs, Queensland, Australia

James Stormon, BPhty, M Health Law

Sydney, New South Wales, Australia

Peter Suffolk, BPhty, MSc

Coordinator, Student Led Physiotherapy and Physiotherapy Clinical Educator,

Faculty of Health Clinics, Health Hub, University of Canberra

Canberra, Australian Capital Territory, Australia

How to use this book

This book is designed to be an adjunct to the training of practitioners attending a accredited Kinesio Taping® course. Its intention is to fill in the gap between symptoms and intervention by providing a resource for assessment and taping techniques of muscles not covered in the official KT1 course. The text is the result of my interpretation of the teachings of recognised experts in the field of length testing and manual muscle testing, and of course the Kinesio Taping® Method.

It is my belief that this book will be of benefit to health professionals throughout their training and into their practice as it relates the joy of anatomy directly to an assessment and intervention technique. At a visual level, the artwork may help students and practitioners to identify with surface anatomy and appreciate the relationship between structures during testing. Other movement-related practitioners may also find the book helpful to analyse, interpret and intervene in movement dysfunction.

The purpose of this book is threefold:

- providing a visual aid in the identification and role of muscle structures
- offering a set of length and strength tests to highlight any deficiencies in particular muscles
- providing practitioners with a basic framework to use and reassess the application of Kinesio® Tape.

Surface anatomy for tape placement has been facilitated with artwork on the bodies of the models, and serves to remind practitioners of the value of anatomical knowledge and the relationship between structures. Basic assessments assist with identifying particular muscular deficits. For the purpose of this text, the practitioner is encouraged to prioritise the muscular taping procedures for an individual client's presentation, rather than only tape for symptoms.

By incorporating the methods in this book, the reader will be encouraged to follow a systematic approach to carry out an assessment for a given joint and to then provide a suitable intervention once an assessment is found to be positive and is prioritised for an intervention; in this case, Kinesio Taping. The taping chapters (chapters 3 to 10) are categorised by joint or area of the body: neck, shoulder, elbow, wrist and thumb, trunk, pelvis, knee and ankle. The examination is organised in a consistent fashion as the reader is taken through anatomy and examination tests designed to differentiate specific musculature and their length and

strength deficits. Coupled with a thorough history and palpation verification, the practitioner is encouraged to find the cause of a problem rather than apply a generic taping application based on a symptomatic diagnosis. The text does not explore skills to take a history or palpate, and the reader is encouraged to access other resources for this.

The examiner is then instructed on length and strength taping interventions with Kinesio Tape and reminded to re-test the intervention by using the testing procedure that indicated the taping intervention, as well as to re-evaluate by reassessing the primary movement dysfunction identified by the client.

Each chapter is concluded with a table to facilitate a systematic approach of assessment around a joint and to also remind practitioners of musculature they may still need to assess or address. The table also serves to help practitioners prioritise the muscular taping procedures for an individual client and reminds the practitioner to intervene with the relevant findings from the functional testing of the individual. Again, the emphasis is on managing the evidence provided by the individual body by considering the muscular contribution to movement dysfunction rather than intervening based on a purely symptomatic diagnosis.

The book therefore facilitates a clinical reasoning approach to assessment and utilisation of the tape based on the presentation and evidence of each individual client.

The book is not intended as a resource for case studies and is not a replacement for the comprehensiveness of training that would otherwise be provided at a training institution. As such, the framework of the book is confined to offering only one or two simple testing procedures for a given muscle. This is done so as to not over-complicate the issue and the reader is reminded of the choice that they have to substitute a test for one that they feel works better given their experience, training and the contextual constraints of the assessment process. Naturally, comprehensive tape-handling procedures cannot be fully demonstrated outside a practical course setting; however, this book can be used as an adjunct to the proper tape-handling experience gained from attending an Accredited Kinesio Taping course.

The book is designed as a teaching aid to incorporate Kinesio Taping techniques into the work of practitioners with their patients, clients or athletes as well as a resource for practitioners already employing the taping techniques. Once the information in this resource has been assimilated and the techniques practised and mastered, the practitioner will have an excellent base upon which to build their taping and treatment repertoire. Those involved in taping regularly will develop the ability to use the principles and adapt the testing and intervention techniques in this text to a myriad of situations.

This book is my first attempt at a project of this magnitude. Any feedback from readers with constructive ideas on how to improve the text would be greatly appreciated.

EVERYDAY PRACTICE

It is intended that the practitioner clinically assesses the origins of the presenting problem and conducts a thorough assessment to best determine the most accurate taping strategy to be used. Additional assessments relevant to the individual practitioner's ability, skill, training and understanding should also be used to formulate a more clear hypothesis of cause. An appropriate referral should be made when an assessment is outside the scope of practice for a Kinesio Taping practitioner.

It is wise to always ask or determine relevant functional limitations for a client. The meaningful task for a particular person is the primary movement measure for which that person has usually sought help. The changes to this task will ultimately be the goal of the treatment and whilst individual applications have their own tests, the overall treatment should be reassessed with respect to the meaningful tasks identified.

Typically a new practitioner may start with general movements at the local site of symptoms and begin an assessment around that joint. If no significant findings are made, the practitioner will look at adjacent joints for significant findings to address. The practitioner should keep in mind the severity of symptoms as the assessment findings should summate to an equivalent amount of significance.

For example: A client presents with a persistent knee pain with squat, the dysfunction is significant to the client yet the practitioner is unable to find 'positive' muscle tests. The practitioner should then conduct further tests at the knee relevant to their training. The intention should be to find significant tests to direct treatment or provide a test to reassess any intervention. If no significant tests are found at the knee, then the cause for the significant dysfunction is unlikely to be entirely at the knee and the practitioner should continue to look at other joints or structures for positive tests. The goal is to seek structures or biomechanical anomalies that would limit the recovery of the knee. It would be more appropriate to manage more significant findings at other relevant joints that affect the knee rather than managing minor muscle deficits that are found local to the knee in this scenario.

Practitioners already familiar with myofascial continuities may skip adjacent joints directly to where they believe the primary driver of a condition to be. Assessments are then conducted around the remote site and treated appropriately; practitioners are reminded that the reassessment process must always involve the local site (of perceived symptoms that are of concern to the client) to demonstrate to the client the relevance of working at a remote site.

KINESIO TAPING WITHIN THE CONTEXT OF CLIENT MANAGEMENT

It is important to understand that the application of tape may have physiological, biomechanical, neurophysiological and psychological ramifications. The taping should not be applied without taking these into account. It is not as simple as applying a piece of sticky tape or bandage over the part that hurts and hoping for the best. Indeed, improper taping or taping for no reason may predispose a client or athlete to injury or add to the severity of an existing injury (Frett & Reilly 1994).

To best serve the client, it is important for any clinician, trainer or therapist to firstly identify the needs of their client. People seek assistance in order to manage or understand a problem themselves. The choice of Kinesio Taping, and for that matter, any therapy, is dependent on the primary needs of the client. Does this person want better function, improved performance, improved endurance, improved power output or other physical changes, or do they want understanding, guidelines for self-management, or management of pain or discomfort? Are these components of function secondary to their true goal of weight loss, fitness, mental health, sport participation, stress management or some other fundamental value?

Whilst these needs cannot easily be grouped for the purpose of research and have at times been considered lower forms of evidence, they are nevertheless *the most important* measure of success as measured by the individual seeking help. They are also the measure by which the client will return for services and advocate for the ability of the service and its provider.

Without first identifying these personalised needs, it becomes very difficult for relevant goals and changes to be measured.

Kinesio Tape then becomes a tool for the practitioner to facilitate change and understanding for the individual client. The content of this text will primarily cover the management of taping applications for our fundamental understanding of muscles.

WHY MANUAL MUSCLE TESTING?

The premise for taping that is targeted over muscles firstly acknowledges that movement dysfunction or non-optimal movement strategies that lead to the presence of symptoms requiring clinician management can be a result of muscular imbalances (Kendall & McCreary 2005, Sahrmann 2002, Janda 1986). When a muscular imbalance, tissue extensibility dysfunction or motor control deficit is identified as the primary source or cause to a presenting problem, then it is appropriate for the practitioner to address these deficits. In breaking down movements to components of muscle length and strength, Kinesio Tape has the potential to be utilised with multiple paradigms of treatment.

The functional efficiency of a muscle is related to its ability to generate tension. The position in range where it generates optimal force efficiency changes to match the subsequent length shortening (Goldspink & Williams 1992). The active component of muscle tension is determined by the number of actin-myosin cross-bridges that are linked at any point in time, the sliding and shortening of these filaments generate mechanical tension that is distributed to all the elements of the cell, as well as the external extra cellular matrix via integrin contact points (Ingber 2010, Chen & Ingber 1999). The passive tension property is largely due to the elastic titin filaments which anchor the myosin chain to the Z-band as well as other connective tissue structures.

Muscles are most efficient and generate optimal force when they function in a mid-range position and have normal resting length. Muscles are less efficient and appear functionally weak when they are required to work in a shortened or lengthened position relative to the resting length because of physiological or mechanical insufficiency (Goldspink & Williams 1992). Physiological insufficiency occurs when a muscle actively shortens into its inner range where the actin filaments overlap each other. As the muscle progressively shortens, there are fewer cross-bridges able to be linked and the muscle is unable to generate optimal force. Mechanical insufficiency occurs when a muscle actively contracts in a lengthened position. In this outer range, the actin-myosin filaments do not adequately overlap; again, there is a reduced number of cross-bridges that are linked (Goldspink & Williams 1992).

When a muscle is chronically functioning at an altered length (this can be either lengthened or shortened) its length–tension relationship adapts accordingly. The position in range in which the maximal force production is achieved changes to match the new length (Goldspink & Williams 1992). The maximal tensional output is achieved in a different range and has implications on the coordination of movement and the output for muscle testing within different ranges (Grossman et al 1982). Muscles habitually short can test strong in their inner range but still be weaker than the normal control (Grossman et al 1982). It is important clinically to always assess with respect to the other limb and reflect on what is contextually 'normal' for the presenting client.

It has also been acknowledged that a muscle can be designed to be involved in more than one functional role; Hodges (2003) suggests that a muscle may have three functional roles: the control of inter-segmental motion, the control of posture and alignment, and the control and production of movement. It is possible that all of these roles are considered to be impacted on when the length–tension ratio of the muscle is altered; the shortening of a muscle to improve its function in one area may adversely affect its function in another (Gibbons 2007). The length and strength tension testing shown in this text is therefore only one testing range option available to a practitioner. A positive test with respect to the testing options provided assumes that this positive test (reflecting an altered length–tension ratio) may impact on the other roles for that muscle. Therefore, it is recommended that the reassessment of the taping intervention be done with respect to all the positive muscle tests performed, as well as the meaningful task in which the identified muscle may in fact be required to operate in a different manner to that of the muscle testing.

The placement of Kinesio Tape to restore length and strength is purposeful and with a directional and tensional significance. Motor perception is determined by neuroreceptors such as Ruffini corpuscles, Pacini corpuscles, Golgi corpuscles and free nerve endings (Schleip 2003). These neuroreceptors are activated by stretch and can only function correctly if they are embedded in tissue that is capable of lengthening (Stecco & Stecco 2009). Furthermore, the sarcomere length within any given muscle may not be uniform along its entire length and there is a necessity for micro sliding to occur at and within the muscle fibre level (Yucesoy 2009). 'Focal adhesions' can develop at actin-myosin filament anchorage sites. These grow in size when mechanical stress is increased and disassemble when the stress is dissipated (Ingber 2003). Thus the restoration of length and the process of assessment to determine where a length or strength deficit exists is fundamental to the application of Kinesio Tape to restore motor function.

The intention of Kinesio Taping to restore length and strength to the muscles primarily focuses on restoration of the functional efficiency of a muscle via stimulation of all the structures below, adjacent and related to the tape placement.

Kinesio Tape is a useful tool to help the clinician to manage specific, identified deficits within the neuro-myofascia related to the condition being managed. Where a strength or length deficit is identified, and when that deficit is disproportional to the level of training, demands of the task, the comparison to the opposite side, or to the client's contextual 'normal', Kinesio Taping may be utilised to address these deficits.

The use of the term 'bias' testing is intentional, so as to acknowledge that any muscle testing cannot implicate one muscle or structure only. That movement is created by a series of coordinated events in the body and that no test provided can implicate one structure (in this case, a muscle) in isolation. All movement testing is in essence a composite testing of the entire movement strategy for the body.

'Bias' testing is therefore undertaken so as to implicate a particular muscle during testing, in preference to (and not necessarily in exclusion to) those around it. The taping itself is over the anatomy of the muscle with respect to its orientation on the client's specific anatomy. The muscle is identified through a length and strength testing process which identifies a deficit when compared to the opposite side or the client's norm. The testing should be conducted as part of a cluster of tests to better confirm and inform the practitioner of the intervention that should be applied.

Whilst this book provides examples of testing options for each muscle, these are by no means definitive and there are many other valid testing variations that can be used.

Depending on where a practitioner is trained or what resource they were trained with, there may be different testing options. The use of Kinesio Taping is therefore a treatment option that follows a practitioner's preferred assessment style. For example, the hip abductors can be assessed in sitting, standing, sidelying, supine or prone positions, depending on what text a practitioner reads and what context he or she is presented with. Undoubtedly there will be new and better testing with and without equipment that will be developed as we better understand the body.

It is not the intention of this text to present *all* the versions of testing that could be available to a practitioner for a given muscle or area but, rather, to present some simple options available to the everyday practitioner who may not have access to expensive testing equipment but will still need to re-evaluate their interventions. Practitioners seeking a detailed level of understanding of musculature and testing for a specific joint are advised to seek specific texts specialising in their region of interest.

It is recommended that practitioners perform testing that they are comfortable and competent with in order to direct muscle taping, and this may be different to what is presented in this resource. With this in mind, it can be useful for a practitioner to use the muscle testing they are familiar with to indicate areas to tape, and to use this resource to assist with areas they are not as familiar with, or to use this resource to add to a 'cluster' of tests that indicate a particular muscle or structure that should be managed. The table at the end of each taping chapter (chapters 3 to 10) can be utilised to remind the therapist to be thorough with testing; however, the therapist can substitute his or her preferred test in the appropriate section.

An experienced practitioner can use alternative tests that they are more familiar with or for which they feel are contextually more appropriate for the given presentation of the client. A client with a lower level of mobility may need to be assessed in whatever position is convenient given the time constraints and the manual handling required. Elite athletes may need alternative strength tests that identify the 5% deficit that is of critical importance to them. An exercise-based practitioner may be better able to assess a weakness in a particular muscle through the evaluation of a client during an exercise on particular equipment.

Once a test is found to be positive, a practitioner should seek to standardise the handling and testing

Isolated muscles vs complex chains

It should be acknowledged that due to the synergistic function of muscles, and because a single alpha motor neuron may innervate fibres in other muscles, no strength testing is completely definitive for one solitary muscle (Stecco 2009). This is not to say that it is useless to conduct muscle testing, but to recognise that it may be appropriate at times to complete a cluster of tests to help formulate a clearer idea of the muscles that should be addressed with the taping intervention. Additional information should be gained from a good history including movement strategies, aggravating movements and relieving strategies, as well as palpation information. The purpose of trying to narrow down testing to implicate the most significant muscles to address is to gain the maximal functional response for an intervention.

procedure for re-evaluation of the success of the intervention. Any variation to the testing procedure should be recorded for replication at subsequent re-evaluation.

The discussion of which test is better than another becomes secondary to the primary intention of testing: to identify (for that client) a test which highlights to the practitioner and the client a deficit which can be used to re-evaluate the success of treatment. Testing serves to rule out areas of involvement and rule in other areas. The muscles associated with each test then provide the practitioner with a postcode on the body for which to deliver his or her therapy, in this case Kinesio Tape. The title of each test therefore informs practitioners of the test that was positive for validation and reassessment. Whilst the testing position aims to be standardised for reassessment, the angle of tape placement and the position of the client during the taping procedure should remain specific to the client and their ability.

TESTING PRINCIPLES

Regardless of the testing procedure that is ultimately used, the same general principles should be applied upon identifying the particular musculature involved in the condition. When a muscle is implicated or suspected, the clinician needs to assess whether the deficit is length-related or strength-related for the muscle-taping procedure.

GENERAL RULES

For a length bias test

The origins and insertions of the muscle are taken apart and assessed for the quality of the end range. Consideration should be noted for the irritable or acute condition where provocation at end range may not be appropriate. Information should be gained from a good history including movement strategies, irritable movements and relieving strategies, as well as gentle palpation information.

For a strength bias test

The origins and insertions of the muscle are approximated and a resistance applied by the examiner to take the origin and insertion apart. Consideration also should be given for irritable or acute conditions where isometric testing may not be appropriate. If a client is unable to hold a start position for testing, it is unnecessary and unwise for an examiner to apply further resistance to the movement as the test is already a positive one.

In a clinical setting the testing is limited by the strength and handling of the practitioner. A strength deficit may be missed by the practitioner if their own strength is less than the client's—and strategies which place the practitioner with a mechanical advantage may need to be considered. The practitioner should also give regard to weight-bearing muscles which may be better tested in weight-bearing or biased in an anti-gravity position depending on the circumstances. Practitioners who feel that the particular muscle deficit would be better assessed in a different loading pattern are encouraged to also do their preferred testing. The intention here is to identify a positive test in order to implicate a muscle that needs to be managed.

Using the testing table

It is recommended that practitioners perform a series of tests around a joint to form a more clear impression of the presenting problem. This also assists in prioritising the intervention. For instance, if the bias testing is positive for length and strength, and if the muscle is irritable on palpation but is otherwise 'asymptomatic' to the client when compared to their painful site, this should be prioritised over the area that is only symptomatic but not indicated in testing.

The structure with the most 'positive' tests—i.e. positive length bias, positive strength bias, irritable on palpation and is also the site of pain—would typically be managed first. Upon completion of the first application it is appropriate to re-assess *all* positive tests to ascertain whether this area has a positive impact on other areas and is therefore higher up in the hierarchy of motor coordination.

Taping guidelines

The tape tension and where to start and finish taping is not an absolute science, as not all clients respond to direction-based receptor stimulation. The guidelines that specify direction of tape application therefore exist for those clients who demonstrate an increase in neural control over muscle activity when the skin is stimulated in one direction, compared to the opposite effect when stimulated in the other direction. The intention of the guidelines for where to start and finish tape is therefore generalised to maximise neural stimulation to achieve a desired goal for those clients with this response. Suffice to say, the instructions for placing tape from origin to insertion for strength and insertion to origin for length may not be as important to non-responders to this stimulus. The Kinesio Taping directional guidelines exist to facilitate a better neural response for a majority of clients without having to additionally instruct practitioners on more extensive Eastern philosophy (Kase 2003).

The guidelines also exist for practitioners to be aware of their intention to treat and to consider the amount of stimulation they are providing and why. For practitioners not so familiar with the subtlety of proprioceptive and lymphatic work, this may be a new concept. For instance, to help a tight or short muscle 'relax and lengthen' again, a body worker may work on the myofascia from proximal to distal with the intention to elongate the tissue (i.e. there is a directional bias to the manual work). However, if the problem is determined to be more lymphatic in nature, the body worker may choose instead to work more superficially from distal to proximal to facilitate the return and processing of lymphatic exudates.

The depth of touch and direction of work is applied with an intention to manage what a practitioner has determined to be the most significant problem. There is an intention to treat with the direction of work and the nature of the touch to address more specifically what they believe is the problem. For much the same reason, Kinesio Taping Inhibition Taping (lengthening application) is applied from insertion to origin as there is an understanding that the tape may have a tendency to recoil towards the starting anchor. It is placed with zero tension and is the first point of fixture; in many novice Kinesio Taping practitioners, it can also typically be the larger anchor as it is placed more intentionally—the recoil of the tape will therefore typically be towards the larger more fixed anchor. When the starting anchor is placed distally, this may give a similar skin stimulating effect on the underlying tissue as holding the distal part of a limb and lengthening it, or conducting manual work with an intention to elongate the soft tissue.

Strength or Facilitation Taping is typically applied from proximal to distal—as the tape recoils towards the starting anchor proximally, there is an intended gathering effect of tissue that may be too long. Apart from the potential stimulus through receptors in the myofascia, the intention is to facilitate the normal overlapping of actin-myosin filaments to restore strength. The higher tension (25–35%) is placed with the intention to provide more stimulation than that of the Inhibition, or Length Taping, in order to 'facilitate and up-regulate' activity of the system. The tension does not exceed 50% as the Kinesio Taping Method recognises that higher tensions may result in compressive forces, a stronger recoil of tape to create changes and a more mechanically corrective intention to treat by using tape (Kase 2006).

The goal of length and strength Kinesio Taping is to create the desired effect without the client being too conscious of the tape or reliant on the tape; in other words, the re-testing is better, but the client is not usually aware of the tape on the body. As with most manual modalities, the exact mechanism is theoretical and yet to be proven, however, the intention to treat remains the same.

Manual glide testing

Practitioners who are familiar with manual glide testing taught at Kinesio Taping courses may use this form of testing to determine where the initial anchor should start specifically for a client. This type of testing determines in which direction the local mechano-receptors would prefer to be stimulated to achieve a desired effect. The starting anchor should be placed where the practitioner intends for the tissue to glide towards (either the origin or insertion of a muscle in this situation). The base and final anchor is placed over the remaining muscle to its bony attachment. The tension on the tape should be consistent with length and strength tensions.

For all muscular taping applications

Regardless of a length or strength application, the skin and fascia around the muscle is placed in a lengthened position (typically the length testing position for that muscle) so that the tension applied on the tape is appropriate to the particular client's full range of motion short of symptoms.

Start and finishing anchors should always be applied with zero tension. This is based on the understanding that some clients have a sensitivity to the shear receptors on their skin. A zone of zero tension is applied with the intention to allow for the shear forces from the tape tension to dissipate.

For a length application (Inhibition Taping)

Length taping is also known as Inhibition Taping as it is understood that a demonstrated shortness in length testing may also be produced by neural excitation or a lack of inhibitory factors to regulate the over-activity in the muscle. The intention of the taping is to stimulate a neural inhibitory effect to restore length and function. The name 'inhibition' is not intended to suggest that the goal should be to produce a 'weaker' muscle on re-testing.

The tissue identified for taping is placed in a lengthened position short of aggravation or provocation, so that the applied tension on the tape is always relative to the maximal range for that client during the time of application. The tape is placed from insertion to origin (distal to proximal) with 15–25% of the available tension applied over the therapeutic zone. The light tension on the tape serves to remind practitioners of their intent to reduce the overlap of actin-myosin filaments or to reduce the over-activity of certain muscular or fascial vectors, with the tape.

An immediate length improvement achieved from the taping is a reflection of the improved neural coordination of the system with regards to that particular movement and in response to an appropriate placement of Kinesio Tape. The practitioner is reminded that Kinesio Taping works on restoring homeostasis to the system and cannot 'restore' neural coordination to an area which is already 'normal'. Researchers evaluating the effectiveness of Kinesio Taping to restore length will find that using a normal subject group will undoubtedly yield non-significant effects. Practitioners who have clients who require more 'flexibility' but are tested to fall within their normal range (that is, right is equal to left or is otherwise normal for the individual) are unlikely to gain a long-term length improvement from Kinesio Taping alone.

For a strength application (Facilitation Taping)

Strength taping is also referred to as Facilitation Taping as it suggests that there may also be cortical inhibitory factors that are being addressed with the tape; the intention of the tape is therefore to facilitate appropriate neural activity.

The tape is typically placed from origin to insertion or the more stable segment relative to a more mobile segment (proximal to distal). The tension on the tape is 25–35% of the available stretch over the therapeutic zone. The slightly higher tension range reminds practitioners of their intent to encourage the overlap of actin-myosin filaments with the tape to restore muscle function.

Muscles that demonstrate both a deficit in strength testing as well as a restriction in length testing are taped with 15-25% tension. The interpretation of these test findings is that the muscle is unable to produce its maximal tension primarily because it is compromised in its length. A restoration of the muscle length should improve the length tension ratio of the muscle and thereby restore strength. A tension of 15-25% of the available stretch is applied to the muscle in its lengthened position in order to restore both the length and strength to the muscle. Re-testing of the muscle should include both strength and length in this scenario.

An immediate 'strength' output achieved from the taping is a reflection of the improved neural coordination of the system with regards to that particular movement and in response to an appropriate placement of Kinesio Tape. The practitioner is reminded that Kinesio Taping works on restoring homeostasis to the system and cannot enhance neural coordination to an area that is already 'normal' and at homeostasis. Researchers evaluating the effectiveness of Kinesio Taping to 'improve' strength to a normal population will undoubtedly find non-significant results. To achieve strength gains for a 'normal' population it is recommended that practitioners conduct interventions which promote muscle hypertrophy for this type of clientele (e.g., gym work).

REHABILITATION

Whilst it is not the purpose of this text to direct the entire process of rehabilitation, it would be appropriate for a client's program to include the length and strength training relevant to the particular muscle which has improved with the Kinesio Tape. If a length application is effective, then a program of dynamic myofascial work to maintain the length achieved is appropriate so that the client is actively engaged with the program, and upon removal of the tape the results are better sustained. If a strength application is effective, then a program of strengthening directed to utilising the taped muscle would be appropriate to better facilitate a normalisation of neural control for when the taping process is ceased.

The goal of the practitioner is to create an opportunity for change with the tape application. Encouraging the client's awareness of the involvement of the particular muscle taped helps to restore normal proprioception and gives an appreciation of the minor adjustments the client is required to make in order to achieve what can be substantial functional gains.

Practitioners are cautioned that each client should be assessed on their individual presentation and the 'evidence' provided by their history and their body rather than receiving a certain application just because it was effective on someone else or effective previously. The effectiveness of Kinesio Tape can only be realised on tissue that demonstrates the need for the intervention. For instance, the primary cause of one sore hip may be different to another sore hip and applying Kinesio Tape to the same structure on each person may yield a benefit for one but not the other.

As the client's function changes, a practitioner cannot assume that the same taping will continue to have the same benefit. Regular assessment is required to direct change in the taping intervention to reflect the changes to function demonstrated by the client. Testing for the individual's deficits and prioritising interventions are encouraged to maximise outcome for each individual during each stage of recovery.

This process of individualised interventions makes the study of Kinesio Taping difficult to research as there is not only one taping process for each symptom or diagnosis; however, this method of assessment and intervention based on the individual and their 'body as evidence' is more clinically relevant and reflective of the changing state of the individual client over time. It acknowledges the multi-factorial and complex causes of pain and dysfunction that is different for each individual, and also aims to relate the interventions back to what is meaningful to the client.

General guidelines

FOR MUSCLES TESTING SHORT (tight, overactive or contains trigger points)

Use a length application (Inhibition Taping):
- The muscle is placed in a lengthened position (typically taking the origin and insertion apart).
- The starting anchor is applied with zero tension on the insertion, the body (base) of the tape is applied with 15–25% tension, the final anchor applied with zero tension on the origin.

FOR MUSCLES TESTING 'WEAK'

Use strength application (Facilitation Taping):
- The muscle is placed in the lengthened position (typically taking the origin and insertion apart).
- The starting anchor is placed with zero tension on the origin, the body (base) of the tape is applied with 25–35% tension and the final anchor applied with zero tension on the insertion.

FOR MUSCLES TESTING BOTH SHORT AND WEAK

The muscle is placed in a lengthened position (typically taking the origin and insertion apart). The starting anchor is applied with zero tension, the body (base) of the tape is applied with 15–25% tension, the final anchor applied with zero tension.

Practitioners need to be aware that optimal force production for a particular muscle may be compromised by changes in the length–tension ratio of a muscle (Goldspink & Williams 1992). For muscles testing both weak and short, an initial application to restore length is recommended first in order to restore the length–tension relationship of the muscle (15-25% tension). Re-evaluation in this instance should include both length and strength bias testing. The expectation is that in restoring normal length, the capacity to produce tension is normalised and therefore an improved 'strength' test should occur.

REFERENCES

Chen, C. S., & Ingber, D. E. (1999). Tensegrity and mechanoregulation: from skeleton to cytoskeleton. *Osteoarthritis and Cartilage, 7*(1), 81–941.

Frett, T. A., & Reilly, T. J. (1994). Athletic taping. In M. B. Mellion (Ed.), *Sports medicine secrets* (pp. 339–392). Philadelphia: Hanley & Belfus.

Gibbons, S. (2007). Clinical anatomy and function of the psoas major and deep sacral gluteus maximus. In A. Vleeming, V. Mooney, & R. Stoekart (Eds.), *Movement, stability and lumbopelvic pain* (pp. 95). Edinburgh: Elsevier.

Goldspink, G., & Williams, P. E. (1992). Muscle fiber and connective tissue changes associated with use and disuse. In L. Ada & C. Canning (Eds.), *Key issues in neurological physiotherapy*. Oxford, United Kingdom: Butterworth and Heinemann.

Grossman, M. R., Sahrmann, S. A., & Rose, S. J. (1982). Review of length associated changes in muscle. *Physical Therapy, 62*(12), 1799–1808.

Hodges, P. W., & Moseley, G. L. (2003). Pain and motor control of the lumbo-pelvic region: effect and possible mechanisms. *Journal of Electromyography and Kinesiology, 13*(4), 361–370.

Ingber, D. E. (2003). Tensegrity II. How structural networks influence cellular information processing networks. *Journal of Cell Science, 116*(8), 1397–1408.

Ingber, D. E. (2010). From cellular mechanotransduction to biologically inspired engineering. *Annals of Biomedical Engineering, 38*(3), 1148–1161.

Janda, V. (1986). Muscle weakness and inhibition (pseudoparesis) in low back pain. In G. P. Grieve (Ed.), *Modern manual therapy of the vertebral column*. Edinburgh: Churchill Livingston.

Kase, K., Hashimoto, T., & Okane, T. (1998). *Kinesio Taping perfect manual: amazing taping therapy to eliminate pain and muscle disorders*. Albuquerque: Kinesio Taping Association.

Kase, K., & Rock Stockheimer, K. (2006). *Kinesio Taping for lymphoedema and chronic swelling.* Albuquerque: Kinesio Taping Association.

Kase, K., Wallis, J., & Kase, T. (2003). *Clinical therapeutic applications of the Kinesio taping methods.* Albuquerque: Kinesio Taping Association.

Kendall, F. P., McCreary, E., Provance, P., Rodgers, M., & Romanic, W. (2005). *Muscles: testing and function with posture and pain.* Baltimore: Lippincott Williams Wilkins.

Sahrmann, S. A. (2002). *Diagnosis and treatment of movement impairment syndromes.* St Louis: Mosby.

Schleip, R. (2003). Fascial plasticity; a new neurobiological explanation. *Journal of Bodywork and Movement Therapies, 7*(1), 11–19.

Stecco, L., & Stecco, C. (2009). *Fascial manipulation: practical part.* Padua, Italy: Piccin (pp. 19–29).

Yucesoy, C. A., & Huijing, P. A. (2007). Substantial effects of epimuscular myofascial force transmission on muscular mechanics have major implications on spastic muscle and remedial surgery. *Journal of Electromyography and Kinesiology 2007, 17*(6), 664–679.

Introduction to Kinesio Taping and the role of muscles within the neuromyofascial-skeletal system

Kinesio Tape has been evolving as a unique treatment tool for trainers, body workers, therapists and medical practitioners since its creation by chiropractor Dr Kenzo Kase in the early 1970s. Under the directorship of Dr Kenzo Kase, the ethos of the Kinesio Taping Method has been to bring into harmony the physiological systems of the body by restoring 'Ku' (space), 'Do' (movement) and 'Rae' (cooling).

In simple terms, a person's compromised physical presentation has an element of:

- space compromise 'Ku': joints are compressed, tissue is restricted and fluid is restricted
- movement compromise 'Do': there are altered movement strategies engaged, and there are restrictions in movement range and in the movement of chemicals and fluids
- thermal compromise (cooling) 'Rae': inflammatory conditions produce heat as do muscles that are required to compensate. Neurological irritations and chemically driven conditions need to be 'cooled' or calmed down.

These elements of harmony are believed to be restored by Kinesio Tape working on various physiological levels to restore the body to homeostasis.

In addition to the physical presentation of a person, Kinesio Taping training takes into account the overall health and wellbeing of a client. Whilst the language of describing this may vary across different therapies, appreciating the importance of this domain and its influence on a person remains consistent amongst most therapies. The physical ability of a person to adapt to stimuli and challenges is influenced by multiple factors: neurological control (the wiring, chemistry and psychological components), the local chemistry of the area and lymphatic exchange, as well as the nutritional support offered to the system for recovery. Dysfunctions in these and other areas may manifest as physical presentations that will need to be addressed in order to achieve more sustainable results. A more holistic management of the person is inherent in the Kinesio Taping Method.

FASCIA

There are several physiological processes by which Kinesio Taping is believed to be working with the body. The key mechanism is considered to be modulation of the fascial system. Fascial plasticity and its responsiveness to stimuli (Findley & Schleip 2007, Schleip 2003, Schleip et al 2012) is fundamental to the effectiveness of the Kinesio Taping Method.

The fascial system is an extensive network throughout the body (Guimberteau 2005, Schleip et al 2012, Myers 2001, Stecco 2004) playing an ectoskeletal role by creating a functional organisation of muscles (Benjamin 2009). The continuum of fascia throughout the body allows it to contribute to a body-wide mechanosensitive signalling system (Langevine 2006) as well as permitting the sliding of structures (Guimberteau 2005, Stecco 2004, Stecco 2012). Fascia should not be considered as an isolated entity; it forms linkages between muscular and non-muscular tissues at several locations in addition to tendon origins and insertions (Yucesoy & Huijing 2007). Small fascial fibres extend to connect to the cell membrane itself (Passerieux et al 2006), and muscular and joint connective tissue should

1

be considered as continuous entities via their fascial continuity (Van Der Wal 2009).

Cutaneous perception (exteroception) and proprioception are located within the fascial system. The superficial fascia allows muscles to slide beneath the skin as they contract, and deep fascia synchronises the activity of the motor units aligned in parallel that actuate the same movement (Stecco & Stecco 2009). Fascia could play an important role in the coordination of proprioception (Findley & Schleip 2007, Schleip 2003) and force transmission (Van der Wal 2009; Huijing 1999, 2001, 2007; Bojsen-Moller et al 2010; Maas & Sandercock 2010). Consequently, it may have an impact on the coordination of complex movements and postures.

When proprioception is diminished, the sense of effort necessary for efficient activation of slow motor units is increased (Grimby & Hannerz 1976); during low load activity, the subject feels that they must try harder to achieve tonic recruitment of motor units. Proprioceptive information from the primary muscle spindle endings is essential for efficient facilitation of tonic or slow motor unit recruitment (Eccles et al 1957, Grimby & Hannerz 1976). The sense of effort has been defined as a judgement on the effort required to generate a force (Enoka & Stuart 1992) and this is processed in higher centres of the central nervous system (CNS) and relates to the mental challenge required to perform a task in the periphery. Restoring or facilitating normal proprioception with Kinesio Tape may offer the individual improved motor function efficiency and improved (reduced) effort for the same task. The opportunity to allow for changes in the CNS with the tape is an exciting area for further research.

Fascia receptors intervene in motor coordination (Stecco et al 2007, Stecco et al 2008, Schleip 2003). Receptors such as muscle spindles and Golgi tendon organs are nerve terminations in myofascia that regulate muscular contraction. Muscle spindles are embedded on the endomysium in parallel with the muscle fibres. The endomysium has a continuity with the connective tissue skeleton and it is this connection that ensures the transmission of the spindle contraction to the entire fascia. These spindles may be activated via the gamma fibre circuit or passively by stretch of the muscle. Both mechanisms can only be activated correctly if the fascia maintains its physiological elasticity. Golgi tendon organs have a web of fibres surrounding their axons. The winding or unwinding of these fibres enables the activation of inhibitory nerve impulses (Stecco & Stecco 2009).

Extensible fibres are therefore necessary for motor perception and thus the goal of Kinesio Taping for length and strength is to restore normal fascia and muscle

physiology. Additionally, the receptors of the deep fascia are all capable of acting as nociceptors whenever they are stretched beyond their normal physiological limit (Stecco et al 2007, Stecco et al 2008); the restoration of muscle physiology may therefore have a positive impact on the experience of pain for the client. The primary role of Kinesio Tape is to return the underlying skin, fascia, lymphatic and neuromuscular activity to a level of homeostasis. The normalisation of these systems is anticipated to result in decreased perceived effort and symptoms during activity, thereby allowing an opportunity for a biological system to change positively.

A basic introduction to three important systems and their relationship is offered below; however, it is recommended that practitioners seek additional education for a more comprehensive understanding of these systems.

1. The myofascial-skeletal (MFS) system

The Kinesio Taping Method embraces the concept that faulty movement can induce pathology (Sahrmann 2002, Lee 2011, Janda 1986, Myers 2009, Stecco et al 2009) and may not just be the result of it. Musculoskeletal pain syndromes are not necessarily caused by isolated events; habitual movements and postures may play an important role in the development of movement dysfunction and the experience of symptoms. The literature has many names to describe aspects of movement faults: substitution strategies (Richardson et al 2004, Jull et al 2008), muscle imbalance (Comerford & Mottram 2001a, Sahrmann 2002), movement impairments (Sahrmann 2002), control impairments (O'Sullivan et al 2005, Dankaerts et al 2009) and maladaptive movements (O'Sullivan et al 2005). The focus of this text is to provide a resource for testing if the source of these movement faults is of a muscular nature and, if so, provide instruction on the management of these with Kinesio Tape.

The physical presentation of a person is directly influenced by the coordination of muscles, and the physical stress and postures placed on the body. The balance of muscles around joints is one of the fundamental forces that impact on the physical and biomechanical presentation of a person. Identifying these movement faults has been the cornerstone of rehabilitation for many years; however, normal or ideal movement can be difficult to define. It is normal to be able to perform any given task in a variety of different ways and with a variety of recruitment strategies (Hodges & Moseley 2003; Moseley & Hodges 2005, 2006). This requires the coordination of many elements of neuromuscular control: central nervous system processing, sensory feedback, and motor coordination. It is also affected by articular, connective tissue, physiological and psychological systems, to name a few. So whilst practitioners recognise that pain is a multidimensional experience (Melzack 1999, Melzack & Wall 1996), the same could be said of dysfunction.

It has been shown that the correction or rehabilitation of the dysfunction can decrease the incidence of pain recurrence (Hides et al 1996, 2001, Jull et al 2002, O'Sullivan et al 1997). Therefore, in this text, the correction of the dysfunction by addressing the myofascial imbalance contributing to the dysfunction is recommended prior to strategies that just relieve symptoms.

Typically, when a client seeks assistance with a 'physical' condition, whether this be an issue with posture, function, mechanics or even 'weight' control, they have an expectation that the work conducted by a practitioner will aim to address or change the myofascial-skeletal (MFS) elements. In order to satisfy the expectations of the client, assessments, interventions and treatments relative to the MFS system need to be conducted at some point in order for the client to validate the interventions and decide whether they have been worthwhile.

The importance of length and strength applications is highlighted by the understanding that it is the myofascial system that creates tension on the skeletal system and it is the balance of myofascial tension around a joint that governs the working function of a joint (Van der Wal 2009). It has also been acknowledged that a muscle can be designed to be involved in more than one functional role. Hodges & Moseley (2003) suggest that a muscle may have three functional roles: the control of inter-segmental motion, the control of posture and alignment, and the control and production of movement. It is possible that all of these roles are considered to be impacted upon when the length–tension ratio of the muscle is altered.

Through coordinated muscle activity, leverage is created on bones and movement is generated. The mismatch of coordination within the myofascia across joints can lead directly to compromised joint positions or increased loading on tissue further away. Where there is fascial tension, a specific pattern of proprioceptor activation occurs which is directly associated with the deep fascia's relationship to a muscle (Benjamin 2009). A lack of movement can also create a stasis in the lymph system which requires muscle pumps to stimulate the movement of deep lymphatics (Kase 2006). It is not difficult to appreciate that many joint-related symptoms that are not traumatic in nature had myofascial causes (Stecco 2009). And it is important to recognise that all chronic conditions will have an element of myofascial compromise that will need to be addressed for long-term relief or management.

2. The neural and psychological system

Whilst function is what practitioners are primarily concerned with, pain is usually the primary concern of a client seeking medical help. The Neuromatrix theory of pain (Melzack & Wall 1996) educates that the experience of pain is in fact an output from the brain and that this can be modified by the sensory experience. Injury can also disrupt the body's normal homeostatic regulation systems by engaging the stress-regulation of systems that give rise to some forms of chronic pain.

The neurological control, or lack of control, of particular MFS units can influence the physical presentation of a person. Fascia is richly innervated (Van Der Wal 2009, Schleip 2003) and can contain several nerve terminal endings of nociceptors capable of detecting stimuli which could be damaging (Mense 2007, 2008). A large number of independent research groups have consistently reported that in the presence of chronic or recurrent pain, patients change the patterns or strategies of synergistic recruitment that are normally used to perform low-load functional movements or postures (Lee 2011, Jull 2000, Sahrmann 2002, Hodges 2003, Hodges & Moseley 2003, Moseley & Hodges 2006, Richardson et al 2004, Dankaerts et al 2006, O'Sullivan et al 2005). Motor function can also be affected by mental stimulation; Schmeid et al (1993) showed that synchronisation of motor units modifies in the presence of visual and auditory feedback.

Pain can affect a client's motivation and adherence to rehabilitation programs. As practitioners, we can observe that in the presence of pain (Hodges & Moseley 2003, Moseley & Hodges 2005), altered motor mechanics may occur; adaptive or maladaptive behaviours or strategies can be demonstrated by the person seeking assistance (Richardson et al 2004, O'Sullivan et al 2005, Comerford & Mottram 2001a, Sahrmann 2002). It is therefore valuable for practitioners to understand the importance of managing symptoms, particularly painful ones, within the context of the interventions that are conducted.

The recruitment of muscles is altered in the presence of pain. Research (Hodges & Moseley 2003, Moseley & Hodges 2005) indicates that, in a pain-free state, the brain and CNS are able to access and utilise a variety of motor control strategies to perform functional tasks and maintain control of movement equilibrium and joint stability. In the presence of pain, the options available to the CNS appear to become limited.

With respect to this, the most reported improvement by clients with the use of Kinesio Tape is that of pain relief (Kase 2003, GonzaLez-Iglesias et al 2008,

1

Lim et al 2013), which is achieved by restoring muscle function, muscle activity, tissue length or lymphatics to homeostasis. It is believed that normal neurophysiological activity is encouraged with purposeful placement of the tape (Kase 2003). Any immediate effect achieved with a Kinesio tape application is indicative of its potential to affect and potentially direct neuroplasticity training with respect to rehabilitation and recovery. Kinesio Taping may provide an opportunity for the client to move within a non-threatening environment within their own body. This critical area of symptomatic relief allows for a new strategy for movement within a compromised system and can create an opportunity for change, particularly in chronic conditions.

Kinesio Taping to restore length and strength aims to restore movement opportunities for the individual. The restoration of muscular efficiencies that may be contributing to dysfunction and symptoms allows an opportunity for change and variability in the system. Options for movement may be offered with specific Kinesio Taping placement allowing for progressions and more rehabilitation options for a practitioner and their client.

Beyond the local stimulus, pain and suffering can be a multifaceted problem with emotional, neuro-inhibitory, social, stress and other factors which all affect the physical presentation of a person, and these systems are also altered or managed by biological and chemical changes (Melzack & Wall 1996). The exact mechanism by which Kinesio Taping works to manage pain and affect function may be as complex as our understanding of pain. It is important for practitioners to appreciate that there may be cognitive or emotional factors that limit the 'physical' progress of therapy and that for some patients, this element will dictate whether they will improve or fail with therapy any physical modality. Thorough questioning and actively engaging with the client during taping interventions may help practitioners decide when an appropriate referral to a specialist should be made.

Understanding the client and being able to connect with them in what is meaningful for them within the context of the problem is of the utmost importance. Given the same painful impairment, injury or diagnosis, no two individuals will have exactly the same experience and behaviour because 'how they manifest the pain or illness is shaped in part by who they are' (Jones & Rivett 2004).

The management of specific neurological patients and conditions is more comprehensively covered in Kinesio Taping speciality courses; however, it is understood that any client who has an immediate length or strength gain with the Kinesio Taping process has in fact had a degree of neurological compromise. The primary mechanism for an immediate change with

a single application of tape would need to have been neurologically modulated at some level.

3. The cellular and lymphatic system

The fascial system has an intimate relationship with lymphatics and local cellular processes; the local chemical exchange in cells and tissue is a direct measure of how a system is able to cope with the load or stress given to it (Kase 2007). This system is also affected by nutritional supply and the body's ability to coordinate the absorption and transportation of nutrients in a chemical state and the elimination of waste. Visceral (Barral 2006) and digestive conditions have long been known to have a strong influence on the lymphatic system (Yoffey 1970).

The loose connective tissue of the fascial system harbours the vast majority of the 15 litres of interstitial fluid (Reed et al 2010, Reed & Rubin 2010) that flow through the extracellular matrix containing fibroblasts, tumour cells, immune cells, adipocytes and other cells. Interstitial fluid regulates nutrient transport to metabolically active cells and plays a crucial role in maintaining healthy tissue (Rutkowski & Swartz 2007). The slightest change in fluid flow can alter the shear stress on a cell surface and alter the biomechanical environment of the cell. Fluid volume is regulated by interstitial hydrostatic and colloidal osmotic pressures which are constantly readjusting due to alterations in capillary filtration and the lymphatics. When muscles contract against a thick, resistant fascial layer, it increases the pressure within a compartment and permits blood and lymphatic fluid to be pumped towards the heart (Benjamin 2009). Conditions where there is an increased pressure within the deep fascial compartment that impairs blood flow can be potentially limb-threatening, as in the case of compartment syndrome (Benjamin 2009).

The lymphatic system relies heavily on active muscle pumps and a gliding fascial system that facilitates an exchange process. Lymphatic endothelial cells of initial lymphatics have anchoring filaments that attach the vessel to the tissue space and assist in opening up the junctions to allow for fluid entry (Leak 1970), the gentle movement of skin engages these initial lymphatic filaments; this characterises manual lymphatic work (Foeldi 2003, Harris 2009, Wittlinger 2004) and the lymphatic applications of Kinesio Tape (Kase 2007). Integrins along the cell wall act as mechanoreceptors that also transmit forces into cells that are converted to intracellular biochemistry and gene expression (Ingber 2003).

A disruption in the superficial lymphatics may require a more superficial Kinesio Taping application technique. It is believed the application of Kinesio Tape on the skin has a direct effect on the underlying and adjacent fascia, often evidenced by convolutions in the tape (Kase 2007). The tape creates tension changes to the skin beneath it, thereby influencing factors such as shear stress, tension and local pressure.

A practitioner may assess that the local muscle pumps are the cause of a lymphatic problem and therefore tape for the muscle activity instead (Kase 2007). In this case, and assessment of length and strength for the local and proximal musculature is appropriate to determine the best taping strategy to apply. Practitioners are cautioned that it is unwise for a practitioner to increase muscular activity and therefore the biological waste in a person without also considering if there is concurrent compromised venous return, or centralised failure such as kidney disease. The increase in muscular waste may add further load on the system if it is not being managed appropriately. It is important for Kinesio Taping practitioners to be aware of these system interactions when choosing to apply the tape.

When muscles contract, the local arterioles rapidly dilate by a mechanism which is not regulated by the skeletal or autonomic nervous system, but rather a direct mechanical connection. Tensile forces from the contracting skeletal muscle alter the conformation of fibronectin fibrils running from the muscle to the nearby arteriole. This pulls open the nitric oxide receptor and causes a local vasodilation (Hocking et al 2008). The normalisation of muscle activity which is the objective of Kinesio Taping for length and strength may have a direct mechanical effect on local lymphatic activity.

Studies indicate that tissue contraction and relaxation can result in a dynamic and body-wide pattern of cellular activity (Langevine et al 2011, Langevine et al 2010). The composition and amount of extracellular matrix is constantly changing which is based not only on the tissue demands but the mechanical environment (Purslow 2010). Mechanical stress can be transferred across cell membranes via integrins that bind to extracellular molecules and anchor them in place. Integrins mediate signals within the cell to modulate growth, remodelling and viability. The mechanical forces on cell surface receptors can immediately alter the organisation and composition of molecules in the cytoplasm and nucleus of cells (Chen & Ingber 1999; Ingber 2003, 2010). Depending on the tensional status of the fascial network, embedded fibroblasts can change from a lamellar to dendritic morphology, and fibroblast activity can respond to mechanical loads with measureable effects such as extracellular calcium influx, calcium-induced release of intracellular calcium stores and the release of ATP (Langevine et al 2010, Langevine et al 2011). The mechanical effect of Kinesio

Taping and the stimulation of fascia is believed to be working to restore homeostasis to various systems, including those at the cellular level.

SYSTEMS INTERACTION

The interaction of the above and other various systems implies that a singular change in one system may have a cascading effect on other systems. Any breakdown in one of the above-mentioned systems has the ability to affect a client's physical presentation. Conversely, the presence of physical symptoms or altered strategies for movement can impact on multiple regions of the body and may also impact on multiple systems. An astute practitioner recognises the interaction between systems and manages conditions with respect to these multiple systems. The following should be considered:

- It is questionable to increase muscle activity in a diatal limb if a proximal lymphatic system disruption is not also addressed.
- In chronic musculoskeletal problems, practitioners may note that clients have been prescribed medication to address chemical imbalances that have developed. Additionally, long-term drug use can have side effects on muscular control. Management of these clients should take into account the relationship of the drugs to the therapy provided.
- Physical improvements may be hampered or delayed if concurrent viral or bacterial aggravators are not managed appropriately.
- If the primary cause of a physical problem is psychological in nature, no amount of taping—or manual therapy, for that matter—will yield a long-term effect unless the client's psychology is concurrently addressed.

Practitioners need to recognise that their expertise has a limit and often a referral to a more experienced and qualified professional is warranted.

Restoration of Ku (space), Do (movement) and Rae (cooling) are at the heart of the Kinesio Taping Method. Treatments by experienced practitioners should be measured and considered; they should aim to balance the systems where possible rather than just optimising one element or system to the detriment of another.

Length and strength tension discrepancies are but one component of the complex nature of non-optimal, failed load transfer or compromised stabilisation strategies. Other taping techniques are available within the Kinesio Taping program, including lymphatic taping, mechanical taping, space taping, functional taping, and epidermis, dermis and fascia taping (EDF), to name a few. These other taping strategies take into account other factors that may be driving the physical

1

symptoms and presentations of a person. They are not covered in this book; however, practitioners should be aware of these alternatives, which are also taught in certified Kinesio Taping courses.

Kinesio Taping for length and strength restoration encourages a clinical reasoning approach that is responsive to new evidence and knowledge both from external research in understanding the body and how it responds to various stimuli, and the emerging evidence from the client's body that may change in response to the work that has been done with the tape and other interventions. This flexible approach allows for change and growth with the continued practice of Kinesio Taping and encourages a practitioner to reflect on the interventions that have been performed with the tape. With improved clinical expertise in using the tape, a practitioner is able to be informed by the external evidence of emerging research and decide whether the external evidence applies to the particular presenting client at all. When the research does apply, a reflective Kinesio Taping practitioner will consider how this information should be integrated into a clinical decision.

Taping the muscles for length and strength can therefore be a useful tool to directly impact on joint mechanics, lymphatics and muscle function through the restoration of normal tissue mechanics and homeostasis. Kinesio Taping can create an opportunity to improve function, mood and attitude by creating an opportunity for change in the experience of pain, symptoms and options for movement.

KINESIO TAPE AND OTHER TAPING TECHNIQUES

As a superficial application on the skin, the benefits that can be offered by Kinesio Tape can be compared to those offered by traditional rigid tape. Taping prophylactically after an area has been treated and rehabilitated can offer the region continued support and may decrease the chance of re-injury (Frett & Reilly 1994). Taping can affect neuromuscular control by altering joint mechanics (Lohrer et al 1999, Wilkerson 2002, Shima et al 2005, Killbreath et al 2006), modulating proprioceptive feedback, and assisting in the restoration of balance (Callaghan et al 2002, Callaghan et al 2012, Refshauge et al 2000, Robbins et al 1995). Taping can assist in changing joint range of motion, decrease the effects of inflammatory exudates and offload tissue, thereby assisting in pain management (Herrington 2006, Simmonds & Keer 2007, McConnell 2000, Felicio et al 2014). Akin to most manual therapy techniques, Kinesio Taping aims to treat the fascial layers by altering the density, tonus, viscosity and movement of fascia (Crane et al 2012, Pohl 2010, Simmonds et al 2012).

Where deficits have been defined in particular musculature and soft-tissue structures, Kinesio Tape over the identified structure has been demonstrated to be beneficial to reduce pain and restore range (GonzaLez-Iglesias et al 2008, Lim et al 2013), restore kinematics (Hsu et al 2009), improve lymphatic clearance (Bialoszewski et al 2009), and improve proprioception and timing (Griebert et al 2014, Tamburella et al 2014, Simon et al 2014, Yeung et al 2015). The reader is reminded that through the mechanisms that Kinesio Tape is believed to be working on the body, Kinesio Tape has no role to play on a 'healthy' population in which no deficits of function have been identified; homeostasis cannot be restored to a system which already has homeostasis. Indeed, research on the effectiveness of Kinesio Taping on a normal population is questionable unless that normal population has been challenged first in such a way that it is no longer under homeostasis, and the effectiveness then has been assessed. Additionally, generic applications without consideration of individual mechanics and positive findings for each individual that are specific to their individual needs will likely yield limited effects.

The primary difference between rigid and Kinesio Taping for length and strength is in the inherent goal to facilitate pain-free range of motion for function. In contrast to rigid taping, which typically has the primary intention to restrict movement by preventing and limiting unwanted movement, Kinesio Tape for length and strength is applied with the tissue in a lengthened position with the intention to facilitate movement without restriction. 'Space' is created by the lifting effect of the tape as it recoils when returned to the neutral position after being placed on the skin in the lengthened position; in this way, local circulation is maintained in contrast to rigid taping. This is particularly evident in the convolutions that can be seen in the tape on various applications.

It is important to recognise that the decision to use Kinesio Tape or rigid tape is not based on a simple argument of one being superior to the other; rather, it is determined by the context and the intended outcome. The purpose of the application of each type of tape may be different, the time a client is required to keep the tape on may be different and each style of tape has its inherent goals and benefits. One taping technique may simply be better tolerated by the client, which would warrant using that type of tape intervention over the other tape—or over some other modality altogether, for that matter.

One can argue that the application of rigid tape may result in poor circulation and skin irritation, but this may be necessary to prevent unwanted movement. If a practitioner wishes to immobilise a limb or a joint, then perhaps Kinesio Tape, which has inherent elastic properties, may not be the most efficient tool to use. Kinesio Tape applications for length and strength aim to maintain full pain-free range of motion by correcting poor muscular strategies and imbalances; the client should not feel any restriction from the tape for these types of Kinesio Tape applications. Of course both Kinesio Taping and rigid taping may be used concurrently to complement each other on the same individual; it is not a matter of Kinesio Taping being applied at the exclusion of other modalities. The combination of various modalities that complement each other to achieve a desired effect particular for an individual and based on the individual's relevant findings reflects good clinical practice.

Another difference in the taping styles is reflected in the Kinesio Taping philosophy of restoring into harmony the elements of Ku, Do and Rae. A change to proprioceptive information is provided to the underlying tissue via Kinesio Tape with the intention to normalise neural activity and muscle function, and restore 'Do'—movement. The goal of restoring 'Ku'—space—is achieved by applying light tension tape over lengthened skin and fascia, aiming to create a decompressive effect when the skin and fascia are lifted from the underlying structures on return to neutral. Skin movement—'Do'—is encouraged by taping and, on return to the neutral position, areas of lower pressure are created where the tape is placed to facilitate lymphatic flow and exchange; this in turn can create 'Rae'—cooling—when inflammatory exudates are removed. With a normalisation in lymphatic flow, fascial gliding and neuromuscular activity, a cascade of benefits can be achieved, including the management of fatigue as well as inflammatory processes associated with poor biomechanics and function. This can offer the client pain relief when systems are restored to homeostasis. A more coordinated system allows for muscles to function efficiently and there is less 'heat' generated by inappropriate muscular and neural activity.

To appreciate how, when and where to apply Kinesio Tape appropriately, practitioners need to understand the relationships between various systems that affect our body. The more comprehensive our understanding of these relationships, the better a practitioner is able to discern how one system affects another and therefore prioritise interventions to target one area over another so that it may have a greater cascade of positive effects for the body rather than just managing one component of the problem.

Traditional training based on Western medical practice has primarily focused on the musculoskeletal system and an assessment of joint mechanics and muscular function local to the symptoms. In the basic training of most institutions, the scope of assessments have been typically topographical—in other words, a knee problem usually has an assessment that involves the joints and muscles of the knee and therefore interventions that primarily concern themselves around this area. This text provides a framework for local muscular tests and interventions for those practitioners that have been trained with this basic medical model.

For practitioners who are experienced in inter-regional relationships and the connectedness of the myofascial-skeletal system, the relationships with adjacent joints and the compensatory requirements of a person as a whole are also relevant, and so additional functional tests will be necessary. Even within this more connected framework it is still important to be able to assess the basic elements of movement and the contribution of each muscle to the required task, to determine the most beneficial and efficient interventions to apply. A minimum of Kinesio Tape intervention for a maximal result should be the ethos for this approach, rather than applying multiple layers of tape. For practitioners who practise a more connected approach, the primary placement of tape may not be over a muscle or structure directly in contact with the area of symptoms or complaints; however, the reassessment process should still directly relate to the symptom and/or function of the area of concern for the client. This approach recognises the relationship between structures and acknowledges that whilst interventions may be applied at a local level, the overall reassessment of the relative success of that intervention should be considered by assessing the impact on the person as a whole and with respect to meaningful functional tasks relevant to the person, and not just the singular tests that identify a deficit in performance.

Taping for the restoration of length and strength can ultimately be a very powerful strategy to offer change to a system. However, with the knowledge of interacting systems, it is only *one* strategy available to practitioners. Practitioners of the Kinesio Taping Method are reminded to respect when an appropriate referral should be made to investigate additional areas if they are suspected to be involved.

Practitioners are encouraged to regularly reflect on clients; how things were done well or may have been done better, consult with other professionals, ask advice from mentors and update their knowledge by attending Kinesio Taping courses and conferences. This will greatly speed up the process of improving a practitioner's level of success and skill using the Kinesio Taping Method.

REFERENCES

Barral, J. P., & Mercier, P. (2006). *Visceral manipulation* (Revised ed.). Seattle: Eastland Press.

Benjamin, M. (2009). The fascia of the limbs and back: a review. *Journal of Anatomy, 214*, 1–18.

Bialoszewski, D., Wozniak, W., & Zarek, S. (2009). Clinical efficacy of Kinesio taping in reducing edema of the lower limbs in patients treated with the Ilizarov method. *Journal of Orthopedics, Traumatology and Rehabilitation, 1*(6), 46–54.

Bosjen-Moller, J., Schwartz, S., Kalliokoski, K. K., Finni, T., & Magnusson, S. P. (2010). Intermuscular force transmission between human plantarflexor muscles in vivo. *Journal of Applied Physiology 109*(6), 1608–1618.

Bravi, R., Quarta, E., Cohen, E. J., Gottard, A., & Minciarcchi, D. (2014). A little elastic for a better performance: kinesiotaping of the motor effector modulates neural mechanisms for rhythmic movement. *Frontiers Systems Neurosci, 8.*

Callaghan, M. J., McKie, S., Richardson, P., & Oldham, J. A. (2012). Effects of patella taping on brain activity during knee joint proprioception tests using functional magnetic resonance imaging. *Physical Therapy, 92*(6), 821–830.

Callaghan, M. J., Selfe, J., Bagley, P. J., & Oldham, J. A. (2002). The effects of patellar taping on knee joint proprioception. *Journal of Athletic Training, 37*(1), 19–24.

Chang, H. Y., Chou, K. Y., Lin, J. J., Lin, C. F., & Wang, C. H. (2010). Immediate effect of forearm Kinesio taping on maximal grip strength and force sense in healthy collegiate athletes. *Phys Ther Sport, 11*(4), 122–127.

Chen, C. S., & Ingber, D. E. (1999). Tensegrity and mechanoregulation: from skeleton to cytoskeleton. *Osteoarthritis and Cartilage, 7*(1), 81–941.

Chinn, L., Dicharry, J., Hart, J. M., Saliba, S., Wilder, R., & Hertel, J. (2014). Gait kinematics after taping in participants with chronic ankle instability. *J Athl Train 49*(3), 322–330.

Comerford, M. J., & Mottram, S. L. (2001). Functional stability retraining: principals and strategies for managing mechanical dysfunction. *Manual Therapy, 6* 3–14.

Crane, J. D., Ogborn, D. I., Cupido, C., Melov, S., Hubbard, A., Bourgeios, J. M., & Tarnopolski, M. A. (2012). Massage therapy attenuates inflammatory signalling after exercise-induced muscle damage. *Science Translational Medicine, 1*(4), 119.

Dankaerts, W., O'Sullivan, P., Burnett, A., & Straker, L. (2006). Altered patterns of superficial trunk muscle activation during sitting in nonspecific low back pain patients: the importance of subclassification. *Spine 31*(17), 2017-2023.

Dankaerts, W., O'Sullivan, P., Burnett, A., Straker, L., Davey, P., & Gupta, R. (2009). Discriminating health controls and two clinical subgroups of non specific chronic low back pain patients using trunk muscle activation and lumbosacral kinematics of postures and movements: a statistical classification model. *Spine, 34*(15), 1610–1618.

Eccles, J. C., Eccles, R. M., & Lundberg, A. (1957). The convergence of monosynaptic excitatory afferents onto many different species of alpha motorneurons. *Journal of Physiology 137*, 22–50.

Enoka, R. M., & Stuart, D. G. (1992). Neurobiology of muscle fatigue. *Journal of Applied Physiology, 72*(5), 1631–1648.

Felicio, L. R., De Lourdes, M. C., Saad, M. C., & Bevilaqua-Degrossi, D. (2014). The effect of a Patella Bandage on postural control of individuals with patellofemoral pain syndrome. *Journal of Physical Therapy Science, 26*(3), 461–464.

Findley, T. W., & Schleip, R. (Eds.). (2007). *Fascia research: the basic science and implications for conventional therapy and healthcare.* Munich: Elsevier Urban and Fischer.

Findley, T. W., & Shalwala, M. (2013). Fascia congress research evidence from the 100 year perspective of Andrew Taylor Still. *Journal of Bodywork and Movement Therapies, 17*(3), 356–364.

Foeldi, M., & Foeldi, E. (2003). *Textbook of lymphology.* Germany: Urban and Fischer.

Frett, T. A., & Reilly, T. J. (1994). Athletic taping. In M. B. Mellion (Ed.), *Sports medicine secrets* (pp. 339–392). Philadelphia: Hanley & Belfus.

González-Iglesias, J., Fernández-de-Las-Peñas, C., Cleland, J. A., Huijbregts, P., & Del Rosario Gutiérrez-Vega, M. (2009). Short-term effects of cervical kinesio taping on pain and cervical range of motion in patients with acute whiplash injury: a randomized clinical trial. *Journal of Orthopedic and Sports Physical Therapy, 39*(7), 515–521.

Griebert, M. C., Needle, A. R., McConnell, J., & Kaminski, T. W. (2014). Lower-leg Kinesio tape reduces the rate of loading in participants with medial tibial stress syndrome. *Physical Therapy in Sport, 18*, 62–67.

Grigg, P. (1994). Peripheral neural mechanisms in proprioception. *Journal of Sport Rehabilitation, 3*, 2–17.

Grimby, L., & Hannerz, J. (1976). Disturbances in voluntary recruitment order of low and high frequency motor units on blockades of proprioception afferent activity. *Acta Physiologica Scandinavia 96*, 207–216.

Guimberteau, J. C. (Writer). (2005). Strolling under the skin. France: Endo Vivo productions.

Guimberteau, J. C., Delage, J. P., & Wong, J. (2010). The role and mechanical behavior of the connective tissue in tendon sliding. *Chirurgie de la Main, 29*(3), 155–166.

Han, J. T., & Lee, J. (2014). Effects of kinesiology taping on repositioning error of the knee joint after quadriceps muscle fatigue. *Journal of Physical Therapy Science, 26*(6), 921–923.

Harris, R. H. (2009). Manual lymphatic drainage. In E. Stillerman (Ed.), *Modalities for massage and bodywork* (pp. 129–147). St Louis: Mosby Elsevier.

Herrington, L. (2006). The effect of corrective taping of the patella on patella position as defined by MRI. *Research in Sports Medicine, 14*, 215–223.

Hides, J. A., Jull, G. A., & Richardson, C. A. (2001). Long term effects of specific stabilizing exercises for first episode low back pain. *Spine, 26*(11), 243–248.

Hides, J. A., Richardson, C., & Jull, G. A. (1996). Multifidus recovery is not automatic after resolution of acute, first episode low back pain. *Spine, 21*(23), 2763-2769.

Hocking, D. C., Titus, P. A., Sumagin, R., & Sarelius, I. H. (2008). Extracellular matrix fibronectin mechanically couples skeletal muscle contraction with local vasodilation. *Circulation Research, 102*(3), 372–379.

Hodges, P. W., & Moseley, G. L. (2003). Pain and motor control of the lumbo-pelvic region: effect and possible mechanisms. *Journal of Electromyography and Kinesiology, 13*(4), 361–370.

Hsu, J., Chen, W., Lin, H., Wang, W. T., & Shih, Y. (2009). The effects of taping on scapular kinematics and muscle performance in baseball players with shoulder impingement syndrome. *Journal of Electromyography and Kinesiology, 19*(6), 1092–1999.

Huijing, P. A. (1999). Muscle as a collagen fibre reinforced composite: a review of force transmission in muscle and whole limb. *Journal of Biomechanics, 32*(4), 329–345.

Huijing, P. A. (2007). Epimuscular myofascial force transmission between antagonistic and synergistic muscles can explain movement limitation in spastic paresis. *Journal of Electromyography and Kinesiology, 17*(6), 708–724.

Huijing, P. A., & Baan, G. C. (2001). Myofasical force transmission causes interaction between adjacent muscles and connective tissue: effect of blunt dissection and compartmental fasciotomy on length force characteristics of rat extensor digitorum longus muscle. *Archives of Physiology and Biochemistry, 109*(2), 97–109.

Ingber, D. E. (2003). Tensegrity II. How structural networks influence cellular information processing networks. *Journal of Cell Science, 116*(8), 1397–1408.

Ingber, D. E. (2010). From cellular mechanotransduction to biologically inspired engineering. *Annals of Biomedical Engineering, 38*(3), 1148–1161.

Janda, V. (1986). Muscle weakness and inhibition (pseudoparesis) in low back pain. In G. P. Grieve (Ed.), *Modern manual therapy of the vertebral column*. Edinburgh: Churchill Livingston.

Jones, M. A., & Rivett, D. A. (2004). *Clinical reasoning for manual therapists*. Edinburgh: Butterworth Heinnemann.

Jull, G., Sterling, M., Falla, D., Treleaven, J., & O'Leary, S. (2008). *Whiplash, headache and neck pain*. Edinburgh: Elsevier.

Jull, G., Trott, P., Potter, H., Zito, G., Niere, K., Shirley, D.,...Richardson, C. (2002). Randomized controlled trial of exercise and manipulative therapy for cervicogenic headache. *Spine, 27*(17), 1835–1843.

Jull, G. A. (2000). Deep cervical flexor muscle dysfunction in whiplash. *Journal of Musculoskeletal Pain, 8*(1/2), 143–154.

Kase, K., & Rock Stockheimer, K. (2006). *Kinesio Taping for lymphoedema and chronic swelling*. Albuquerque: Kinesio Taping Association.

Kase, K., Wallis, J., & Kase, T. (2003). *Clinical therapeutic applications of the Kinesio taping methods*. Albuquerque: Kinesio Taping Association.

Kendall, F. P., McCreary, E., Provance, P., Rodgers, M., & Romanic, W. (2005). *Muscles: testing and function with posture and pain*. Baltimore: Lippincott Williams Wilkins.

Killbreath, S. L., Perkins, S., Crosbie, J., & McConnell, J. (2006). Gluteal taping improves hip extension during stance phase of walking following stroke. *Australian Journal of Physiotherapy, 52*(1), 53–56.

Langevine, H. M. (2006). Connective tissue: a body-wide signalling network? *Medical Hypothesis, 66*, 1074–1077.

Langevine, H. M., Bouffard, N. A., Fox, J. R., Palmer, B. M., Wu, J., Iatridis, J. C., . . . Howe, A. K. (2011). Fibroblast cytoskeletal remodeling contributes to connective tissue tension. *Journal of Cellular Physiology, 226*(5), 1166–1175.

Langevine, H. M., Storch, K. N., Snapp, R. R., Bouffard, N. A., Badger, G. J., Howe, A. K., & Taatjes, D. J. (2010). Tissue stretch induces nuclear remodeling in connective tissue fibroblasts. *Histochemistry and Cell Biology, 133*(4), 405–415.

Leak, L. V. (1970). Electron microscopic observations on lymphatic capillaries and the structural components of the connective tissue-lymph interface. *Microvascular Research, 2*, 361–391.

Lee, D. (Ed.) (2011). *The pelvic girdle: an integration of clinical expertise and research* (4th ed.). Edinburgh: Churchill Livingstone.

Lee, D. G. (2008). *The pelvic girdle* (4th ed). Edinburgh: Elsevier.

Lim, C., Park, Y., & Bae, Y. (2013). The effect of the Kinesio taping and spiral taping on menstrual pain and premenstrual syndrome. . *Journal of Physical Therapy Science, 25*(7), 761–764.

Lohrer, H., Alt, W., & Gollhofer, A. (1999). Neuromuscular properties and functional aspects of taped ankles. *The American Journal of Sports Medicine, 27*, 69–75.

McConnell, J. (2000a). A novel approach to pain relief, pre-therapeutic exercise. *Journal of Science and Medicine in Sport, 3*. http://dx.doi.org/10.1016/S1440-2440(00)80041-9

McConnell, J. (2000b). Management of patellofemoral problems. *Manual Therapy, 1*(2), 60–66.

Maas, H., & Sandercock, T. G. (2010). *Force Transmission between Synergistic Skeletal Muscles through Connective Tissue Linkages. Journal of Biomedicine and Biotechnology*, Article ID 575672.

Melzack, R. (1999). Pain and stress: a new perspective. In R. J. Gatchel & D. C. Turk (Eds.), *Psychosocial factors in pain* (pp. 89–106). New York: Guildford Press.

Melzack, R. (2001). Pain and the neuromatrix in the brain *Journal of Dental Education, 65*(12), 1378–1382.

Melzack, R., & Wall, P. (1996). *The challenge of pain*. London: Penguin Science.

Mense, S. (2007). *Neuroanatomy and neurophysiology of low back pain*. Paper presented at the First International Fascia Research Congress, Boston.

Mense, S. (2008). Muscle pain: mechanisms and clinical significance. *Deutsches Arzteblatt International, 105*(2), 214–219.

Moseley, G. L., & Hodges, P. (2005). Are the changes in postural control associated with low back pain caused by pain interference? *Clinical Journal of Pain, 21*(4), 323–329.

Moseley, G. L., & Hodges, P. (2006). Reduced variability of postural strategy prevents normalization of motor changes induced by back pain: a risk factor for chronic trouble? *Behavioural Neuroscience, 120*(2), 474–476.

Myers, T. W. (2009). *Anatomy trains myofascial meridians for manual and movement therapists* (2nd ed.). Edinburgh: Churchill Livingstone.

O'Sullivan, P. (2005). Diagnosis and classification of chronic low back pain disorders: maladaptive movement and motor control impairments as underlying mechanisms. *Manual Therapy, 10*(4), 242–255.

O'Sullivan, P., Phyty, G. D., Twomey, L., & Allison, G. (1997). Evaluation of specific stabilizing exercises in the treatment of chronic low back pain with radiological diagnosis of spondylosis or spondylolisthesis. *Spine, 22*(24), 2959–2967.

Passerieux, E., Rossingnol, R., Chopard, A., Carnino, A., Marinin, J. F., Letellier, T., & Delage, J. P. (2006). Structural reorganisation of the perimysium in bovine skeletal muscle: junctional plates and associated intracellular subdomains. *Journal of Structural Biology, 154*(2), 27–34.

Pohl, H. (2010). Changes in the structure of collagen distribution in the skin caused by a manual technique. *Journal of Bodywork and Movement Therapies, 14*(1), 27–34.

Purslow, P. (2009). The structure and functional significance of variations in the connective tissue within muscle. In P. A. Huijing, P. Hollander, T. W. Findley, & R. Schleip (Eds.), *Fascia research II: basic science and implications for conventional and complementary health care*. Munich: Elsevier Urban and Fischer.

Reed, R. K., Liden, A., & Rubin, K. (2010). Edema and fluid dynamics in connective tissue remodelling. *Journal of Molecular and Cellular Cardiology, 48*(3), 518–523.

Reed, R. K., & Rubin, K. (2010). Transcapillary exchange: role and importance of the interstitial fluid pressure and the extracellular matrix. *Cardiovascular Research, 87*(2), 211–217.

Refshauge, K. M., Kilbreath, S. L., & Raymond, J. (2000). The effects of recurrent ankle inversion sprains and taping on proprioception at the ankle. *Medicine and Science in Sports and Exercise, 32*, 10–14.

Richardson, C., Hodges, P., & Hides, J. (2004). *Therapeutic exercise for lumbopelvic stabilization: a motor control approach for the treatment and prevention of low back pain*. Edinburgh: Elsevier.

Robbins, S., Waked, E., & Rappel, R. (1995). Ankle taping improves proprioception before and after exercise in young men. *British Journal of Sports Medicine, 29*, 242–247.

Rutkowski, J. M., & Swartz, M. A. (2007). A driving force for change: interstitial flow as a morphoregulator. *Trends in Cell Biology, 17*(1), 44–50.

Sahrmann, S. A. (2002). *Diagnosis and treatment of movement impairment syndromes*. St Louis: Mosby.

Schleip, R. (2003). Fascial plasticity; a new neurobiological explanation. *Journal of Bodywork and Movement Therapies, 7*(1), 11–19.

Schleip, R., Findley, T. W., Chaitow, L., & Huijing, P. A. (Eds.). (2012). *Fascia, the tensional network of the human body: the science and clinical applications in manual and movement therapies*. Edinburgh: Elsevier Churchill and Livingstone.

Schleip, R., Klinger, W., & Lehmann- Horn, F. (2006). *Fascia is able to contract in a smooth muscle-like manner and thereby influence muscle mechanics*. Paper presented at the 5th World Congress of Biomechanics, Germany.

Schleip, R., Naylor, I. L., Ursa, D., Melzer, W., Zorn, A., Wilke, H. J., . . . Klinger, W. (2006). Passive muscle stiffness may be influenced by active contractility of intramuscular connective tissue. *Medical Hypothesis, 66*(1), 66–71.

Schmied, A., Ivarsson, C., & Fetz, E. E. (1993). Short term synchronization of motor units in human extensor digitorum communis muscle: relation to contractile properties and voluntary control. *Experimental Brain Research, 97*, 169–172.

Schwind, P. (2006). *Fascial and membrane technique: a manual for comprehensive treatment of the connective tissue system.* Edinburgh: Elsevier.

Sharmann, S. A. (2002). *Diagnosis and treatment of movement impairment syndromes.* St Louis: Mosby.

Shima, M., Maeda, A., & Hirosashi, K. (2005). Delayed latency of peroneal reflex to sudden inversion with ankle taping and bracing. *International Journal of Sports Medicine, 26*, 476–480.

Simmonds, J. V., & Keer, R. J. (2007). Hypermobility and hypermobility syndrome. *Manual Therapy, 12*(4).

Simmonds, N., Miller, P., & Gemmell, H. (2012). A theoretical framework for the role of fascia in manual therapy. *Journal of Bodywork and Movement Therapies, 16*(1), 83–93.

Simon, J., Garcia, W., & Docherty, C. L. (2014). The effect of kinesio tape on force sense in people with functional ankle instability. *Clinical Journal of Sports Medicine, 24*(4), 289–294.

Smeulders, M. J., Kreulen, M., Hajj, J. J., Huijing, P. A., & Van der Horst, C. M. (2005). Spastic muscle properties are affected by length changes of adjacent structures. *Muscle Nerve, 32*(2), 208–215.

Stecco, C. (2012). *Fascial anatomy overview.* Paper presented at the Third International Fascia Research Congress, Vancouver.

Stecco, C., Gagey, O., Bellonic, A., Pazzoulia, A., Porzionatoc, A., Macchic, V., . . . V., D. (2007). Anatomy of the deep fascia of the upper limb. Second part: study of innervation. *Morphologie 91*, 38–43.

Stecco, C., Porzionato, A., Lancerotto, L., Stecco, A., Macchi, V., Day, J. A., & De Caro, R. (2008). Histological study of the deep fasciae of the limbs. *Journal of Bodywork and Movement Therapies 12*, 225–230.

Stecco, L. (2004). *Fascial manipulation.* Padua, Italy: Piccin.

Stecco, L., & Stecco, C. (2009a). *Fascial manipulation: practical part.* Padova: Piccin (pp. 19–29).

Stecco, L., & Stecco, C. (2009b). *Fascial manipulation: practical part.* Padua, Italy: Piccin.

Tamburella, F., Scivoletto, G., & Molinari, M. (2014). Somatosensory inputs by application of Kinesio Taping: Effects on spasticity, balance and gait in patients with chronic spinal cord injury. *Frontiers in Human Neuroscience, 8*, 367.

Tsai, H. J., Hung, H. C., Yang, J. L., Huang, C. S., & Tsauo, J. Y. (2009). Could Kinesio Tape replace the bandage in decongestive lymphatic therapy for breast-cancer related lymphedema? A pilot study. *Support Care Cancer, 17*(11), 1353–1360.

Van der Wal, J. (2009). The architecture of the connective tissue in the musculoskeletal system: an often overlooked functional parameter as to proprioception in the locomotor apparatus. *Journal of Therapeutic Massage and Bodywork, 4*(2), 9–23.

Voglar, M., & Sarabon, N. (2014). Kinesio tape in young healthy subjects does not affect postural reflex reactions and anticipatory postural adjustments of the trunk. A pilot study. *Journal of Sports Science & Medicine, 13*(3), 673–679.

Whittlinger, H., Harris, R. H., & McKillop- Thrift, K. (1993). Dr Vodder's manual lymphatic drainage: current perspectives. *Massage Therapy Journal, 32*(2), 46–53.

Wittlinger, H., Wittlinger, G., Wittlinger, A., & Wittlinger, M. (2004). *Dr Vodder's manual lymph drainage.* Heidelberg: Thieme.

Wilkerson, G. B. (2002). Biomechanical and neuromuscular effects of ankle taping and bracing. *Journal of Athletic Training, 37*(4), 436–445.

Yeung, S. S., Yeung, E. W., Sakunkaruna, Y., Mingsoongnern, S., Hung, W. Y., Fan, Y. L., & Iao, H. C. (2015). Acute effect of Kinesio taping on knee extensor peak torque and electromyographic activity after exhaustive isometric knee extension in healthy young adults. *Clinical Journal of Sport Medicine, 25*(3), 284–290.

Yoffey, J. M., & Courtice, F. C. (1970). *Lymphatics: lymph and the lymphomyeloid complex.* London: Academic Press.

Yucesoy, C. A., & Huijing, P. A. (2007). Substantial effects of epimuscular myofascial force transmission on muscular mechanics have major implications on spastic muscle and remedial surgery. *Journal of Electromyography and Kinesiology, 17*(6), 664–679.

CHAPTER 2

Kinesio Taping basics

GENERAL PRINCIPLES OF APPLICATION

- 'Anchors' are used at each end of a Kinesio Taping application in order to help disperse the shear forces created by the tension used in the tape.
- These anchors are applied with zero tension. Due to the fact that the Kinesio Tape has a 10% pre-tension applied whilst it is on the backing paper, the practitioner needs to remove the backing from the tape and allow it to settle (for only a second or two) before applying it to skin.
- Tape anchors are typically applied above and below a target zone. This zone between the anchors should have the appropriate therapeutic tension applied with the tape.
- The tape can be left on the skin for 3–5 days. It is easier to remove after this, as the top layer of skin cells will shed in approximately that amount of time. It is not recommended to leave the tape on for longer.
- Be careful not to use a hair dryer over a taped area as the excess heat can cause the glue to become overly activated and stick excessively to the skin.
- If there is any skin irritation or sensitivity, carefully remove the tape immediately. For clients with known skin-sensitivity issues, use a small test patch of Kinesio Tape for 24 hours prior to undertaking a full application. Whilst most clients who may have sensitivities to other types of taping will be comfortable with Kinesio Tape, there are still some who will have a skin irritation.

- Small amounts of hair (particularly if it is fine or sparse) will not significantly limit the effectiveness of a Kinesio Taping application. However, the tape does need to stick to the skin and so more dense or matted hair should be clipped or shaved first.

KNOWING THE LIMITATIONS OF TAPE

Braces can range from extreme support to minimal compression and, likewise, tape can either be restrictive, as in the case of rigid tape, or allow for greater mobility with the intention of facilitating biomechanics, as with the application of Kinesio Tape for length and strength. The practitioner should therefore be realistic in their expectation of Kinesio Tape and its inherent elastic properties. When there has been severe damage such as a fracture the primary intention of management may be to limit all ranges of movement and therefore plaster of Paris, fibreglass casts and cam boots may be more suitable to achieving this purpose. In this situation, Kinesio tape may be used instead to aid lymphatic movement underneath these stabilising tools.

CONTRAINDICATIONS

- **Fragile or healing skin**: There is a risk of tearing (or re-tearing) the skin during tape removal.
- **Malignant sites**: Due to the enhanced lymphatic movement promoted by the use of Kinesio Tape, there is a risk of assisting in the spread of a

malignancy. Ensure that appropriate consultations with specialists and medical management are taken.

- **Cellulitis or infected areas**: As with malignancies, an active infection may be spread by a Kinesio Taping application. Ensure that the client is under medical management to control the infection.
- **Known tape allergies**: If a client has known allergies to tape, and specifically to Kinesio Tape, seek an alternative form of treatment.

PRECAUTIONS

In the presence of the following conditions, Kinesio Taping can be used effectively; however, care and consideration of the extraneous issues needs to be kept in mind and an 'ideal' taping application may need to be modified accordingly.

- Diabetes
- Kidney disease
- Congested heart failure
- Asthma
- High or low blood pressure
- Primary lymphoedema
- Swelling of internal organs
- Open wounds
- Pregnancy

REMOVING THE TAPE

Tape should be removed with care. In areas of high tissue mobility (e.g. the neck) removal is best undertaken by 'tapping' the skin away from the tape rather than pulling the tape from the skin. This minimises skin irritation as the tape is removed. In areas where hair has been taped, sensitivity can be reduced by applying pressure to, or rubbing, the tape and skin whilst the tape is being removed. This provides a more 'normal'

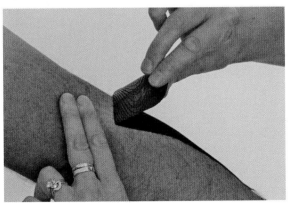

Removal — taping

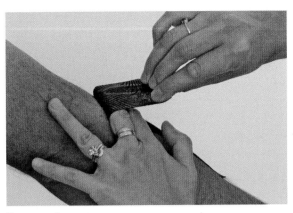

Removal — pressure

stimulus to the thalamus and avoids painful thresholds being reached during the tape removal process.

Removing in the direction of hair growth is desirable to limit the sensation of hairs being pulled during the removal process.

For sensitive skin (or for tape placed on a child), it can be beneficial to remove the tape when it is saturated during a bath or shower.

It is desirable to let the skin rest at least 24 hours after removal before a new Kinesio Taping application is made over the same area. This also allows practitioners to ascertain whether changes have been sustained.

SKIN PREPARATION

Ensure skin is clean, free from any oils or creams and dry. Clip or shave any dense or matted hair.

KINESIO TAPING TERMINOLOGY

- **I-strip**: The tape is a single strip with rounded ends. The appropriate therapeutic tension is focused within the 'therapeutic' zone directly over the target tissue.

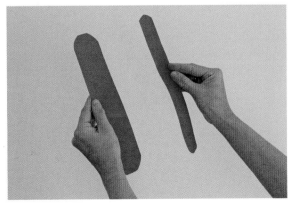

I-strip

2

- **Y-strip**: The tape is cut down the middle with one anchor remaining as a whole. All the edges are rounded off. The tension is applied on each tail over the target tissue.

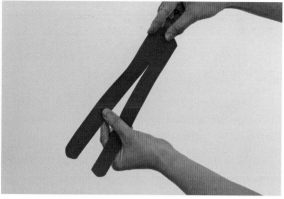

Y-strip

- **X-strip**: The tape is folded in half. The tape is cut down the middle at the open ends and the last component of the tape is left as a whole. The edges are rounded and the tape is then unfolded for applications. The tension is placed in the centre of the X directly over the target tissues with each of the four ends being an anchor.

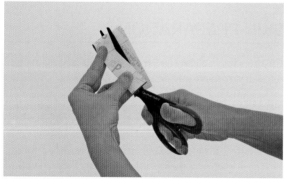

X-strip cut 1

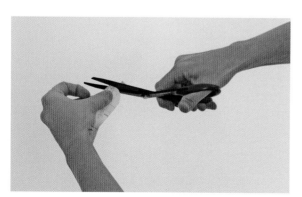

X-strip cut 2

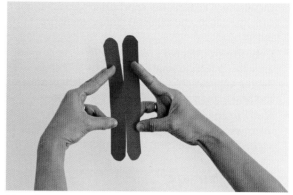

X-strip cut 3

- **Fan cut**: The tape is cut down its length using the dotted lines on the Kinesio Tape substrate for guidance leaving a common anchor at the end. More fingers of tape will have a more superficial impact on tissue.

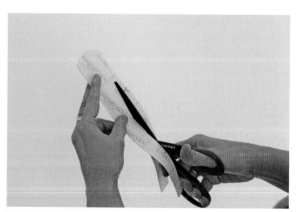

Fan cut 1

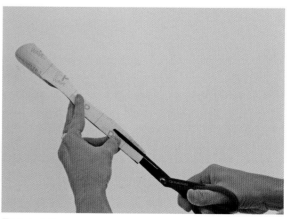

Fan cut 2

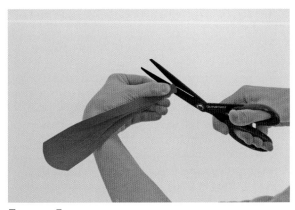

Fan cut 3

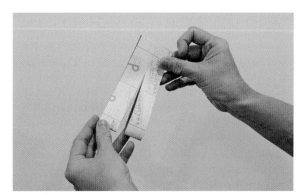

Web cut 1

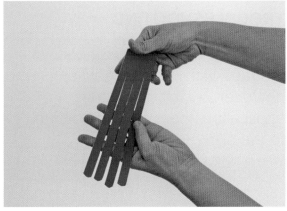

Fan cut 4

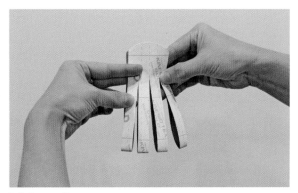

Web cut 2

- **Web cut:** The tape is folded in half and the two ends (anchors) lined up. From the folded end, the tape is cut down the middle using the dotted line on the backing to assist with cutting straight. Only cut up to the anchor — do not cut right through the full length of the piece of tape. Additional cuts can be made to make the webbing smaller by cutting down the length of the tape again using the dotted lines as a guide. The edges are rounded off whilst the tape is folded together. On opening up the tape, there are two identical sized anchors created. The therapeutic tape tension is applied in the 'web' zone between the two anchors.

TENSION

The precise tension applied to a Kinesio Taping application is of critical importance to obtaining a desired result.

It is not sufficient to simply 'stretch it a bit' before placing it on the skin. The consideration of the tape tension with respect to the intended effect is an

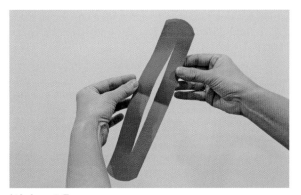

Web cut 3

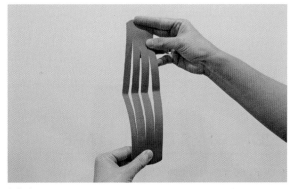

Web cut 4

important component of the Kinesio Taping method. It reflects the clinical reasoning of a practitioner and their intention to treat or manage a condition. It identifies why a specific application type has been chosen for a particular client. The tension on the tape, it's 'intention' on the body and the re-assessment of whether this intention has been achieved with the tape, allows practitioners to reflect on how effective they have been with their assessment and intervention.

Over many years and with the input of thousands of practitioners, the Kinesio Taping Association International (KTAI) has determined that specific responses are obtained from the following tensions:

- 0–15%: lymphatic and pain applications
- 15–25%: muscle lengthening/relaxation. Also appropriate for restoring muscle strength when a muscle is both short and weak on testing
- 25–35% muscle strengthening/facilitation
- 50–75%: mechanical correction techniques
- 75–100%: ligament techniques

The percentages stated above are the proportion of the *available stretch* that a strip of Kinesio Tape has. It is *not* the proportion of the length of tape itself.

For example, a 10 cm strip of Kinesio Tape will stretch approximately an extra 5 cm (the precise number depends on how thinly it is cut). Therefore, 100% tension is that extra 5 cm. Fifty per cent tension would be stretching that 10 cm strip of tape by an extra 2.5 cm and 25% tension would be to stretch it by an extra 1.25 cm.

It is such an important point that restating it is warranted: the precise tension applied to a Kinesio Taping application is of critical importance to obtaining a desired result, as a practitioner should have an intention to treat and reassess with any application of Kinesio Tape.

For example, if a muscle relaxation outcome is required, and the tape is stretched beyond the 15–25% boundary then the muscle may not be relaxed—and in fact may be stimulated in such a way as to 'activate' even more, thus worsening the existing problem. Higher tension applications (greater than 50%) imply that a practitioner is aware that these higher tensions may also have compressive effects on the tissue below and in some cases can lead to greater tissue trauma. Further instructions on the use of high tensions during Kinesio Taping applications can be found in official Kinesio Taping courses.

PROPERTIES OF THE TAPE

- Kinesio Tape is made of 100% cotton, and is latex-free and breathable.

- The acrylic adhesive is 100% medical grade and is heat activated.
- The tape is applied to the paper backing with a pre-stretch of 10%.
- The tape stretches along the longitudinal axis only and extends to about an extra 40–60% of its resting length depending on the width of the tape.
- The thickness and weight of Kinesio Tape has been designed to mimic human skin and there are no medicinal properties in the tape.
- The tape has water resistant properties that allow it to be used in water (showering, swimming, etc). Simply pat the tape dry afterwards, being careful not to rub and catch edges or corners of the tape.

TROUBLESHOOTING

The client has previously had the tape with no skin reactions; however, on this particular application, there was a reaction to the skin

When a client is not sensitive to the glue on a test patch but still develops a skin reaction, it is likely that the reaction is due to excessive tension on the tape. With higher tape tensions, there is an increased risk of tissue trauma as the tape recoils across the skin. Alternatively, the reaction can be a response to an over-stimulus of mechanoreceptors at the site. In both cases, decreasing the tension on the tape is appropriate.

There is a skin reaction to the tape at the anchor only

The client is unlikely to be allergic to the glue on the tape. It is more likely that the anchor has been applied with tension; rather than dispersing tape tension, the anchor pulls the skin causing a skin reaction. Ensure that anchors are applied with zero tension.

There is a skin reaction to the tape in one segment only

The client is unlikely to be allergic to the glue on the tape. The reaction is more likely to be a reaction to the over-stimulus of mechanoreceptors at that site. Taping tension may not be uniform throughout the application resulting in a local response along the tape. Ensure that the correct tension is placed on the tape over the therapeutic zone and decrease the tension on the tape if an over-stimulus of mechanoreceptors is suspected.

The tape is rolling off earlier than usual

Always check that the tape is rubbed on to activate the glue. If other products such as creams and ointments are used prior to the tape application, these may affect the glue's adhesiveness. Clean and dry the skin prior to tape application and rub the tape to activate the glue.

The client did not have any issues with the tape whilst it was on but noticed a skin reaction after the tape was removed

Improper removal of the tape can lead to tissue trauma; if the tape is removed earlier than the rate at which natural skin cells are shed, or is pulled off aggressively, the top layer of epithelial cells may be removed, exposing the tissue underneath. The exposed tissue is more sensitive and may react to other products, materials and soaps that come into contact with the tissue after the tape is removed. Educate clients on the safe removal of tape.

The tape is rolling off at the anchor

Ensure that the glue on the anchor is activated by rubbing the tape. To avoid rubbing the anchor off, the backing of the tape or the client's clothes may be placed over the tape anchors during the activation process. Alternatively, apply a small strip of micropore or hypoallergenic tape over the anchors or areas of high wear to hold down the edges whilst awaiting body heat to activate the glue. If this sacrificial tape rolls off, it can be replaced as needed.

The client's reaction to the tape appears to be seasonal

Clients who typically experience allergies may have heightened sensitivities during allergy season. The skin may already be sensitised and irritable prior to the application of tape. Clients should consult their medical practitioner as to whether antihistamines may be useful to manage exaggerated responses to stimulus. Ensure that the allergy or inflammatory condition is being managed medically. Proper skin preparation is necessary to remove any allergens on the skin prior to the tape application.

I would like to use Kinesio Tape on my client but they are typically allergic to tape and have strong allergic responses

The use of some skin preparations may be beneficial to use under the tape. Commercial products can be obtained with consultation of a pharmacist and applied on the skin prior to the tape application. Use a test patch in addition to the skin preparation and use lighter tensions on the tape.

My client's skin had a reaction on this occasion and I am aware of how to avoid this irritation in future with correct handling; how do I manage the skin response in the meantime?

Milk of magnesia available commercially at a pharmacy may assist in settling the skin, as may other anti-inflammatory skin products. The client should consult a pharmacist for the best product for their skin type and medical history.

BIBLIOGRAPHY

Kase, K., Hashimoto, T., & Okane, T. (1998). *Kinesio Taping perfect manual: amazing taping therapy to eliminate pain and muscle disorders*. Albuquerque: Kinesio Taping Association.

Kase, K., & Rock Stockheimer, K. (2006). Kinesio Taping for lymphoedema and chronic swelling. Albuquerque: Kinesio Taping Association.

Kase, K., Wallis, J., & Kase, T. (2003). *Clinical therapeutic applications of the Kinesio Taping methods*. Albuquerque: Kinesio Taping Association.

Techniques for testing and taping the neck

Sternocleidomastoid (SCM)

Scalenes

Splenius capitis

Splenius cervicis

Levator scapula

Upper trapezius

ANATOMY
Sternocleidomastoid (SCM)

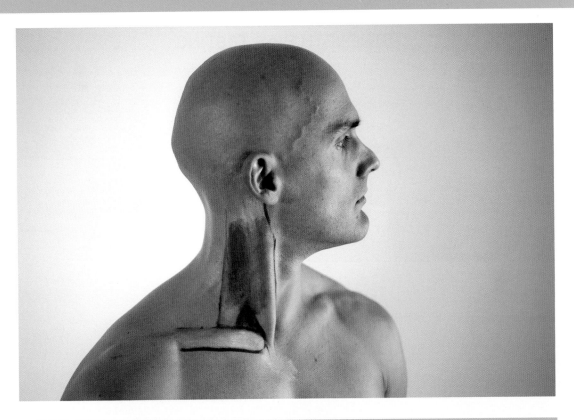

Sternocleidomastoid (SCM)

Origin:	Manubrium of the sternum and medial ⅓ of the clavicle
Insertion:	Mastoid process of the temporal bone and the lateral ½ of the superior nuchal line of the occiput
Nerve supply:	Accessory nerve (cranial nerve XI). Ventral rami of C2, C3
Function:	Flexes the lower cervical spine and extends the upper cervical spine. Laterally flexes and contralaterally rotates the head and neck. Elevates the sternum at the clavicle

MUSCLE TESTING
Sternocleidomastoid (SCM)

STRENGTH BIAS TESTING

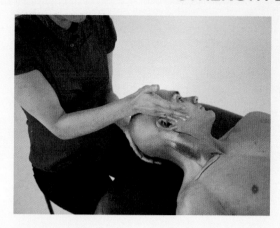

Client position
The client is lying supine with the head in full rotation to the contralateral side.

Instruction to client
The client is instructed to maintain the rotated head position whilst lifting the head off the bed.

Examiner position and notes
The examiner sits at the top of the bed with the testing hand positioned over the head above the level of the ear and the supporting hand under the occiput in case the client is unable to hold the position at the start or fatigues. The examiner should note if the client is attempting to rotate the head back to neutral as a compensatory strategy.

Resistance
The examiner places the hypothenar eminence above the ear and applies a force from one ear to the other in the direction down towards the bed. Resistance using the hypothenar eminence reminds the examiner to be careful, controlled and less aggressive with the testing of the neck. Practitioners are encouraged to use the hypothenar eminence to first learn the test in order to avoid accidental or excessive pressure on the ears and/or neck; practitioners familiar with aggressive handling during treatments are also less likely to apply excessive force when using the less familiar hypothenar eminence during testing. Naturally, once the examiner is comfortable with the appropriate resistance to apply, the hand position can be modified.

MUSCLE TESTING
Sternocleidomastoid (SCM)

LENGTH BIAS TESTING

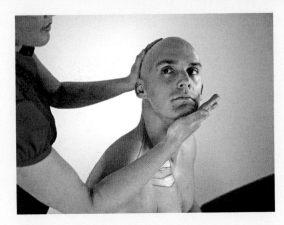

Client position
The client is seated with neutral lordosis and with the feet supported.

Instruction to client
The client is instructed to relax the neck in order for the examiner to move the neck into extension, lateral flexion and rotation to the side being tested.

Examiner position and notes
The examiner stands behind and to the side of the muscle being tested on the client. The examiner's outside forearm rests over the lateral aspect of the client's shoulder and stabilises it whilst the examiner assesses for compensatory movements. The fingertips of this upper limb are positioned over the client's chin in order to direct movement. The other hand is placed on the occiput of the client to direct movement and assess for resistance at the end of range.

Whilst stabilising the lateral shoulder, the client is first taken into cervical extension, then lateral flexion away and then rotation to the same side.

The SCM and scalenes have very similar movement functions and so the determination to tape one muscle in preference to the other is identified by the bias with which each muscle is taken into the lengthened position. The SCM being more anteriorly placed is 'wound' up first by taking the neck into extension. As the primary movement vector for the SCM is lower cervical spine flexion and upper cervical extension, the process of first lengthening the muscle by taking the lower cervical spine into extension implicates SCM length restrictions over scalenes if the tension is earlier in the movement. Palpation of the muscles also helps to prioritise an intervention of SCM or scalenes.

3

KINESIO TAPING
Sternocleidomastoid (SCM)

STRENGTH TAPING

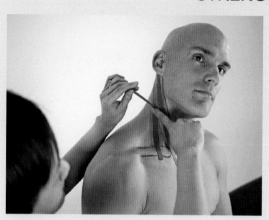

Client position

The client is seated with the neck held in extension and lateral flexion away from the side being taped. Rotate the neck so that the chin is facing up to the ceiling.

Measurement of tape

Measure a length of tape from the mastoid process to the sternum. Cut this tape down the centre into two strips, each 2.5 cm-wide; the second strip can be applied to the other side or used for a subsequent application. Cut the 2.5 cm-wide strip in two again and round out the edges of both strips of tape. Alternatively, cut the mastoid anchor into a crescent shape and cut the remaining tape into a Y-strip. Finally, round both anchors at the end of the Y-strip.

Tape application

Sternal head: apply the starting anchor to the sternum with zero tension. Place the tissue in the lengthened position and apply the base of the tape over the muscle with 15–25% tension towards the mastoid process. Apply the final anchor on the mastoid with zero tension.

Clavicular head: apply the starting anchor on the clavicle with zero tension. Place the tissue in the lengthened position and apply the base of the tape over the muscle with 15–25% tension towards the mastoid process. Apply the final anchor on the mastoid process with zero tension.

Alternative Y application: apply the mastoid anchor to the mastoid process with zero tension. Place the tissue in the lengthened position and tear the backing of the tape so that each tail can be applied separately. Apply each tail down to the sternal and clavicular origins respectively with 25–35% tension. Apply each anchor over the sternum or clavicle with zero tension.

STRENGTH TAPING

Additional notes

When applying a Y-strip it is more practical to start at the common anchor and apply the two tails on to the skin with the appropriate tension and the correct position rather than start at two anchors and attempt to come to a common point from different start positions, as this may in fact adversely affect the tension of the application.

The hairline may be a sensitive area or may require a special cut of the tape in order to tape higher into the neck line. It is often more practical to start the tape at the hairline and apply the tape with the appropriate tension to achieve results, rather than start in the reverse direction and find that the tape is too long and have to trim the tape near hair. For the initial application, it can be more practical to apply a Y-strip to determine an appropriate length of tape. Once an ideal length of tape is confirmed, practitioners may start at the sternum for subsequent applications and use two separate I-strips.

Reassessment

Reassess your client for changes in strength, tonal changes, functional changes and symptoms.

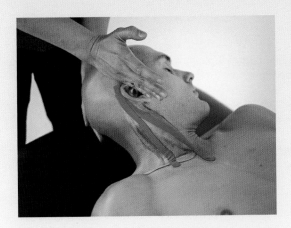

KINESIO TAPING
Sternocleidomastoid (SCM)

LENGTH TAPING

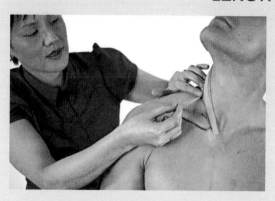

Client position

The client is seated with the neck held in extension and lateral flexion away from the side being taped. Rotate the neck so that the chin is facing up to the ceiling.

Measurement of tape

Measure a length of tape from the mastoid process to the sternum. Cut this tape down the centre into two strips, each 2.5 cm-wide; the second strip can be applied to the other side or used for a subsequent application. Cut the mastoid anchor into a crescent shape and cut the remaining tape into a Y-strip. Finally, round both anchors at the end of the Y-strip.

Tape application

Apply the mastoid anchor to the mastoid process with zero tension. Place the tissue in the lengthened position and tear the backing of the tape so that each tail can be applied separately. Run each tail down to the sternal and clavicular origins respectively with 15–25% tension. Apply each anchor over the sternum or clavicle with zero tension. Rub the tape to activate the glue.

Additional notes

As the neck is a sensitive area, tension towards the lower side of the spectrum is recommended.

Reassessment

Reassess your client for changes in length, strength, tonal changes, functional changes and symptoms.

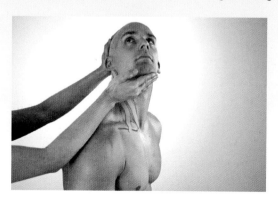

ANATOMY
Scalenes

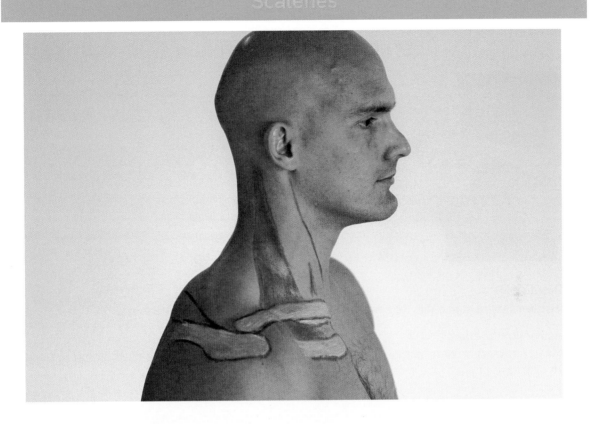

Anterior scalene

Origin:	First rib at the scalene tubercle
Insertion:	Transverse process C3–6
Nerve supply:	Ventral rami of C4–6
Function:	Flexes, laterally flexes and contralaterally rotates the neck. Elevates the first rib when acting from above

Middle scalene

Origin:	First rib lateral to the tubercle of the first rib
Insertion:	Transverse process C2–7
Nerve supply:	Ventral rami C3–8
Function:	Laterally flexes and flexes the neck. Elevates the first rib when acting from above

Posterior scalene

Origin:	Second rib behind the tubercle for the serratus anterior
Insertion:	Transverse process C5–7
Nerve supply:	Ventral rami C6–8
Function:	Laterally flexes the neck. Elevates the second rib when acting from above

MUSCLE TESTING
Scalenes

3

STRENGTH BIAS TESTING A

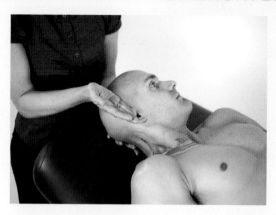

Client position

The client is lying supine with the head in 30 degrees rotation to the contralateral side.

Instruction to client

The client is instructed to maintain the rotated head position whilst lifting the head off the bed and laterally flexing towards the ipsilateral clavicle.

Examiner position and notes

The examiner sits at the top of the bed with the testing hand positioned over the head above the level of the ear and the supporting hand under the occiput in case the client is unable to hold the position for the start or fatigues. The examiner should note if the client is attempting to rotate the head back to neutral as a compensatory strategy.

If the client is unable to hold the head against gravity, if there is a lag in the hold of the head once the supporting hand is removed, or if there are increases in symptoms, this is indicative of a positive test and additional resistance applied by the examiner is unnecessary and unwise.

This test offers a convenience to testing and comparing to the sternocleidomastoid without having to move the client. As these two muscles act as synergists, if there is no distinct difference in testing between the scalenes and SCM, or the examiner is unsure, the alternative testing position may be more appropriate as it more effectively biases the testing towards the scalenes because it works more directly against gravity. Completing both tests gives further confirmation of the value of this muscle with regards to the client's problem.

Resistance

Apply resistance with the hypothenar eminence in an oblique direction in the line of one ear to the other.

Resistance using the hypothenar eminence reminds the examiner to be careful, controlled and less aggressive with the testing of the neck. Practitioners are encouraged to use the hypothenar eminence to first learn the test in order to avoid accidental or excessive pressure on the ears and/or neck; practitioners familiar with aggressive handling during treatments are also less likely to apply excessive force by using the less familiar hypothenar eminence during testing. Naturally, once the examiner is comfortable with the appropriate resistance to apply, the hand position can be modified.

MUSCLE TESTING
Scalenes

STRENGTH BIAS TESTING B

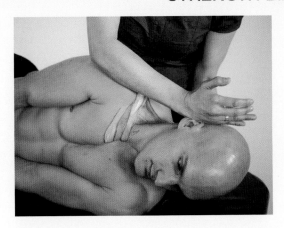

Client position

The client is sidelying with the side being tested uppermost. The head is slightly forward and the neck is rotated to look down to the bed (approximately 30 degrees rotation away from neutral).

Instruction to client

Instruct the client to lift the head off the bed against gravity in the forward flexed position whilst keeping the neck in the rotated position.

Examiner position and notes

The examiner is positioned at the top of the bed with the testing hand positioned over the head above the level of the ear and the supporting hand under the head in case the client fatigues.

If the client is unable to lift their head against gravity, or if there are increases in symptoms, this is indicative of a positive test and additional resistance applied by the examiner is unnecessary and unwise.

Resistance using the hypothenar eminence reminds the examiner to be careful, controlled and less aggressive with the testing of the neck. The palm of the hand is not used here in order to avoid accidental or excessive pressure on the ears; practitioners familiar with aggressive handling during treatments are also less likely to apply excessive force by using the less familiar hypothenar eminence during testing.

The sidelying testing position implicates the scalenes muscles as the prime mover over the SCM as the scalenes are better placed to work against gravity.

Resistance

If lifting against gravity is not significant, the examiner may then apply resistance with the heel of the hand over the occiput in the direction of returning the head to the bed (resisting the lateral flexion component of the test).

MUSCLE TESTING
Scalenes

LENGTH BIAS TESTING

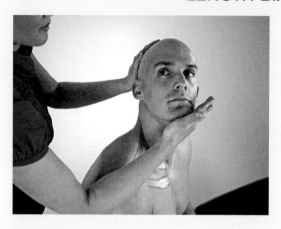

Client position

The client is upright sitting with the feet supported.

Instruction to client

The client is instructed to relax the neck in order for the examiner to move the neck into lateral flexion away from the side tested, extension, and rotation towards the side being tested.

Examiner position and notes

The examiner is standing behind and to the side of the muscle being tested on the client. The outside forearm rests over the lateral aspect of the client's shoulder and stabilises it whilst the examiner assesses for compensatory movements. The fingertips of this upper limb are positioned over the client's chin in order to direct movement. The other hand is placed on the occiput of the client to direct movement and assess for resistance at the end of range.

Whilst stabilising the lateral shoulder, the client is first taken into cervical lateral flexion away from the side tested, then extension and then rotation to the same side.

As the scalene and SCM have very similar movement functions, the determination to tape one muscle in preference to the other is identified in the bias of how each muscle is taken into the lengthened position. The scalenes being more laterally placed is 'wound' up first by taking the neck into lateral flexion. The rotation and extension elements of the length test can be swapped to further indicate a positive test to the examiner. An earlier end point when lateral flexion is wound up prior to extension indicates taping for scalenes. Palpation of the muscles also helps to prioritise an intervention of SCM or scalenes.

KINESIO TAPING
Scalenes

STRENGTH TAPING

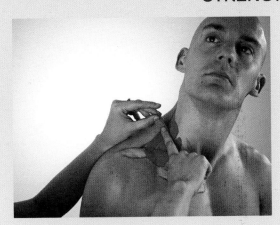

Client position

The client is seated with the neck held in extension and lateral flexion away from the side being taped. Add rotation of the neck to maximise tissue stretch.

Measurement of tape

Measure a length of tape from under the border of upper trapezius and sternocleidomastoid (C3) to the clavicle. Cut the tails of the tape so as to fit in the triangle created between the border of the upper trapezius, the sternocleidomastoid and the clavicle. Round out the triangular anchor and cut the remaining tape into a fan strip of three or more tails. Round the edges of the tails.

For clients with smaller muscles, the length of tape can be halved into a 2.5 cm-wide tape and fans cut from this (the width of the tails of the fan will naturally be thinner and this is appropriate for smaller clients).

Tape application

Apply the common anchor to the clavicle. With the tissue in a lengthened position, apply the tails up towards C3 below the border of the SCM and upper trapezius with 25–35% tension. For each tail, ensure that maximal tissue stretch is achieved by changing the angle of the neck. Apply the final anchors with zero tension.

Additional notes

As the neck is a sensitive area, tension towards the lower side of the spectrum is recommended. The tape should be handled very lightly.

STRENGTH TAPING

Reassessment

Reassess the client for change in strength, tonal changes, functional changes and symptoms.

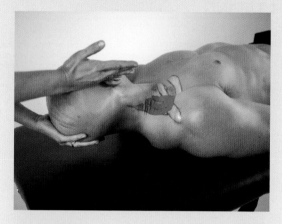

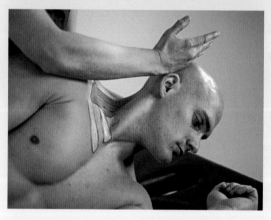

3

KINESIO TAPING
Scalenes

LENGTH TAPING

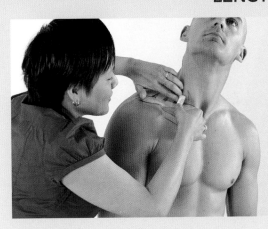

Client position

The client is seated with the neck held in extension and lateral flexion away from the side being taped. Add rotation of the neck to maximise tissue stretch.

Measurement of tape

Measure a length of tape from under the border of upper trapezius and sternocleidomastoid (C3) to the clavicle. Cut this tape diagonally so as to fit in the triangle created between the border of the upper trapezius, the sternocleidomastoid and the clavicle. Round out the triangular anchor and cut the remaining tape into a fan strip of three or more tails depending on the area needing to be covered. Round the edges of the tails.

For clients with smaller muscles, the length of tape can be halved into a 2.5 cm-wide tape and fans cut from this (the width of the tails of the fan will naturally be thinner and this is appropriate for smaller clients).

Tape application

Apply the common anchor to C3 below the border of the SCM and upper trapezius. With the tissue in a lengthened position, apply the tails down to the clavicle with 15–25% tension. For each tail, ensure that maximal tissue stretch is achieved by changing the angle of the neck. Apply the final anchors with zero tension over the clavicle and ribs.

Additional notes

As the neck is a sensitive area, tension towards the lower side of the spectrum is recommended. The tape should be handled very lightly.

LENGTH TAPING

Reassessment

Reassess your client for changes in length, strength, tonal changes, functional changes and symptoms.

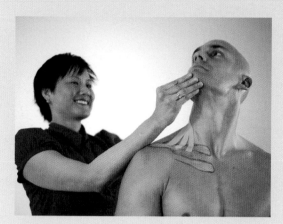

3

ANATOMY
Splenius capitis

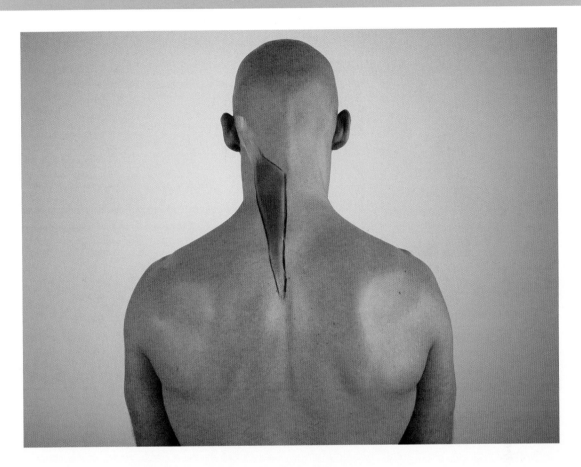

Splenius capitis	
Origin:	Nuchal ligament from C3–C6 and spinous process of C7–T4
Insertion:	Mastoid process of the temporal bone at the lateral ⅓ of the superior nuchal line of the occiput
Nerve supply:	Suboccipital nerve (C1)
Function:	Extends, laterally flexes and ipsilaterally rotates the head and neck

MUSCLE TESTING
Splenius capitis

STRENGTH BIAS TESTING

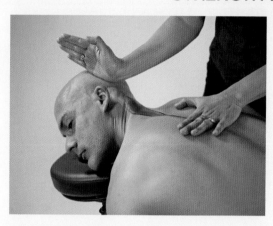

Client position
The client is lying prone on the bed.

Instruction to client
The client is instructed to turn to the side being tested with full rotation and extend the neck off the bed.

Examiner position and notes
The examiner stands at the top of the bed with the testing hand positioned over the head, the stabilising hand is applied to the thoracic spine to examine for compensatory activity in the trunk.

The examiner should note if the client is unable to maintain full rotation and is attempting to rotate the head back to the neutral position during testing, this would indicate a positive test as the client is compromised in their strategy.

Resistance
The examiner applies resistance over the head in the direction of the floor.

MUSCLE TESTING
Splenius capitis

LENGTH BIAS TESTING

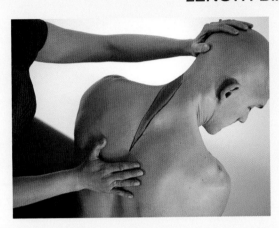

Client position
The client is seated in neutral lordosis and with the feet supported.

Instruction to client
Instruct the client to rotate away from the side being tested and then to flex and laterally flex the neck away from the side being tested. At the completion of the neck movement, remind the client to maintain a chin tuck. This stretch is identical to the levator scapula stretch except that there is no need to hold the scapula down (scapular depression).

Examiner position and notes
The examiner stands behind the client and can apply overpressure by stabilising the thoracic spine whilst applying an upward force on the occiput to lengthen the tissue.

KINESIO TAPING
Splenius capitis

STRENGTH TAPING

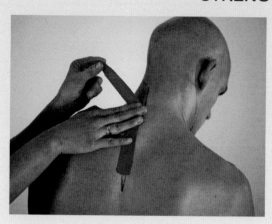

Client position

The client is seated with the neck held in flexion, full rotation and lateral flexion away from the side being taped. The chin is tucked in.

Measurement of tape

Measure a length of tape from the mastoid process to C7 protuberance or further to T4. Cut the tape down the centre to create a 2.5 cm-wide I-strip; the second strip can be used for a subsequent application or the other side. Cut one anchor into a crescent shape to fit behind the ear onto the mastoid process.

Tape application

Apply the anchor at the C7 protuberance or lower to T4, with zero tension. With the tissue in the lengthened position, apply the tape obliquely towards the mastoid process with 25–35% tension. Apply the final anchor with zero tension. Rub the tape to activate the glue.

Additional notes

As the neck is a sensitive area, tension towards the lower side of the spectrum is recommended.

Because the hairline may be a sensitive area or may require a special cut of the tape in order to tape higher into the neck line, it can be more practical to start the tape at the hairline on the mastoid process and then apply the tape with the appropriate tension towards the spine to achieve results. Starting at C7 and finding that the tape is too long and having to trim the tape near hair may not be ideal for a client, particularly on the first application. Once an ideal length has been calculated, practitioners may commence taping with the initial anchor at the spine on subsequent strength applications.

STRENGTH TAPING

Reassessment

Reassess your client for change in strength, tonal changes, functional changes and symptoms.

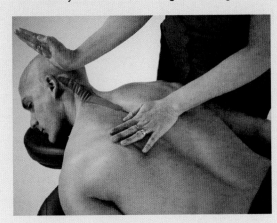

KINESIO TAPING
Splenius capitis

LENGTH TAPING

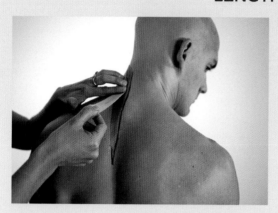

Client position

The client is seated with the neck held in flexion, full rotation and lateral flexion away from the side being taped. The chin is tucked in.

Measurement of tape

Measure a length of tape from the mastoid process to C7 protuberance or further to T4. Cut the tape down the centre to create a 2.5 cm-wide I-strip; the second strip can be used for a subsequent application or the other side. Cut one anchor into a crescent shape to fit behind the ear onto the mastoid process.

Tape application

Apply the anchor at the mastoid process with zero tension. With the tissue in the lengthened position apply the tape obliquely towards the C7 protuberance with 15–25% tension. Apply the final anchor with zero tension. Rub the tape to activate the glue.

Additional notes

As the neck is a sensitive area, tension towards the lower side of the spectrum is recommended.

Reassessment

Reassess your client for changes in length, strength, tonal changes, functional changes and symptoms.

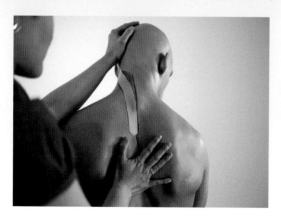

ANATOMY
Splenius cervicis

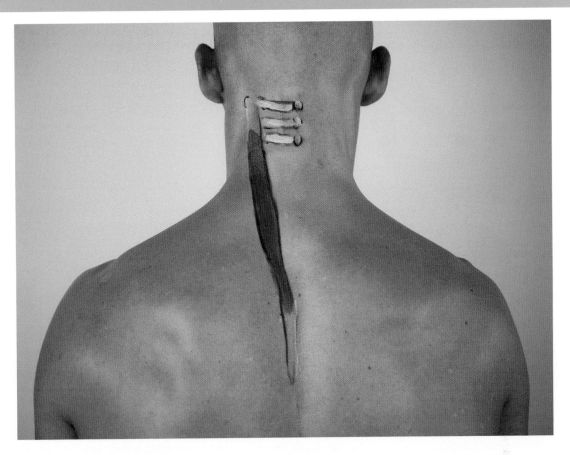

Infraspinatus

Origin:	Spinous process T3–6
Insertion:	Transverse process of C1–3
Nerve supply:	Lateral branches of the lower dorsal primary rami of the spinal nerves
Function:	Extends, laterally flexes and ipsilaterally rotates the neck

MUSCLE TESTING
Splenius cervicis

STRENGTH BIAS TESTING

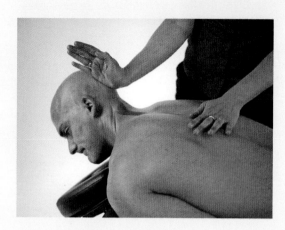

Client position
The client is lying prone on the bed.

Instruction to client
The client is instructed to slightly rotate the head (30 degrees) to the side being tested and extend the neck off the bed.

Examiner position and notes
The examiner stands at the top of the bed with the testing hand positioned over the head above the level of the ear and the stabilising hand is applied to the thoracic spine to examine for compensatory activity in the trunk. The examiner should note if the patient is attempting to rotate the head fully or is unable to maintain the rotated position.

Resistance
The examiner applies resistance over the head in the direction of the floor.

MUSCLE TESTING
Splenius cervicis

LENGTH BIAS TESTING

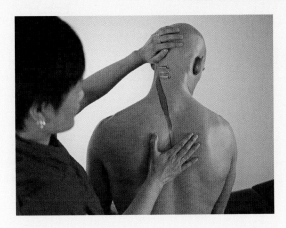

Client position

The client is seated in neutral lordosis and with the feet supported.

Instruction to client

The client is instructed to rotate the head slightly away from the side being tested (approximately 30 degrees) and flex the neck. The chin should be tucked in.

Examiner position and notes

The examiner stands behind the client and can apply overpressure by stabilising the thoracic spine whilst applying an upward force on the occiput to lengthen the tissue.

KINESIO TAPING
Splenius cervicis

STRENGTH TAPING

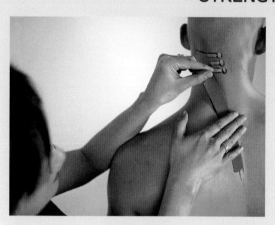

Client position

The client is seated with the neck held in flexion, slight rotation and lateral flexion away from the side being taped. The chin is tucked in.

Measurement of tape

Measure a length of tape from under the hairline to the mid-thoracic spine. Cut the tape down the centre to create a 2.5 cm-wide I-strip; the second strip can be used for a subsequent application or on the other side. Cut one anchor to fit into the shape of the hairline.

Tape application

Apply the anchor with zero tension at the mid-thoracic spine. With the muscles in a lengthened position, apply the tape over the paraspinal muscles with 25–35% tension towards the hairline. Apply the final anchor under the hairline with zero tension. Rub the tape to activate the glue.

Additional notes

As the neck is a sensitive area, tension towards the lower side of the spectrum is recommended.

Because the hairline may be a sensitive area or may require a special cut of the tape in order to tape higher into the neck line, it may more practical to start the tape at the hairline for the first application and apply the tape with the appropriate tension towards the thoracic spine to achieve results, rather than start in the reverse direction and find that the tape is too long and having to trim the tape near hair. Once an ideal length is determined, a practitioner can start on the thoracic spine for subsequent strength applications.

STRENGTH TAPING

Reassessment
Reassess your client for change in strength, tonal changes, functional changes and symptoms.

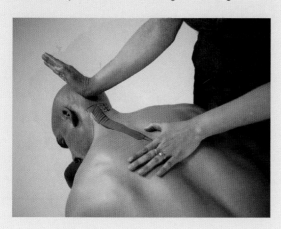

3

KINESIO TAPING
Splenius cervicis

LENGTH TAPING

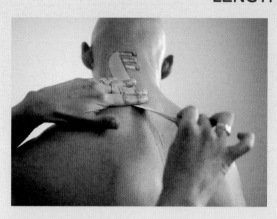

Client position

The client is seated with the neck held in flexion, slight rotation and lateral flexion away from the side being taped. The chin is tucked in.

Measurement of tape

Measure a length of tape from under the hairline to the mid-thoracic spine. Cut the tape down the centre to create a 2.5 cm-wide I-strip; the second strip can be used for a subsequent application or on the other side. Cut one anchor to fit into the shape of the hairline.

Tape application

Apply the anchor under the hairline with zero tension. With the tissue in the lengthened position, apply the tape over the paraspinal muscles with 15–25% tension towards the middle of the thoracic spine. Apply the final anchor on the thoracic spine with zero tension. Rub the tape to activate the glue.

Additional notes

As the neck is a sensitive area, tension towards the lower side of the spectrum is recommended.

Reassessment

Reassess your client for changes in length, strength, tonal changes, functional changes and symptoms.

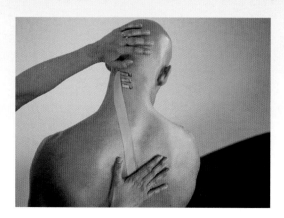

ANATOMY
Levator scapula

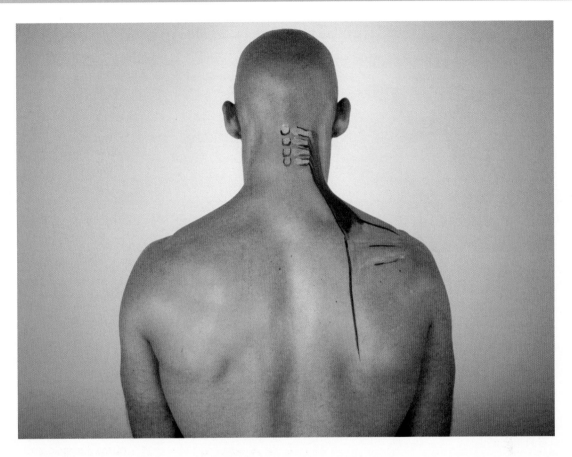

Levator scapula

Origin:	Transverse process of C1–C4
Insertion:	Medial border of the scapula, from the root of the spine to the superior angle
Nerve supply:	Nerve root C3–5
Peripheral nerve:	Dorsal scapular nerve, C3, C4
Function:	Elevates, adducts and downwardly rotates the scapula at the scapulocostal joint. Extends, laterally flexes and ipsilaterally rotates the neck at the spinal joints

MUSCLE TESTING
Levator scapula

STRENGTH BIAS TESTING

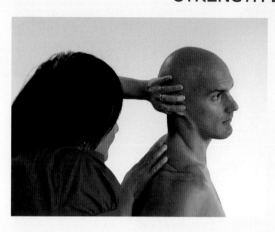

Client position

The client is seated in neutral lordosis and with the feet supported.

Instruction to client

The client is instructed to tilt the head back to the side being tested and to elevate the shoulder blade by bringing the elbows back so that the occiput approaches the medial border of the scapula.

Examiner position and notes

The examiner is positioned behind the client on the side being tested. The heel of the hand is placed on the occiput facing superiorly. The other hand is placed on the shoulder with the forearm resting on the client's humerus.

Resistance

Apply resistance to the scapula by applying a force along the humerus to move the shoulder towards flexion and upward rotation of the scapula. Concurrently apply a force through the heel of the hand on the occiput towards cervical flexion to the opposite side being tested.

MUSCLE TESTING
Levator scapula

LENGTH BIAS TESTING

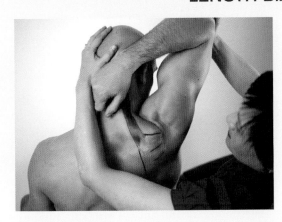

Client position

The client is seated in neutral lordosis and with the feet supported.

Instruction to client

Cervical component: The client is instructed to flex the neck, laterally flex and rotate away from the side being tested.

Scapula component: The client is instructed to place the hand behind the head in order to engage scapular upward rotation, depression of the medial border of the scapula and abduction of the inferior scapular angle.

Examiner position and notes

The examiner should note any shoulder compensations or if symptoms are produced which would indicate the end of range has been reached or that the alternative testing position is more appropriate. End range resistance can be assessed by moving the elbow up (to increase upward rotation and abduction of the scapula) or adding cervical lateral flexion and flexion at the occiput.

Additional notes

If clients have limited shoulder range, an alternative test is to maintain shoulder depression by holding the bench. The examiner can apply overpressure to assess for restriction at the occiput or scapula.

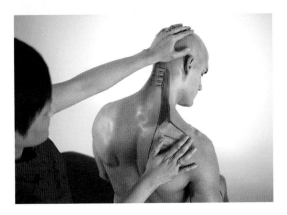

3

KINESIO TAPING
Levator scapula

STRENGTH TAPING

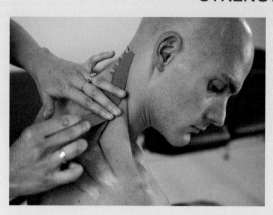

Client position

The client is seated in neutral lordosis and with the feet supported. The client is instructed to flex the neck, laterally flex and rotate away from the side being taped. Maintain shoulder depression by reaching down and holding the bench.

Measurement of tape

Measure a length of tape from under the hairline to the medial spine of the scapula. Cut down the length of the tape to create a 2.5 cm-wide tape. Trim one of the anchors to match the hairline.

Tape application

Place the starting anchor with zero tension just underneath the occiput below the hairline. With the tissue in the lengthened position, apply the tape down towards the medial scapular spine with 25–35% tension. Complete the taping by applying the anchor onto the medial superior scapula with zero tension. Rub the tape to activate the glue.

Additional notes

As the neck is a sensitive area, tension towards the lower side of the spectrum is recommended.

Reassessment

Reassess your client for change in strength, tonal changes, functional changes and symptoms.

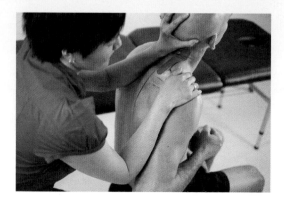

KINESIO TAPING
Levator scapula

LENGTH TAPING

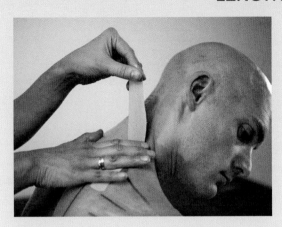

Client position

The client is seated in neutral lordosis and with the feet supported. The client is instructed to flex the neck, laterally flex and rotate away from the side being tested. Maintain shoulder depression by reaching down and holding the bench.

Measurement of tape

Measure a length of tape from under the hairline to the medial spine of the scapula. Cut down the length of the tape to create a 2.5 cm-wide tape. Trim one of the anchors to match the hairline.

Tape application

Place the starting anchor with zero tension over the medial scapular spine. With the tissue in a lengthened position, apply the tape up towards the occiput with 15–25% tension. Complete the taping by applying the anchor onto the hairline with zero tension. Rub the tape to activate the glue.

Additional notes

As the neck is a sensitive area, tension towards the lower side of the spectrum is recommended.

The hairline may be a sensitive area or may require a special cut of the tape in order to tape higher into the neck line. For the first application, it can be more practical to start the tape at the hairline and apply the tape with the appropriate tension towards the scapula to achieve results. Starting at the scapula and finding that the tape is too long and having to trim the tape near hair may be avoided. Once an ideal length has been determined, a practitioner may commence taping at the scapula on subsequent length applications.

LENGTH TAPING

Reassessment

Reassess your client for changes in length, strength, tonal changes, functional changes and symptoms.

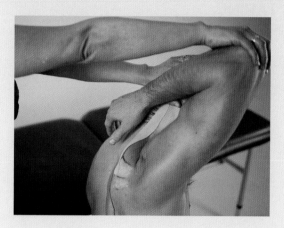

ANATOMY
Upper trapezius

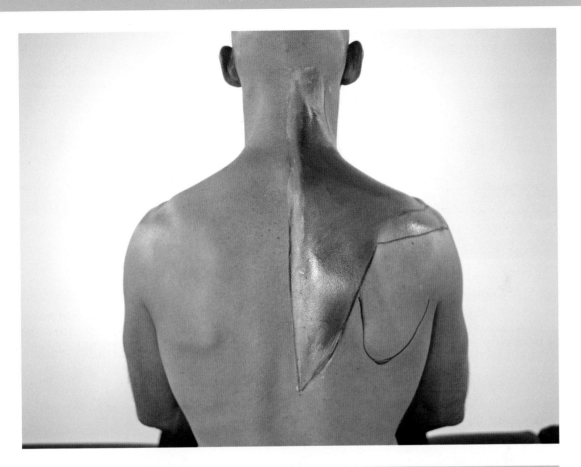

Upper trapezius

Origin:	External occipital protuberance, medial ⅓ superior nuchal line, ligamentum nuchae, spinous processes of C7
Insertion:	Lateral ⅓ clavicle, acromion process, lateral ⅓ of spine of the scapula
Nerve supply:	Nerve root C1–5.
Peripheral nerve:	Spinal portion of the accessory nerve (cranial nerve XI); ventral rami of C3, C4
Function:	Elevates, retracts, upwardly rotates the scapula at the scapulocostal joint. Extends, laterally flexes and contralaterally rotates the head and neck at the spinal joints

MUSCLE TESTING
Upper trapezius

STRENGTH BIAS TESTING

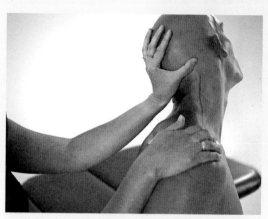

Client position

The client is seated in neutral lordosis and with the feet supported. The hands and back should not be in contact with the supporting surface. Laterally flex the client's neck to the side being tested and rotate the head away, elevate the acromioclavicular joint of the shoulder towards the ear. The shoulder may abduct to assist in this movement.

Instruction to client

The client is instructed to maintain shoulder abduction and elevation relative to the head position against the resistance applied by the examiner.

Examiner position and notes

During function testing, the examiner is positioned behind the client and towards the side being tested.

Resistance

Apply resistance simultaneously over the lateral shoulder in the direction of shoulder depression and over the posterior aspect of the occiput in the direction of anterior and contralateral neck flexion.

MUSCLE TESTING
Upper trapezius

LENGTH BIAS TESTING

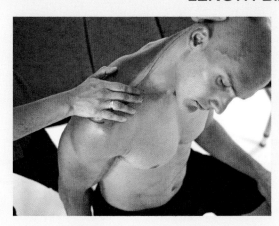

Client position
The client is seated in neutral lordosis and with the feet supported

Instruction to client
The client is instructed to forward flex the neck and laterally flex away from the side tested, then rotate the head back to the same side. The client is to maintain scapular stability by holding under the bench or their leg on the side being tested.

Examiner position and notes
The examiner is positioned standing behind the client in order to assess for range of the movement and quality of the movement. Palpate the trapezius near its insertion at the clavicle for resting tone.

Overpressure can be applied if the client is not irritable to assess for the quality of the end feel. One hand is placed on the acromion to stabilise it whilst the other hand is placed under the occiput to apply a force in the direction for flexion and lateral flexion.

The examiner should note any symptoms that are reproduced during the testing for re-evaluation after the intervention. Range should be compared to the non-affected side for a baseline of normal range when available.

KINESIO TAPING
Upper trapezius

STRENGTH TAPING

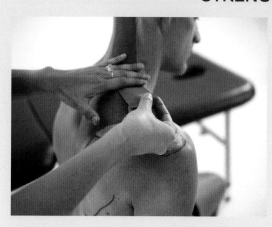

3

Client position

The client is seated with the neck flexed forward and laterally flexed to the contralateral side and rotated to the ipsilateral side so as to obtain maximal tissue stretch over the area.

Measurement of tape

Measure a length of tape from under the hairline to the acromion.

Tape application

Apply the anchor under the hairline with zero tension. Place the tissue in the lengthened position and apply the tape with 25–35% tension following the line of the upper trapezius. Complete the taping by applying the anchor onto the acromioclavicular joint with zero tension. Rub the tape to activate the glue. As the neck is a sensitive area, tension towards the lower side of the spectrum is recommended.

Reassessment

Reassess your client for change in strength, tonal changes, functional changes and symptoms.

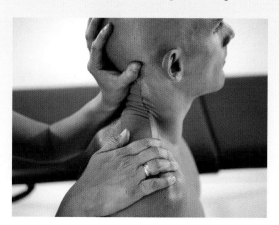

KINESIO TAPING
Upper trapezius

LENGTH TAPING

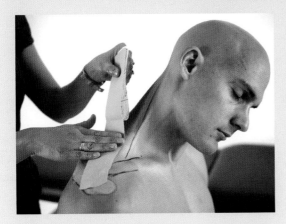

Client position

The client is seated with the neck flexed forward and laterally flexed to the contralateral side and rotated to the ipsilateral side so as to obtain maximal tissue stretch over the area.

Measurement of tape

Measure a length of tape from under the hairline to the acromion. The tape can be left as an I-strip or cut into a Y to combine taping for the middle trapezius and also allow for a better angle as the tape travels up towards the occiput.

Tape application

Apply the anchor over the acromioclavicular joint with zero tension. Place the tissue in the lengthened position and apply the tape with 15–25% tension. Complete the taping by applying the anchor under the occiput with zero tension. Rub the tape to activate the glue.

Additional notes

As the neck is a sensitive area, tension towards the lower side of the spectrum is recommended.

The hairline may be a sensitive area or may require a special cut of the tape in order to tape higher into the neck line. It can be more practical on the first application to start the tape at the hairline and apply the tape with the appropriate tension to achieve results, rather than start in the reverse direction and find that the tape is too long and have to trim the tape near hair. Once an appropriate length of tape has been determined, a practitioner may choose to start the taping process at the acromion on subsequent applications.

LENGTH TAPING

Reassessment

Reassess your client for changes in length, strength, tonal changes, functional changes and symptoms.

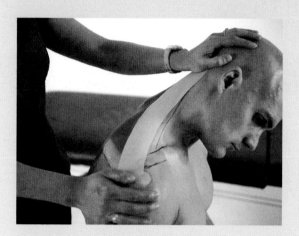

NECK ASSESSMENT SHEET

Clinic: .... Date: ....

Client name: ....

Functional review

Functional limitation	Pre-test measure	Post-test measure

Muscle testing

Tested priority	Muscle	Strength		Length		Comments
		Right	Left	Right	Left	
	Sternocleidomastoid					
	Anterior scalene					
	Middle scalene					
	Posterior scalene					
	Splenius capitis					
	Splenius cervicis					
	Levator scapula					
	Upper trapezius					

Treatment

Intervention	Re-test measures	Plan

Practitioner: .... Signature: ....

BIBLIOGRAPHY

Berryman Reese, N. M. (2012). *Muscle and sensory testing*. Missouri: Elsevier-Saunders.

Berryman Reese, N., & Bandy, W. D. (2010). *Joint range of motion and muscle length testing*. Missouri: Saunders Elsevier.

Calais-Germain, B. (1993). *Anatomy of movement* (12 ed.). Seattle: Eastland Press.

Comerford, M., & Mottram, S. (2012). *Kinetic control: the management of uncontrolled movement*. Sydney, Australia: Elsevier.

Kase, K., Hashimoto, T., & Okane, T. (1998). *Kinesio Taping perfect manual: amazing taping therapy to eliminate pain and muscle disorders*. Albuquerque: Kinesio Taping Association.

Kase, K., & Rock Stockheimer, K. (2006). *Kinesio Taping for lymphoedema and chronic swelling*. Albuquerque: Kinesio Taping Association.

Kase, K., Wallis, J., & Kase, T. (2003). *Clinical therapeutic applications of the Kinesio taping methods*. Albuquerque: Kinesio Taping Association.

Kendall, F. P., McCreary, E., Provance, P., Rodgers, M., & Romanic, W. (2005). *Muscles: testing and function with posture and pain*. Baltimore: Lippincott Williams Wilkins.

Standring, S., Borely, N., Collings, P., Crossman, A., Gatzoulis, M., Healy, J., … Wigley, C. (2008). *Gray's anatomy: the anatomical basis of clinical practice* (S. Susan Ed. 40 ed.). London, United Kingdom: Churchill Livingstone Elsevier.

3

Techniques for testing and taping the shoulder

CHAPTER 4

Upper trapezius

Middle deltoid

Middle trapezius

Anterior deltoid

Lower trapezius

Teres major

Coracobrachialis

Latissimus dorsi

Rhomboid

Supraspinatus

Levator scapula

Infraspinatus and teres minor

Serratus anterior

Pectoralis major

Posterior deltoid

Pectoralis minor

ANATOMY
Upper trapezius

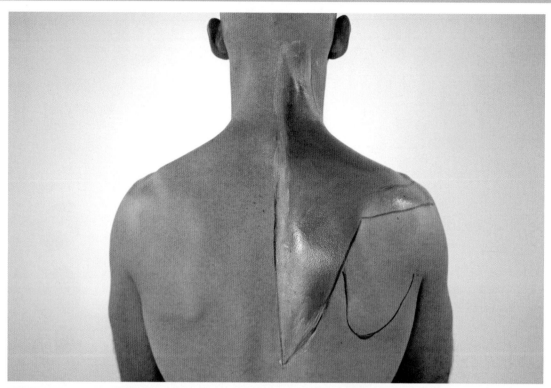

4

Upper trapezius	
Origin:	External occipital protuberance, medial ⅓ superior nuchal line, ligamentum nuchae, spinous processes of C7
Insertion:	Lateral ⅓ clavicle, acromion process, lateral ⅓ of the spine of the scapula
Nerve supply:	Nerve root: C1–5 Peripheral nerve: spinal portion of the accessory nerve (CN XI); ventral rami of C3, C4
Function:	Elevates, retracts, upwardly rotates the scapula at the scapulocostal joint. Extends, laterally flexes and contralaterally rotates the head and neck at the spinal joints

MUSCLE TESTING
Upper trapezius

STRENGTH BIAS TESTING

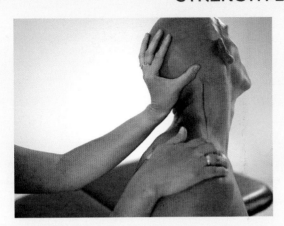

Client position
The client is seated in neutral lordosis and with the feet supported. The hands and back should not be in contact with the supporting surface. Laterally flex the client's neck to the side being tested and rotate the head away. Elevate the acromioclavicular joint of the shoulder towards the ear; the shoulder may abduct to assist in this movement.

Instruction to client
The client is instructed to maintain shoulder abduction and elevation relative to the head position against the resistance applied by the examiner.

Examiner position and notes
During function testing, the examiner is positioned behind the client and towards the side being tested.

Resistance
Apply resistance simultaneously over the lateral shoulder in the direction of shoulder depression and over the posterior aspect of the occiput in the direction of anterior and contralateral neck flexion.

MUSCLE TESTING
Upper trapezius

LENGTH BIAS TESTING

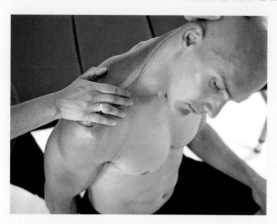

4

Client position

The client is seated in neutral lordosis and with the feet supported.

Instruction to client

The client is instructed to forward flex the neck and laterally flex away from the side tested, then rotate the head back to the same side. The client is to maintain scapular stability by holding under the bench or their leg on the side being tested.

Examiner position and notes

The examiner is positioned standing behind the client in order to assess for range and quality of the movement. Palpate the trapezius near its insertion at the clavicle for resting tone.

Overpressure can be applied if the client is not irritable to assess for the quality of the end feel. One hand is placed on the acromion to stabilise it whilst the other hand is placed under the occiput to apply a force in the direction for flexion and lateral flexion.

The examiner should note any symptoms that are reproduced during the testing for re-evaluation after the intervention. Range should be compared to the non-affected side for a baseline of normal range when available.

KINESIO TAPING
Upper trapezius

STRENGTH TAPING

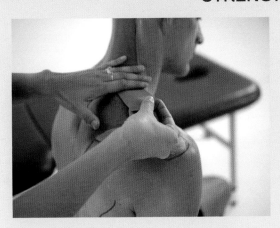

Client position
The client is seated in neutral lordosis with the neck flexed forward and laterally flexed to the contralateral side and rotated to the ipsilateral side so as to obtain maximal tissue stretch over the area.

Measurement of tape
Measure a length of tape from under the hairline to the acromion.

Tape application
Apply the anchor under the hairline with zero tension. With the tissue in a lengthened position, apply the tape with 25–35% tension following the line of the upper trapezius. Complete the taping by applying the anchor onto the acromioclavicular joint with zero tension. Rub the tape to activate the glue. As the neck is a sensitive area, tension towards the lower side of the spectrum is recommended.

Reassessment
Reassess your client for changes in strength, tonal changes, functional changes and symptoms.

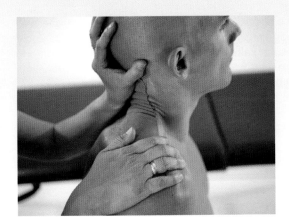

KINESIO TAPING
Upper trapezius

LENGTH TAPING

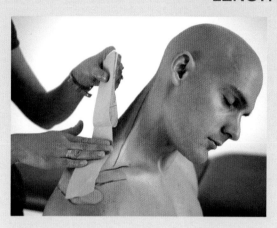

Client position

The client is seated in neutral lordosis with the neck flexed forward and laterally flexed to the contralateral side and rotated to the ipsilateral side so as to obtain maximal tissue stretch over the area.

Measurement of tape

Measure a length of tape from under the hairline to the acromion. The tape can be left as an I-strip or cut into a Y to combine taping for the middle trapezius and also allow for a better angle as the tape travels up towards the occiput.

Tape application

Apply the anchor over the acromioclavicular joint with zero tension. With the tissue in a lengthened position, apply the tape with 15–25% tension. Complete the taping by applying the anchor under the occiput with zero tension. Rub the tape to activate the glue.

Additional notes

As the neck is a sensitive area, tension towards the lower side of the spectrum is recommended.

The hairline may be a sensitive area or may require a special cut of the tape in order to tape higher into the neck line. It can be more practical on the first application to start the tape at the hairline and apply the tape with the appropriate tension to achieve results, rather than start in the reverse direction and find that the tape is too long and have to trim the tape near hair. Once an appropriate length of tape has been determined a practitioner may choose to start the taping process at the acromion on subsequent applications.

LENGTH TAPING

Reassessment

Reassess your client for changes in length, strength, tonal changes, functional changes and symptoms.

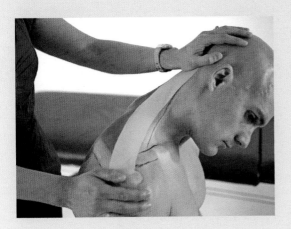

4

ANATOMY
Middle trapezius

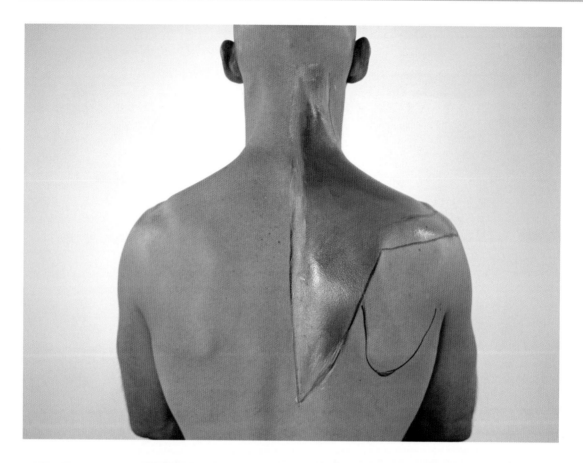

Middle trapezius

Origin:	Spinous process of T1–5 and intervening supraspinal ligament
Insertion:	Medial border of the acromion process of the scapula, spine of the scapula
Nerve supply:	Nerve root: C1–5 Peripheral nerve: spinal portion of the accessory nerve (CN XI); ventral rami of C3, C4
Function:	Retracts the scapula (scapular adduction) at the scapulocostal joint

MUSCLE TESTING
Middle trapezius

STRENGTH BIAS TESTING

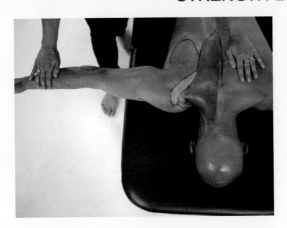 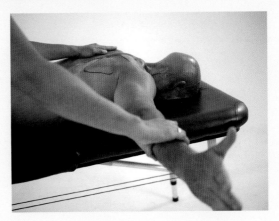

Client position

The client is lying prone with the upper limb at 90 degrees abduction and complete external rotation (thumb is pointing to the ceiling). The client's head is in a neutral position or rotated to the opposite side if a head hole is unavailable.

Instruction to client

The examiner is positioned to the side of the plinth on the side that is to be tested. The client is instructed to pull the shoulder blade towards the spine (scapular retraction) whilst taking the thumb to the ceiling. The examiner stabilises the thorax and palpates the middle trapezius. The effort should come from the attempt to draw the shoulder blade towards the spine.

Examiner position and notes

In the presence of middle trapezius weakness, it is common to substitute posterior deltoid activity in order to generate abduction on the humerus; care should be taken to observe scapular movement so that the abduction of the humerus is not mistaken for scapular adduction.

Resistance

Whilst stabilising the opposite thorax, resistance can be applied over the dorsum of the distal forearm in the direction of horizontal adduction (towards the floor). The emphasis of testing is on the ability of the client to maintain the scapula (as opposed to the humerus) position during resistance.

MUSCLE TESTING
Middle trapezius

LENGTH BIAS TESTING

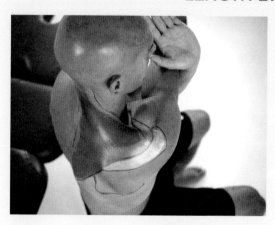

Client position

The client is seated in neutral lordosis and with the feet supported.

Instruction to client

The client is instructed to horizontally adduct the upper arm keeping the trunk facing forward, bend both elbows and protract the shoulder by taking the elbow forward whilst maintaining the shoulder depression.

Examiner position and notes

The examiner is positioned standing behind the client in order to assess for the range and quality of the movement. Palpate the trapezius above the spine of the scapula for tone. Overpressure can be applied if the client is not irritable to assess for the quality of the end feel. The examiner should note any symptoms that are reproduced during the testing for re-evaluation after the intervention. Range should be compared to the non-affected side for a baseline of normal range when available.

KINESIO TAPING
Middle trapezius

STRENGTH TAPING

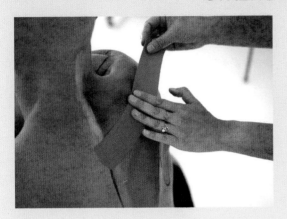

Client position
The client is seated in neutral lordosis with the feet supported. The shoulder is horizontally adducted and protracted with the assistance of the other upper limb.

Measurement of tape
Measure a length of tape from T1 or T5 to the spine of the scapula just proximal to the acromion process. After allowing for the anchors at the spine and at the acromion, the length of the therapeutic zone of the tape is calculated by reducing the remaining length of tape by ¼. This minimises error when the correct tension in the tape is applied to the muscle whilst on stretch. When a practitioner is in doubt as to how long to make a piece of tape, it is recommended to err on the side of excess length as muscles operate in units and the additional length of tape can provide beneficial stimulus to adjacent muscles.

Tape application
Apply the anchor at the spine with zero tension. With the tissue in a lengthened position, apply the tape with 25–35% tension. Complete the taping by applying the anchor onto the lateral spine of the scapula with zero tension. Rub the tape to activate the glue.

Reassessment
Reassess your client for changes in strength, tonal changes, functional changes and symptoms.

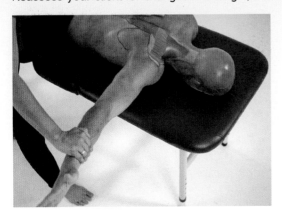

KINESIO TAPING
Middle trapezius

LENGTH TAPING

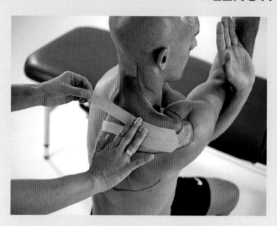

Client position

The client is seated in neutral lordosis with the feet supported. The shoulder is horizontally adducted and protracted with the assistance of the other upper limb.

Measurement of tape

Measure a length of tape from T1 or T5 to the spine of the scapula just proximal to the acromion process. The tape can be cut into a Y to cover the bulk of the middle trapezius or kept as an I-strip to address specific fibres.

Tape application

Apply the anchor at the lateral spine of the scapula with zero tension. With the tissue in a lengthened position, apply the tape with 15–25% tension towards the spine. Complete the taping by applying the anchor onto the spine with zero tension. Rub the tape to activate the glue.

Reassessment

Reassess your client for changes in length, strength, tonal changes, functional changes and symptoms.

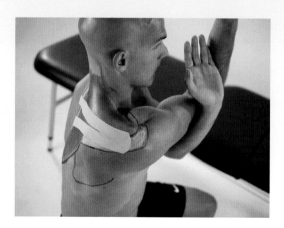

ANATOMY
Lower trapezius

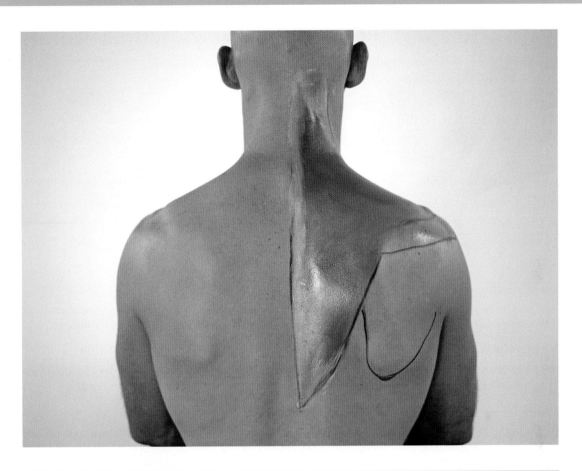

Lower trapezius

Origin:	Spinous process of T6–12 and intervening spinal ligaments
Insertion:	Tubercle on the medial end of the scapular spine
Nerve supply:	Nerve root: C1–5 Peripheral nerve: spinal portion of the accessory nerve (CN XI); ventral rami of C3, C4
Function:	Depresses, retracts and upwardly rotates the scapula at the scapulocostal joint

MUSCLE TESTING
Lower trapezius

STRENGTH BIAS TESTING

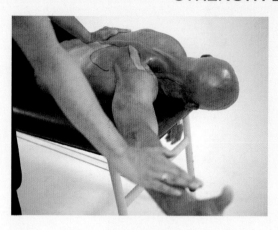

Client position

The client is lying prone with the upper limb at 130 degrees abduction and complete external rotation. The client's head is rotated to the opposite side if no head hole is available on the bed for testing.

Instruction to client

The client is instructed to elevate the arm towards the ceiling by taking the thumb to the ceiling and in doing so will perform depression and adduction of the scapula in the upwardly rotated position.

Examiner position and notes

The examiner is positioned on the side of the plinth on the contralateral side when resistance is applied to the scapula, OR standing on the ipsilateral side if resistance is applied to the forearm. This testing also involves significant middle trapezius activity and when resistance is applied at the distal forearm, the functional test may also implicate involvement of the deltoid muscles.

Resistance

Whilst stabilising the thorax, apply resistance over the lateral aspect of the scapula in the direction of scapular abduction and elevation (the client attempts to depress and adduct in response to this). If greater leverage is required, apply resistance at the distal forearm towards the floor.

MUSCLE TESTING
Lower trapezius

LENGTH BIAS TESTING

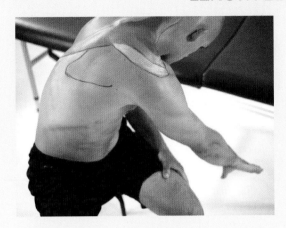

Client position
The client is seated in neutral lordosis and with the feet supported.

Instruction to client
The client is instructed to pronate the forearm, reach towards or past the opposite knee and round out the spine to protract and elevate the scapula.

Examiner position and notes
The examiner is positioned to assess for the range and quality of the movement. Overpressure can be applied if the client is not irritable to assess for the quality of the end feel. The examiner should note any symptoms that are reproduced during the testing for re-evaluation after the intervention. Range should be compared to the non-affected side for a baseline of normal range when available.

KINESIO TAPING
Lower trapezius

STRENGTH TAPING

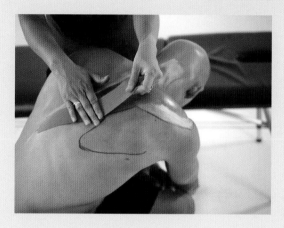

Client position

The client is seated in neutral lordosis with the spine flexed, the shoulder protracted and reaching to the opposite lower limb, with the forearm pronated (thumb pointing down).

Measurement of tape

Measure an I-strip of tape from T12 to the medial ⅓ of the scapular spine.

Tape application

Apply the anchor on the spine at T12 with zero tension. With the tissue in the lengthened position, apply the tape with 25–35% tension towards the medial ⅓ of the scapular spine. Complete the taping by applying the anchor onto the scapular spine with zero tension. Rub the tape to activate the glue.

Reassessment

Reassess your client for changes in strength, tonal changes, functional changes and symptoms.

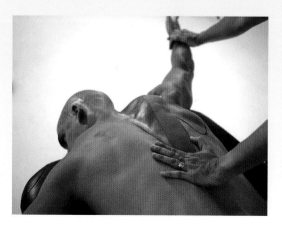

KINESIO TAPING
Lower trapezius

LENGTH TAPING

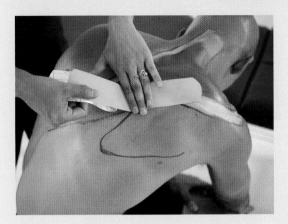

Client position
The client is seated in neutral lordosis with the spine flexed, the shoulder protracted and reaching to the opposite lower limb, with the forearm pronated (thumb pointing down).

Measurement of tape
Measure an I-strip of tape from T12 to the medial ⅓ of the scapular spine.

Tape application
Apply the anchor on the medial spine of the scapula with zero tension. With the tissue in a lengthened position, apply the tape with 15–25% tension towards T12. Complete the taping by applying the anchor onto the spine with zero tension. Rub the tape to activate the glue.

Reassessment
Reassess your client for changes in length, strength, tonal changes, functional changes and symptoms.

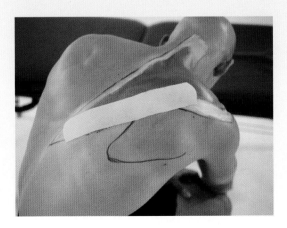

ANATOMY

4

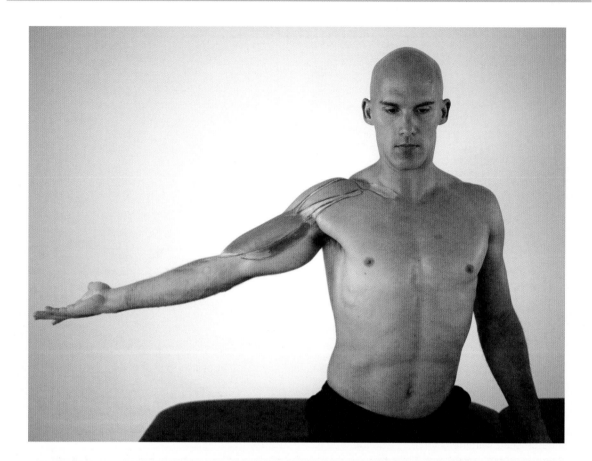

Coracobrachialis

Origin:	Coracoid process of the scapula
Insertion:	Middle ⅓ of the medial shaft of the humerus
Nerve supply:	Nerve root: C6, C7 Peripheral nerve: musculocutaneous nerve
Function:	Flexes, adducts and horizontally flexes the arm at the shoulder joint

MUSCLE TESTING
Coracobrachialis

STRENGTH BIAS TESTING

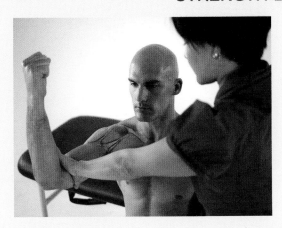

Client position
The client is seated in neutral lordosis and with the feet supported.

Instruction to client
The client is instructed to flex the elbow to 90 degrees and the shoulder to 90 degrees and then take the shoulder into slight adduction. The client is instructed to attempt to maintain the position during testing.

Examiner position and notes
The examiner stands to the front of the client and to the side. Place the testing hand proximal to the bent elbow (shoulder being tested) and the stabilising hand on the opposite shoulder. Coracobrachialis is differentiated with the biceps for its function at the shoulder by testing the shoulder flexion for the biceps with the elbow in extension and with the resistance placed distal to the elbow. The biceps also function as an elbow flexor and can be further implicated with strength testing for elbow flexion.

Resistance
Resist the client's flexion and horizontal adduction of the arm at the shoulder joint by applying a force to the distal end of the upper arm just proximal to the elbow joint in the direction of the shoulder abduction and extension. Once the muscle is activated, the stabilising hand can be removed so the practitioner can feel for the contraction of the coracobrachialis at the medial-proximal ½ of the arm.

MUSCLE TESTING
Coracobrachialis

LENGTH BIAS TESTING

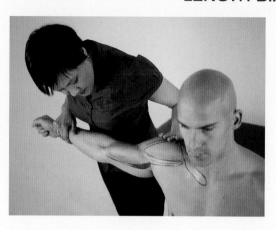

Client position

The client is seated in neutral lordosis and with the feet supported.

Instruction to client

The client is instructed to abduct the shoulder to 90 degrees, with the elbow extended and the forearm facing forward. The client is then instructed to horizontally abduct the shoulder so that the upper limb is behind the body.

Examiner position and notes

The examiner stands to the side of the client. The stabilising hand is placed on the posterior shoulder whilst the other hand is positioned above the wrist to feel for end range.

KINESIO TAPING
Coracobrachialis

STRENGTH TAPING

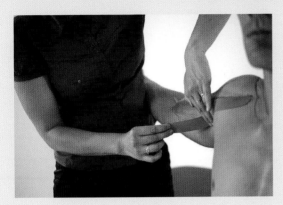

Client position

The client is seated with the shoulder in horizontal abduction. The practitioner may add further length to the tissue by applying overpressure with their trunk. Alternatively, the client may rest the arm on a high bed or the wall.

Measurement of tape

Measure a length of tape from the middle of the medial shaft of the humerus to the coracoid process. Cut the tape down its length to create a 2.5 cm-wide tape. The second piece can be used for subsequent applications.

Tape application

Apply the starting anchor on to the coracoid process with zero tension. With the tissue in the lengthened position, apply the base of the tape with 25–35% tension anterior to the medial intermuscular septum and towards the middle of the humeral shaft. Complete the taping by applying the anchor onto the humeral shaft with zero tension. Rub the tape to activate the glue.

Reassessment

Reassess your client for changes in strength, tonal changes, functional changes and symptoms.

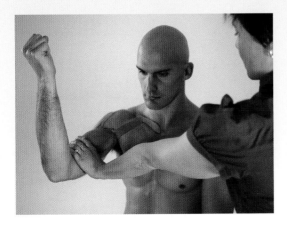

KINESIO TAPING
Coracobrachialis

LENGTH TAPING

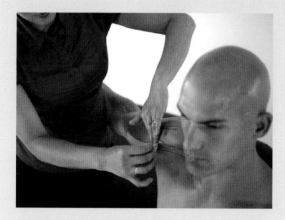

Client position

The client is seated with the shoulder in horizontal abduction. The practitioner may add further length to the tissue by applying overpressure with their trunk. Alternatively, the client may rest the arm on a high bed or the wall.

Measurement of tape

Measure a length of tape from the middle of the medial shaft of the humerus to the coracoid process. Cut the tape down its length to create a 2.5 cm-wide tape. The second piece can be used for subsequent applications.

Tape application

Apply the starting anchor onto the medial shaft of the humerus with zero tension. With the tissue on stretch, apply the base of the tape with 15–25% tension anterior to the medial intermuscular septum and towards the coracoid process. Complete the taping by applying the anchor onto the coracoid with zero tension. Rub the tape to activate the glue.

Reassessment

Reassess your client for changes in length, strength, tonal changes, functional changes and symptoms.

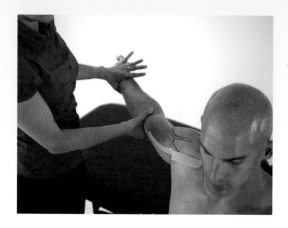

ANATOMY
Rhomboid

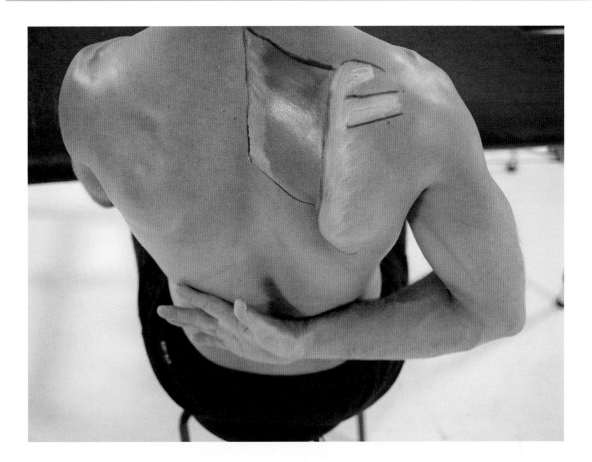

Rhomboid	
Origin:	Spinous process of C7–T5 and intervening spinous ligament
Insertion:	Medial border of the scapula from the spine of the scapula to the inferior border of the scapula
Nerve supply:	Nerve root: C5 Peripheral nerve: dorsal scapular nerve
Function:	Retracts, elevates and downwardly rotates the scapula at the scapulocostal joint

MUSCLE TESTING
Rhomboid

STRENGTH BIAS TESTING

TESTING A

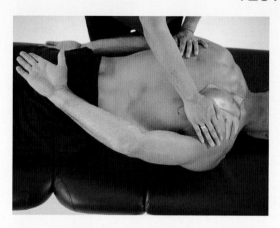

Client position

The client is lying prone with the upper limb held behind the back.

Instruction to client

The client is instructed to keep the dorsum of the hand off the body whilst reaching down and towards the opposite buttocks. The hand is reaching obliquely back and down to the gluteal region in order to create scapular retraction and downward rotation. The client should attempt to maintain the scapular position during the testing.

Examiner position and notes

The examiner is positioned on the contralateral side of the bed. With one hand stabilising the thorax, first palpate the rhomboid between the border of the scapula and spinous process C7–T5.

Resistance

The examiner applies a resistance to the medial inferior border of the scapula in the direction of scapular abduction and upward rotation.

4

TESTING B

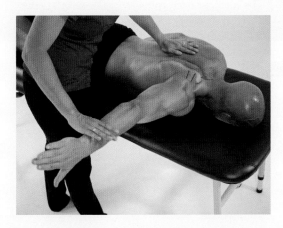

Client position

The client is lying prone with the upper limb in abduction at 90 degrees and the scapula retracted; this movement may be assisted by the examiner for the client to appreciate the scapula movement being tested. The client's thumb is pointed down towards the floor to bias the testing for rhomboids over the middle trapezius; the rhomboid muscle downwardly rotates the scapula whereas the middle trapezius upwardly rotates the scapula.

Instruction to client

The client is instructed to attempt to maintain the abducted shoulder position with the thumb pointing down to the floor during testing. The focus of the work should be coming from the scapula rather than the upper limb.

Examiner position and notes

The examiner is positioned on the ipsilateral side of the bed. With one hand stabilising the thorax, resistance is applied over the forearm. The distal application of the force allows better mechanical leverage for the examiner; however, care should be taken to note strategies arising from the posterior deltoid and/or triceps muscles. Whilst the examiner is applying the resistance distally, the focus of the test is on the movement of the scapula and the ability of the client to maintain the scapular position. It is easier for the examiner to note movement that occurs at the inferior angle of the scapula.

Resistance

The examiner applies a resistance to the distal forearm towards the floor.

MUSCLE TESTING
Rhomboid

LENGTH BIAS TESTING

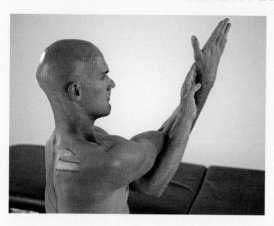

Client position

The client is seated in neutral lordosis and with the feet supported.

Instruction to client

The client's arm is held across the body by the opposite upper limb and the client is asked to protract the shoulder by reaching the elbow forward whilst maintaining depression of the scapula.

Examiner position and notes

The examiner is positioned to assess for range and quality of the movement. It is not usually necessary for the examiner to apply overpressure as this is done by the client's opposite arm. The examiner should note any symptoms that are reproduced during the testing for re-evaluation after the intervention. Range should be compared to the non-affected side for a baseline of normal range when available.

KINESIO TAPING
Rhomboid

STRENGTH TAPING

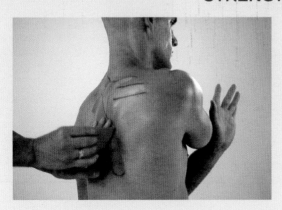

Client position

The client is seated with the upper limb horizontally adducted and the arm held by the opposite arm; the scapula is protracted by reaching further forward.

Measurement of tape

Measure a length of tape from T2 to the inferior border of the scapula whilst it is protracted. This can be left as an I-strip to address specific fibres or cut into an X-strip to allow for more tissue coverage.

Tape application

For an I-strip application, apply the starting anchor on the spine at the level of T2 with zero tension. With the tissue in a lengthened position, apply the tape towards the inferior angle of the scapula with 25–35% tension. Complete the taping by applying the anchor onto the scapula with zero tension. Rub the tape to activate the glue.

For an X-strip application, tear the tape in the middle of the X and apply 25–35% tension into the middle of the tape. With tissue in the lengthened position, place the stretched tape onto the skin. Complete the taping by applying the anchors onto the spine and scapula with zero tension. Rub the tape to activate the glue.

Reassessment

Reassess your client for changes in strength, tonal changes, functional changes and symptoms.

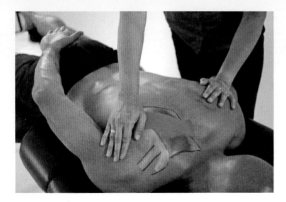

KINESIO TAPING
Rhomboid

LENGTH TAPING

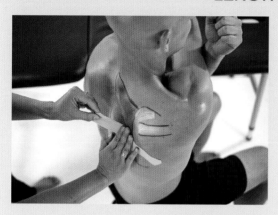

4

Client position

The client is seated with the upper limb horizontally adducted and the arm held by the opposite arm; the scapula is protracted by reaching further forward.

Measurement of tape

Measure a length of tape from T2 to the inferior border of the scapula whilst it is protracted. This can be left as an I-strip to address specific fibres or cut into an X-strip to allow for more tissue coverage.

Tape application

For an I-strip application, apply the starting anchor with zero tension on the inferior angle of the scapula. With the tissue in the lengthened position, apply the tape towards T2 with 15–25% tension. Complete the taping by applying the anchor onto the spine with zero tension. Rub the tape to activate the glue.

For an X-strip application, tear the tape in the middle of the X and apply 15–25% tension into the middle of the tape. With tissue in the lengthened position, place the stretched tape onto the skin. Complete the taping by applying the anchors onto the spine and scapula with zero tension. Rub the tape to activate the glue.

Reassessment

Reassess your client for changes in length, strength, tonal changes, functional changes and symptoms.

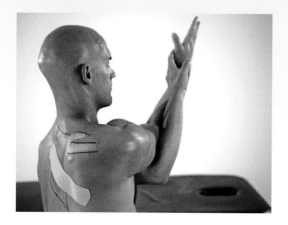

ANATOMY
Levator scapula

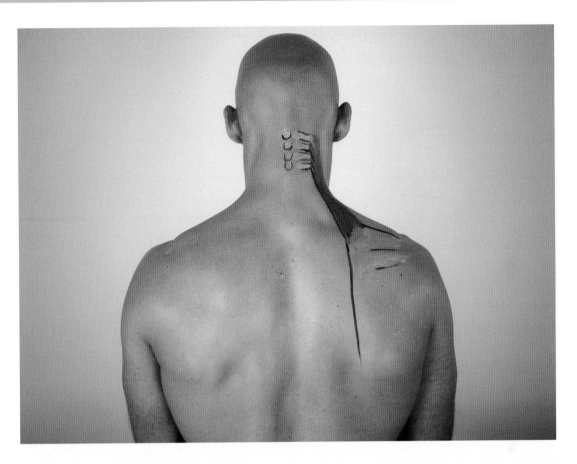

Levator scapula

Origin:	Transverse process of C1–4
Insertion:	Medial border of the scapula, from the root of the spine to the superior angle
Nerve supply:	Nerve root: C3–5 Peripheral nerve: dorsal scapular nerve, C3, C4
Function:	Elevates, adducts and downwardly rotates the scapula at the scapulocostal joint. Extends, laterally flexes and ipsilaterally rotates the neck at the spinal joints

MUSCLE TESTING
Levator scapula

STRENGTH BIAS TESTING

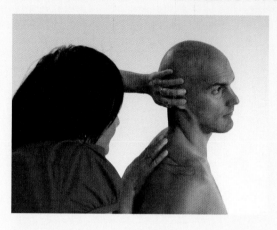

Client position
The client is seated in neutral lordosis and with the feet supported.

Instruction to client
The client is instructed to tilt the head back to the side being tested and to elevate the shoulder blade by bringing the elbows back so that the occiput approaches the medial border of the scapula.

Examiner position and notes
The examiner is positioned behind the client on the side being tested. The heel of the hand is placed on the occiput facing superiorly. The other hand is placed on the shoulder with the forearm resting on the client's humerus.

Resistance
Apply resistance to the scapula by applying a force along the humerus to move the shoulder towards flexion and upward rotation of the scapula. Concurrently apply a force through the heel of the hand on the occiput towards cervical flexion to the opposite side being tested.

MUSCLE TESTING
Levator scapula

LENGTH BIAS TESTING

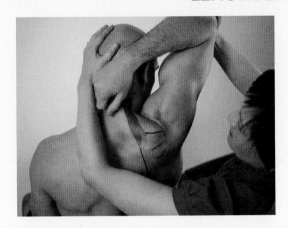

Client position

The client is seated in neutral lordosis and with the feet supported.

Instruction to client

Cervical component: The client is instructed to flex the neck, laterally flex and rotate away from the side being tested.

Scapula component: The client is instructed to place the hand behind the head in order to engage scapular upward rotation, depression of the medial border of the scapula and abduction of the inferior scapular angle.

Examiner position and notes

The examiner should note any shoulder compensations or if symptoms are produced which would indicate the end of range has been reached or that the alternative testing position is more appropriate. End range resistance can be assessed by moving the elbow up (to increase upward rotation and abduction of the scapula) or adding cervical lateral flexion and flexion at the occiput.

Alternatively, if clients have limited shoulder range, they may maintain shoulder depression by holding the bench. The examiner can apply overpressure to assess for restriction at the occiput or scapula.

ALTERNATIVE TESTING

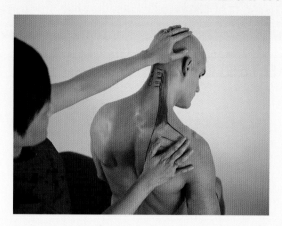

KINESIO TAPING
Levator scapula

STRENGTH TAPING

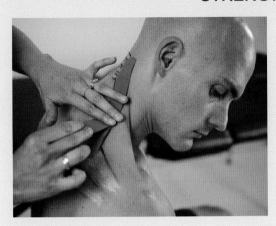

Client position

The client is seated in neutral lordosis and with the feet supported. The client is instructed to flex the neck, laterally flex and rotate away from the side being taped. Maintain shoulder depression by reaching down and holding the bench.

Measurement of tape

Measure a length of tape from under the hairline to the medial spine of the scapula. Cut down the length of the tape to create a 2.5 cm-wide tape. Trim one of the anchors to match the hairline.

Tape application

Place the starting anchor with zero tension just underneath the occiput below the hairline. With the tissue in the lengthened position, apply the tape down towards the medial scapular spine with 25–35% tension. Complete the taping by applying the anchor onto the medial superior scapula with zero tension. Rub the tape to activate the glue.

Additional notes

As the neck is a sensitive area, tension towards the lower side of the spectrum is recommended.

STRENGTH TAPING

Reassessment

Reassess your client for changes in strength, tonal changes, functional changes and symptoms.

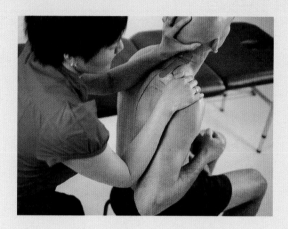

4

KINESIO TAPING
Levator scapula

LENGTH TAPING

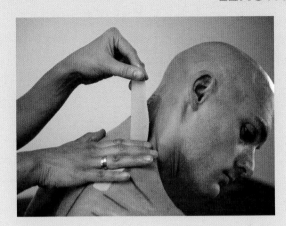

Client position

The client is seated in neutral lordosis and with the feet supported. The client is instructed to flex the neck, laterally flex and rotate away from the side being tested. Maintain shoulder depression by reaching down and holding the bench.

Measurement of tape

Measure a length of tape from under the hairline to the medial spine of the scapula. Cut down the length of the tape to create a 2.5 cm-wide tape. Trim one of the anchors to match the hairline.

Tape application

Place the starting anchor with zero tension over the medial scapular spine. With the tissue in a lengthened position, apply the tape up towards the occiput with 15–25% tension. Complete the taping by applying the anchor onto the hairline with zero tension. Rub the tape to activate the glue.

Additional notes

As the neck is a sensitive area, tension towards the lower side of the spectrum is recommended.

The hairline may be a sensitive area or may require a special cut of the tape in order to tape higher into the neck line. For the first application, it can be more practical to start the tape at the hairline and apply the tape with the appropriate tension towards the scapula to achieve results. Starting at the scapula and finding that the tape is too long and having to trim the tape near hair may be avoided. Once an ideal length has been determined, a practitioner may commence taping at the scapula on subsequent length applications.

LENGTH TAPING

Reassessment

Reassess your client for changes in length, strength, tonal changes, functional changes and symptoms.

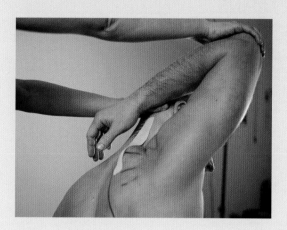

ANATOMY
Serratus anterior

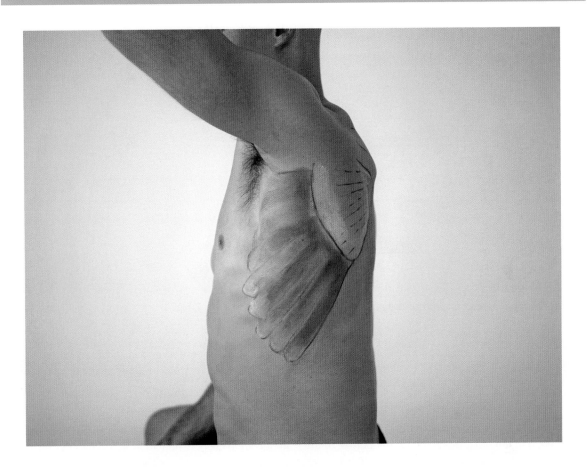

Serratus anterior

Origin:	Anterior surface of ribs 1–9
Insertion:	Anterior surface of entire medial border of the scapula
Nerve supply:	Nerve root: C5–7 Peripheral nerve: long thoracic nerve
Function:	Protracts and upwardly rotates the scapula at the scapulocostal joint. Upper fibres elevate the scapula, lower fibres depress the scapula

MUSCLE TESTING
Serratus anterior

STRENGTH BIAS TESTING

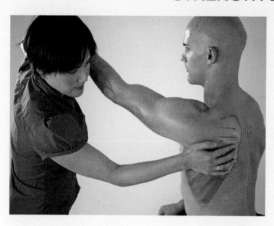

Client position

The client is seated in neutral lordosis and with the feet supported.

Instruction to client

The client is instructed to flex the shoulder to approximately 125 degrees and in doing so performs scapular upward rotation. The client is then instructed to push the fist forward as if sustaining a punch in the air, thereby protracting the scapula.

Examiner position and notes

The examiner is positioned in front and to the side of the client. Place one testing hand over the fist of the client and the other along the lateral border of the scapula. If the client is unable to achieve the position or maintain the position, this is a positive test.

Resistance

Apply resistance along the shaft of the upper limb through the fist; simultaneously apply resistance to the inferior angle of the scapula in the direction of downward rotation.

MUSCLE TESTING
Serratus anterior

LENGTH BIAS TESTING

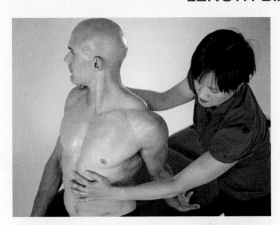

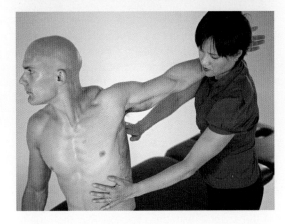

Client position

The client is seated in neutral lordosis and with the feet supported.

Instruction to client

The client is instructed to reach behind the back and rest the hands on the bed, or hold onto the back of the seat at chest height or, alternatively, the examiner may support the shoulder at an appropriate height. The client is then instructed to rotate the body to the opposite side which causes a retraction of the scapula. As the serratus anterior attaches to the ribs at various angles, it may be appropriate to test the length and tone of muscle through an arc of the shoulder range.

Examiner position and notes

The examiner is positioned to assess for range and quality of the movement. Palpate the tone of the muscle at the lateral ribs, and assess for any distinct variations from one rib to the next. The examiner should note any symptoms that are reproduced during the testing for re-evaluation after the intervention. Range should be compared to the non-affected side for a baseline of normal range when available.

KINESIO TAPING
Serratus anterior

STRENGTH TAPING

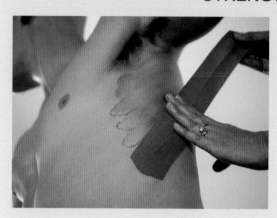

Client position

The client is seated in neutral lordosis and with the feet supported. The client is instructed to reach behind the back and rest the hands on the bed, or hold onto the back of the seat at chest height or, alternatively, the practitioner may support the shoulder at an appropriate height. The client is then instructed to rotate the body to the opposite side which causes a retraction of the scapula. Alternatively, instruct the client to place their hand on the head and retract the shoulders back by rotating the elbow back.

Measurement of tape

Measure a length of tape from the medial border of the scapula to the anterolateral ribs.

Tape application

Apply the starting anchor onto the lateral rib with zero tension. With the tissue in a lengthened position, apply the tape to the ribs and up the medial border of the scapula with 25–35% tension. Complete the taping by applying the anchor onto the medial border of the scapula with zero tension. Rub the tape to activate the glue.

Reassessment

Reassess your client for changes in strength, tonal changes, functional changes and symptoms.

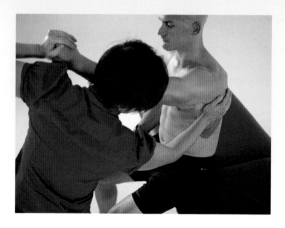

KINESIO TAPING
Serratus anterior

LENGTH TAPING

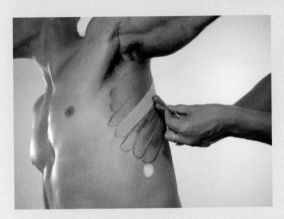

Client position

The client is seated in neutral lordosis and with the feet supported. The client is instructed to reach behind the back and rest the hands on the bed, or hold onto the back of the seat at chest height or, alternatively, the examiner may support the shoulder at an appropriate height. The client is then instructed to rotate the body to the opposite side causing a retraction of the scapula. Alternatively, instruct the client to place their hand on the head and retract the shoulders back by rotating the elbow back.

Measurement of tape

Measure a length of tape from the medial border of the scapula to the anterolateral ribs. Trim the tape into a Y cut or into a fan cut.

Tape application

Apply the starting anchor onto the lateral border of the scapula. With the tissue in a lengthened position, apply each tail with 15–25% tension towards the rib. Complete the taping by applying the anchor onto the rib with zero tension. Rub the tape to activate the glue.

Reassessment

Reassess your client for changes in length, strength, tonal changes, functional changes and symptoms.

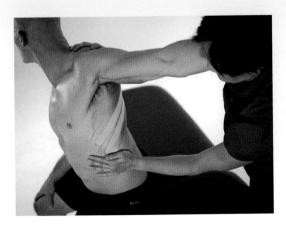

ANATOMY

Posterior deltoid

4

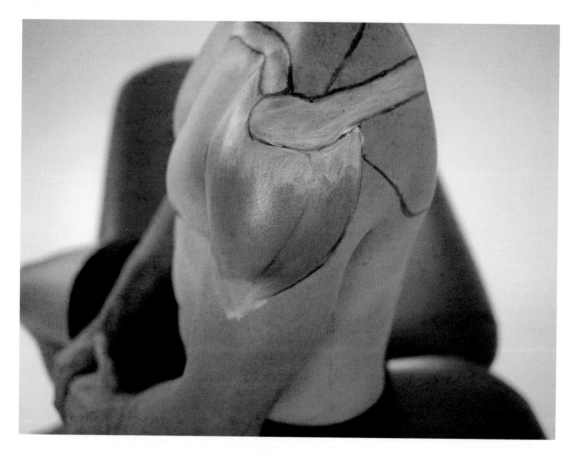

Posterior deltoid

Origin:	Lateral ⅓ of the spine of the scapula
Insertion:	Deltoid tuberosity of the humerus
Nerve supply:	Nerve root: C5, C6 Peripheral nerve: axillary nerve
Function:	Extends, abducts and laterally rotates the upper arm. Horizontally extends the arm at the shoulder joint

MUSCLE TESTING
Posterior deltoid

STRENGTH BIAS TESTING

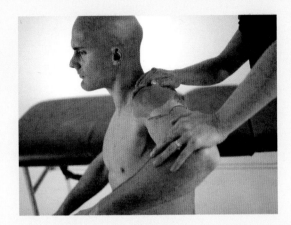

Client position
The client is seated in neutral lordosis and with the feet supported.

Instruction to client
With the elbow flexed to 90 degrees, the client is instructed to abduct the shoulder to 90 degrees along the scapular plane and orientate the forearm so that it is pointing to the ground at a 45-degree angle. Take the shoulder from this point into slight horizontal abduction/extension.

Examiner position and notes
The examiner stands to the back of the client and on the same side to be tested. The stabilising hand is placed on the shoulder to be tested with the testing hand placed proximal to the elbow.

Resistance
Apply a force on the humerus in a direction following the shaft of the forearm (45 degrees towards the floor). The examiner should utilise their body weight to lean in to the testing to protect their own body.

4

MUSCLE TESTING
Posterior deltoid

LENGTH BIAS TESTING

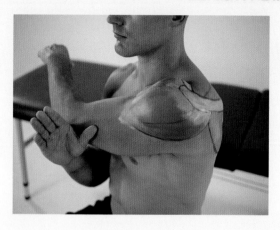

Client position

The client is seated in neutral lordosis and with the feet supported.

Instruction to client

The client is instructed to horizontally adduct the upper arm and pull the arm in towards the chest with the opposite upper limb whilst keeping the trunk facing forward.

Examiner position and notes

The examiner is positioned to assess for range and quality of the movement. The examiner should note any symptoms that are reproduced during the testing for re-evaluation after the intervention. Range should be compared to the non-affected side for a baseline of normal range when available.

KINESIO TAPING
Posterior deltoid

STRENGTH TAPING

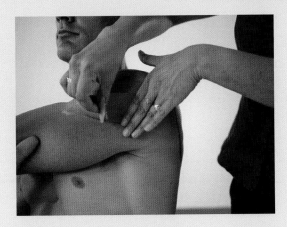

Client position
The client is seated in neutral lordosis and with the feet supported. The client is instructed to horizontally adduct the upper arm and hold this position with the other arm whilst keeping the trunk facing forward.

Measurement of tape
Measure a length of tape from the deltoid tuberosity to the lateral spine of the scapula.

Tape application
Apply the starting anchor on the lateral spine of the scapula with zero tension. With the tissue in a lengthened position, apply the base of the tape with 25–35% tension towards the deltoid tuberosity. Complete the taping by applying the anchor with zero tension. Rub the tape to activate the glue.

Reassessment
Reassess your client for changes in strength, tonal changes, functional changes and symptoms.

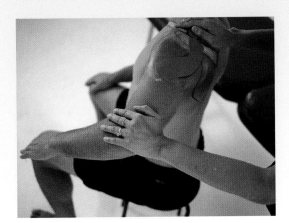

KINESIO TAPING
Posterior deltoid

LENGTH TAPING

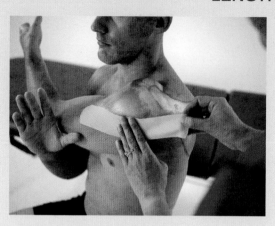

Client position

The client is seated in neutral lordosis and with the feet supported. The client is instructed to horizontally adduct the upper arm and hold this position with the other arm whilst keeping the trunk facing forward.

Measurement of tape

Measure a length of tape from the deltoid tuberosity to the lateral spine of the scapula.

Tape application

Apply the starting anchor on the deltoid tuberosity with zero tension. With the tissue in a lengthened position, apply the base of the tape with 15–25% tension up towards the lateral spine of the scapula. Complete the taping by applying the anchor with zero tension. Rub the tape to activate the glue.

Reassessment

Reassess your client for changes in length, strength, tonal changes, functional changes and symptoms.

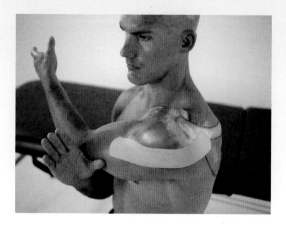

ANATOMY
Middle deltoid

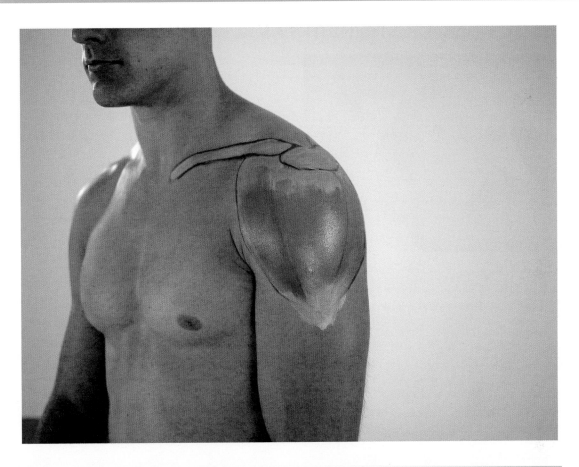

Middle deltoid

Origin:	Acromion process of the scapula
Insertion:	Deltoid tuberosity of the humerus
Nerve supply:	Nerve root: C5, C6 Peripheral nerve: axillary nerve
Function:	Abducts the humerus

MUSCLE TESTING
Middle deltoid

STRENGTH BIAS TESTING

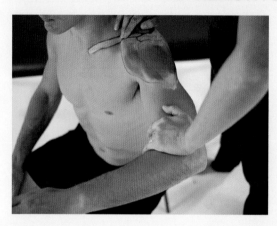

Client position

The client is seated in neutral lordosis and with the feet supported.

Instruction to client

With the elbow flexed to 90 degrees, the client is instructed to abduct the shoulder to 90 degrees along the scapular plane.

Examiner position and notes

The examiner stands to the back of the client and on the same side to be tested. The stabilising hand is placed on the shoulder to be tested with the testing hand placed proximal to the elbow.

Resistance

Apply a force over the distal humerus towards the floor. The force applied is perpendicular to the client's forearm and floor. The examiner should utilise their body weight to lean in to the testing to protect their own body.

MUSCLE TESTING
Middle deltoid

LENGTH BIAS TESTING

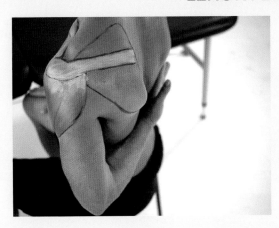

4

Client position
The client is seated in neutral lordosis and with the feet supported.

Instruction to client
Length bias testing of the muscle is difficult as the trunk is in the way. Instruct the client to reach behind the back and depress the shoulder to maximise tissue stretch.

Examiner position and notes
For this muscle, it is useful to palpate the resting tone of the muscle as length bias testing may be unclear.

KINESIO TAPING
Middle deltoid

STRENGTH TAPING

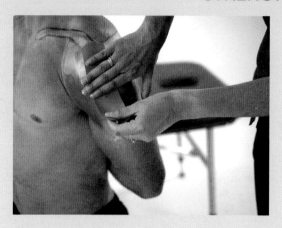

Client position
The client is seated in neutral lordosis and is instructed to reach the hand up and behind the back, and depress the shoulder to maximise tissue stretch.

Measurement of tape
Measure a length of tape from the deltoid tuberosity to the acromion process.

Tape application
Apply the starting anchor on the acromion with zero tension. With the tissue in a lengthened position, apply the base of the tape with 25–35% tension towards the deltoid tuberosity. Complete the taping by applying the anchor with zero tension. Rub the tape to activate the glue.

Reassessment
Reassess your client for changes in strength, tonal changes, functional changes and symptoms.

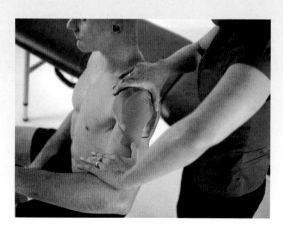

KINESIO TAPING
Middle deltoid

LENGTH TAPING

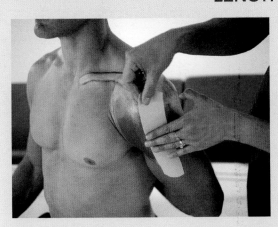

Client position

The client is seated in neutral lordosis and instructed to reach the hand up and behind the back, and depress the shoulder to maximise tissue stretch.

Measurement of tape

Measure a length of tape from the deltoid tuberosity to the acromion process.

Tape application

Apply the starting anchor on the deltoid tuberosity with zero tension. With the tissue in a lengthened position, apply the base of the tape with 15–25% tension up towards the acromion process. Complete the taping by applying the anchor with zero tension. Rub the tape to activate the glue.

Reassessment

Reassess your client for changes in length, strength, tonal changes, functional changes and symptoms.

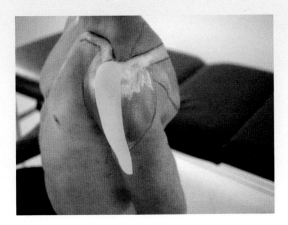

109

ANATOMY
Anterior deltoid

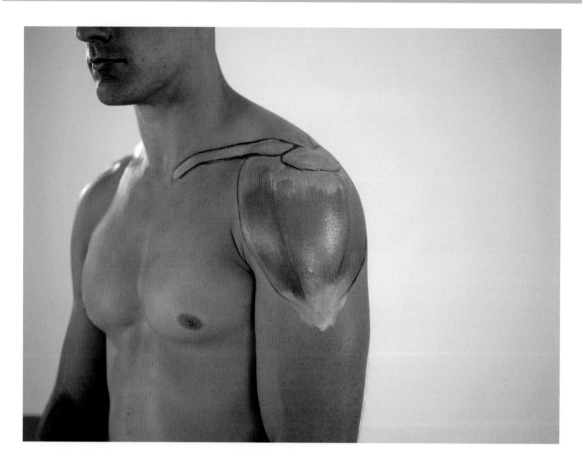

Anterior deltoid	
Origin:	Lateral ⅓ to ½ of the clavicle
Insertion:	Deltoid tuberosity of the humerus
Nerve supply:	Nerve root: C5, C6 Peripheral nerve: axillary nerve
Function:	Flexes, abducts and medially rotates the humerus. Horizontally flexes the upper arm

MUSCLE TESTING
Anterior deltoid

STRENGTH BIAS TESTING

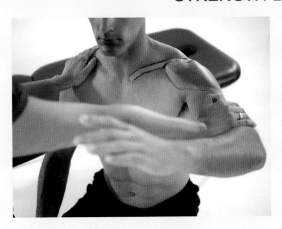

Client position
The client is seated in neutral lordosis and with the feet supported.

Instruction to client
With the elbow flexed to 90 degrees, the client is instructed to abduct the shoulder along the scapular plane and then orientate the forearm so that it is obliquely pointing to the ceiling (placed at a 45-degree angle towards the ceiling). Take the shoulder from this point into slight flexion.

Examiner position and notes
The examiner stands to the front of the client and to the side, placing the testing hand proximal to the bent elbow (shoulder being tested) and the stabilising hand on the opposite shoulder.

Resistance
Apply a force on the humerus obliquely towards the floor in a direction that follows the shaft of the forearm (placed at a 45 degree-angle towards the ceiling). The examiner should utilise their body weight to lean in to the testing to protect their own body.

MUSCLE TESTING
Anterior deltoid

LENGTH BIAS TESTING

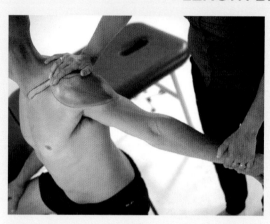

Client position
The client is seated in neutral lordosis and with the feet supported.

Instruction to client
The client is instructed to take the upper limb back behind the body, with the thumb pointing behind to externally rotate the shoulder.

Examiner position and notes
The examiner stands behind the client. One hand stabilises the client's shoulder whilst the other assesses for end feel by applying overpressure at the wrist. The examiner should note any symptoms that are reproduced during the testing for re-evaluation after the intervention. Range should be compared to the non-affected side for a baseline of normal range when available.

KINESIO TAPING
Anterior deltoid

STRENGTH TAPING

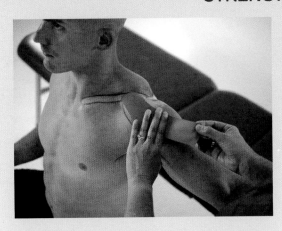

Client position
The client is seated with the shoulder in extension and external rotation with the arm resting behind the body.

Measurement of tape
Measure a length of tape from the deltoid tuberosity to the lateral clavicle.

Tape application
Apply the starting anchor on the lateral clavicle with zero tension. With the tissue in a lengthened position, apply the base of the tape with 25–35% tension towards the deltoid tuberosity. Complete the taping by applying the anchor with zero tension. Rub the tape to activate the glue.

Reassessment
Reassess your client for changes in strength, tonal changes, functional changes and symptoms.

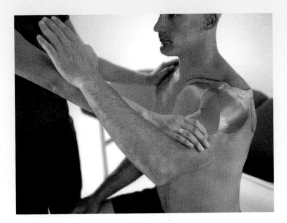

KINESIO TAPING
Anterior deltoid

LENGTH TAPING

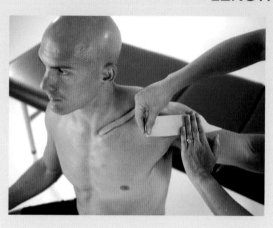

Client position

The client is seated with the shoulder in extension and external rotation with the arm resting behind the body.

Measurement of tape

Measure a length of tape from the deltoid tuberosity to the lateral clavicle.

Tape application

Apply the starting anchor on the deltoid tuberosity with zero tension. With the tissue in a lengthened position, apply the base of the tape with 15–25% tension up towards the lateral clavicle. Complete the taping by applying the anchor with zero tension. Rub the tape to activate the glue.

Reassessment

Reassess your client for changes in length, strength, tonal changes, functional changes and symptoms.

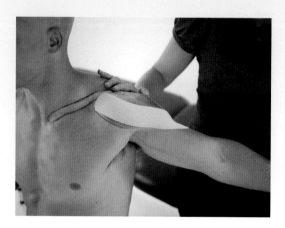

ANATOMY
Teres major

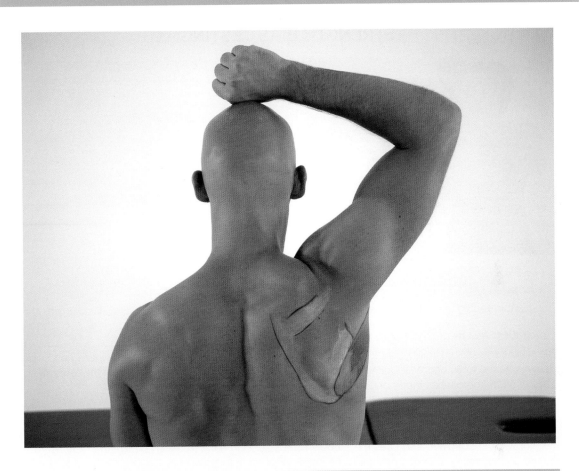

Teres major

Origin:	Inferior angle and dorsal inferior ⅓ of the lateral border of the scapula
Insertion:	Medial lip of the bicipital groove of the humerus
Nerve supply:	Nerve root: C5, C6 Peripheral nerve: lower subscapular nerve
Function:	Medially rotates, adducts and extends the upper arm. Upwardly rotates the scapula at the glenohumeral and scapulocostal joints. Has a role in minimising translatory forces at the glenohumeral joint during flexion and extension tasks

MUSCLE TESTING
Teres major

STRENGTH BIAS TESTING

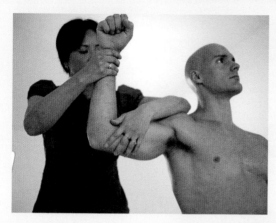

Client position
The client is seated in neutral lordosis and with the feet supported.

Instruction to client
The shoulder is placed in 90 degrees abduction and the elbow is supported by the examiner's hand. The elbow is flexed to 90 degrees. During the test the client is instructed to attempt to rotate the forearm so that the palm approaches the floor.

Examiner position and notes
The examiner stands behind the client and rests the elbow on the client's shoulder whilst supporting the elbow. The examiner also uses the elbow of the stabilising hand to ascertain whether any hitching occurs during testing and then maintains the shoulder position if this occurs. The testing hand is placed proximal to the wrist joint.

Resistance
The examiner resists the client's rotation towards the floor by applying a force in the direction of lateral/external rotation.

MUSCLE TESTING
Teres major

LENGTH BIAS TESTING

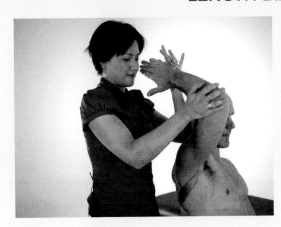

Client position
The client is seated in neutral lordosis and with the feet supported.

Instruction to client
With the elbow flexed to 90 degrees, the client is instructed to flex the shoulder to the overhead position (forearm on head position). Once in full flexion, the client is instructed to attempt to rotate the forearm out whilst keeping the elbow position (lateral rotation of the humerus).

Examiner position and notes
The examiner stands behind the client and stabilises the lateral elbow whilst assessing for range and resistance by applying overpressure to the hand in a direction of lateral rotation. The examiner should note any symptoms that are reproduced during the testing for re-evaluation after the intervention. Range should be compared to the non-affected side for a baseline of normal range when available.

KINESIO TAPING
Teres major

STRENGTH TAPING

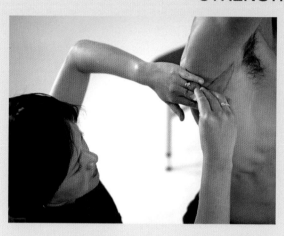

Client position

The client is seated and instructed to take the arm into lateral rotation and flexion in the overhead position (forearm on head position). The position is held with the assistance of the client's opposite hand at the elbow as they attempt to further externally rotate the shoulder by turning the wrist outwards.

Measurement of tape

Measure a length of tape from the inferior border of the scapula to the medial aspect of the axilla.

Tape application

Apply the starting anchor on the inferior border of the scapula with zero tension. With the tissue in the lengthened position, apply the base of the tape with 25–35% tension towards the medial intermuscular septum just under the axilla. Complete the taping by applying the anchor adjacent to the axilla.

Reassessment

Reassess your client for changes in strength, tonal changes, functional changes and symptoms.

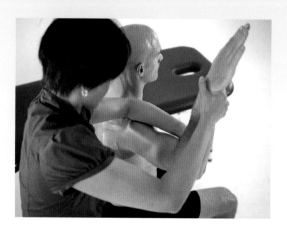

KINESIO TAPING
Teres major

LENGTH TAPING

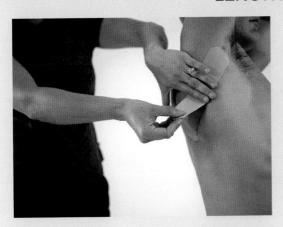

Client position

The client is seated and instructed to take the arm into lateral rotation and flexion in the overhead position (forearm on head position). The position is held with the assistance of the client's opposite hand at the elbow as they attempt to further externally rotate the shoulder by turning the wrist outwards.

Measurement of tape

Measure a length of tape from the inferior border of the scapula to the medial aspect of the axilla.

Tape application

Apply the starting anchor adjacent to the axilla with zero tension. With the tissue in the lengthened position, apply the base of the tape with 15–25% tension towards the inferior border of the scapula. Complete the taping by applying the anchor onto the scapula with zero tension. Rub the tape to activate the glue.

Reassessment

Reassess your client for changes in length, strength, tonal changes, functional changes and symptoms.

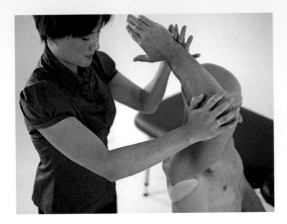

ANATOMY
Latissimus dorsi

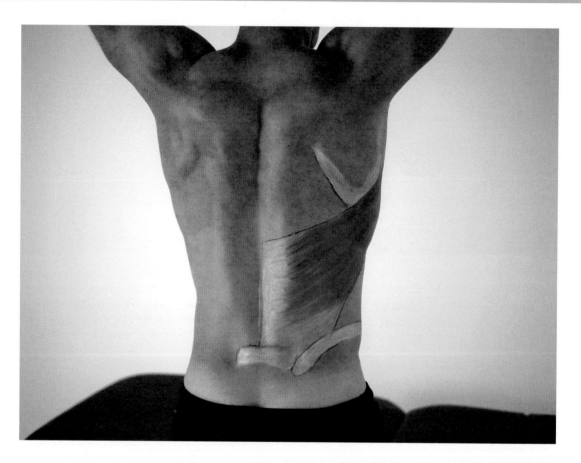

Latissimus dorsi

Origin:	Via the thoracolumbar fascia; spinous process T7–L5, posterior sacrum, posterior iliac crest, lowest three to four ribs and the inferior angle of the scapula
Insertion:	Medial lip of the bicipital groove of the humerus
Nerve supply:	Nerve root: C6–8 Peripheral nerve: thoracodorsal nerve
Function:	Extends, adducts and medially rotates the arm at the shoulder joint

MUSCLE TESTING
Latissimus dorsi

STRENGTH BIAS TESTING

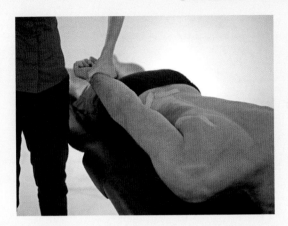

Client position

The client is prone with the shoulder held in internal rotation with the palm facing upwards. The shoulder is also in extension and adduction behind the back but without resting on the body.

Instruction to client

The client is instructed to resist the force applied by the examiner by maintaining the shoulder and upper limb position in internal rotation, extension and adduction without trying to hold against the back or buttocks during the testing.

Examiner position and notes

The examiner is positioned to the side of the client. The testing hand is placed proximal to the wrist compromised strategy which can be indicated with trunk rotation, alternative leg lifting and shoulder hitching.

Resistance

The examiner applies resistance in the direction of shoulder flexion and abduction to clear the trunk.

MUSCLE TESTING
Latissimus dorsi

LENGTH BIAS TESTING

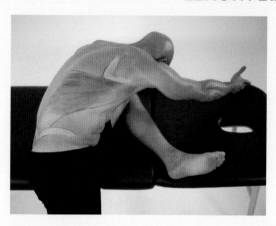

Client position

The client is sitting sideways on a plinth, the opposite hip is abducted and the trunk flexed and laterally flexed away from the side being tested. The arm is reaching forward diagonally across the body with the forearm supinated.

Instruction to client

The client is instructed to take the arm into lateral rotation, flexion and adduction in the overhead position in front of the body whilst also performing trunk flexion, lateral flexion and rotation away from the side being tested.

Examiner position and notes

The examiner is positioned to assess for range and quality of the movement. The examiner should note any symptoms that are reproduced during the testing for re-evaluation after the intervention. Range should be compared to the non-affected side for a baseline of normal range when available.

4

KINESIO TAPING
Latissimus dorsi

STRENGTH TAPING

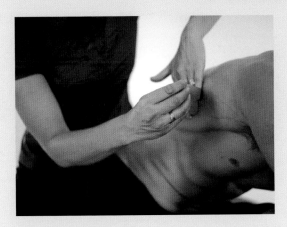

Client position
The client is sitting sideways on a plinth, the opposite hip is abducted and the trunk flexed and laterally flexed away from the side being tested. The arm is reaching forward diagonally across the body with the forearm supinated.

Measurement of tape
Measure a length to tape from the sacrum to the medial aspect of the axilla. Fold the tape in two and cut down in the style of a web cut, leaving a 5 cm anchor at both ends.

Tape application
Apply the starting anchor at the sacrum with zero tension. With the tissue in the lengthened position, lightly apply the base of the tape with 25–35% tension towards the axilla. Apply the anchor onto the axilla with zero tension and then lift the base of the tape and apply at appropriate angles to cover the muscle, its rib attachments and its scapular attachments. Rub the tape to activate the glue.

Reassessment
Reassess your client for changes in strength, tonal changes, functional changes and symptoms.

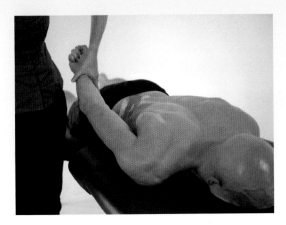

KINESIO TAPING
Latissimus dorsi

LENGTH TAPING

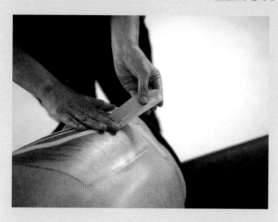

Client position

The client is sitting sideways on a plinth, the opposite hip is abducted and the trunk flexed and laterally flexed away from the side being tested. The arm is reaching forward diagonally across the body with the forearm supinated.

Measurement of tape

Measure a length to tape from the sacrum to the medial aspect of the axilla. Fold the tape in two and cut down in the style of a web cut, leaving a 5 cm anchor at both ends.

Tape application

Apply the starting anchor adjacent to the axilla with zero tension. With the tissue in the lengthened position, lightly lay the base of the tape with 15–25% tension towards the sacrum. Apply the anchor onto the sacrum with zero tension and then lift the base of the tape and apply at appropriate angles to cover the muscle, its rib attachments and its scapular attachments. Rub the tape to activate the glue.

Reassessment

Reassess your client for changes in length, strength, tonal changes, functional changes and symptoms.

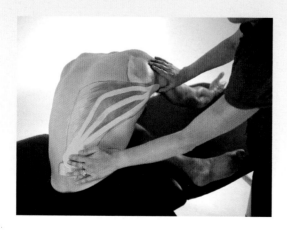

ANATOMY
Supraspinatus

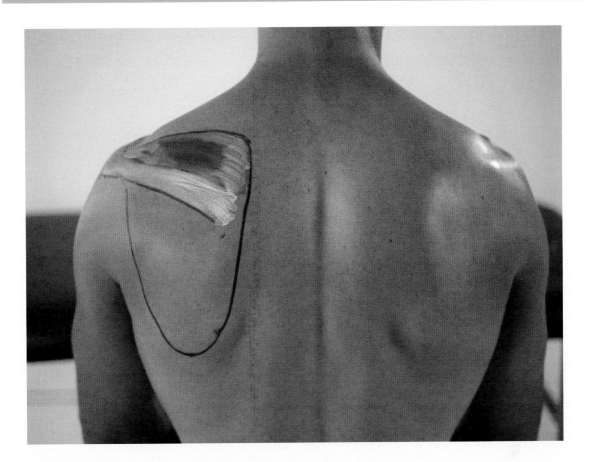

Supraspinatus

Origin:	Supraspinous fossa of the scapula
Insertion:	Greater tubercle of the humerus
Nerve supply:	Nerve root: C5 Peripheral nerve: suprascapular nerve
Function:	Abduction and flexion of the shoulder along the scapular plane. Laterally rotates the shoulder. Has a primary role in stabilising the humeral head with respect to the glenoid fossa throughout range

MUSCLE TESTING
Supraspinatus

STRENGTH BIAS TESTING

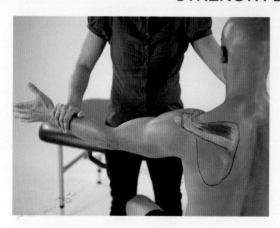

Client position
The client is seated in neutral lordosis and with the feet supported.

Instruction to client
The shoulder is placed in lateral rotation with the elbow in extension (the thumb faces upwards). The client is instructed to flex the shoulder in the scapular plane (approximately 30 degrees to the frontal plane) to 90 degrees. This testing can also be done in lower scaption ranges to implicate taping over this muscle.

Examiner position and notes
The examiner is positioned to the side of the client and in front. The stabilising hand is placed on the ipsilateral shoulder and the testing arm is placed proximal to the wrist (proximal to the elbow in the case of elbow pathology).

Resistance
The examiner applies resistance in the direction of extension and adduction towards the trunk.

MUSCLE TESTING
Supraspinatus

LENGTH BIAS TESTING

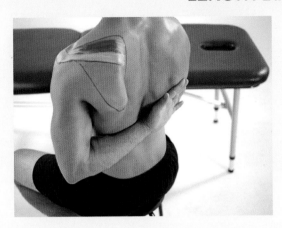

4

Client position
The client is seated in neutral lordosis and with the feet supported.

Instruction to client
The client places the hand behind the back and reaches up the back.

Examiner position and notes
For this muscle, it is useful to palpate the resting tone of the muscle above the spine of the scapula or observe for wasting in this area.

KINESIO TAPING
Supraspinatus

STRENGTH TAPING

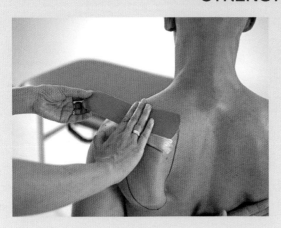

Client position

The client is seated in neutral lordosis and with the feet supported. The client places their hand behind their back and reaches up the back and their hand.

Measurement of tape

Measure a length of tape above the spine of the scapula (the supraspinous fossa) to the greater tuberosity of the humerus.

Tape application

Apply the anchor with zero tension above the medial spine of the scapula. With the tissue in the lengthened position, apply the base with 25–35% tension over the supraspinous fossa above the spine of the scapula. Complete the taping by applying the anchor onto greater tuberosity of the humerus with zero tension. Rub the tape to activate the glue.

Reassessment

Reassess your client for changes in strength, tonal changes, functional changes and symptoms.

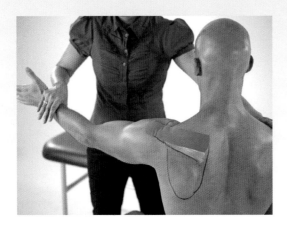

KINESIO TAPING
Supraspinatus

LENGTH TAPING

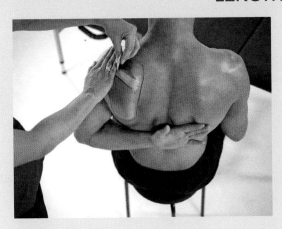

Client position
The client is seated in neutral lordosis and with the feet supported. The client places their hand behind their back and their hand reaches up the back.

Measurement of tape
Measure a length of tape above the spine of the scapula (the supraspinatus fossa) to the greater tuberosity of the humerus.

Tape application
Apply the anchor with zero tension on the greater tuberosity of the humerus. With the tissue in the lengthened position, apply the base with 15–25% tension over the supraspinous fossa above the spine of the scapula. Complete the taping by applying the anchor over the medial border of the scapula with zero tension. Rub the tape to activate the glue.

Reassessment
Reassess your client for changes in length, strength, tonal changes, functional changes and symptoms.

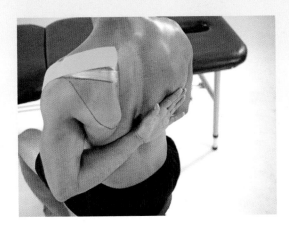

ANATOMY

Infraspinatus and teres minor

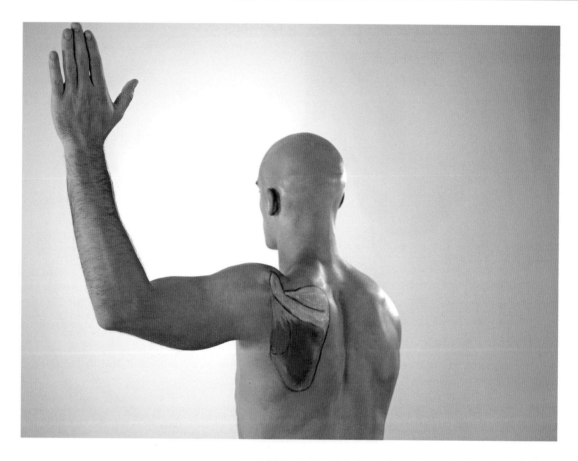

Infraspinatus

Origin:	Infraspinous fossa of the scapula
Insertion:	Greater tubercle of the humerus
Nerve supply:	Nerve root: C5, C6 Peripheral nerve: suprascapular nerve
Function:	Laterally rotates the upper arm and is more active during medium to higher load

Teres minor

Origin:	Superior ⅔ of the dorsal surface of the scapula at the lateral border
Insertion:	Greater tubercle of the humerus
Nerve supply:	Nerve root: C5 Peripheral nerve: axillary nerve
Function:	Laterally rotates and adducts the upper arm. Has a role in minimising translatory forces at the glenohumeral joint during flexion and extension tasks

MUSCLE TESTING
Infraspinatus

STRENGTH BIAS TESTING

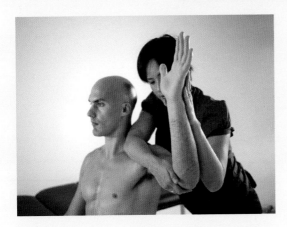

Client position
The client is seated in neutral lordosis and with the feet supported.

Instruction to client
The shoulder is placed in 90 degrees abduction and the elbow is supported by the examiner's hand. The elbow is flexed to 90 degrees. The client is instructed to rotate the forearm so that the palm faces the ceiling.

Examiner position and notes
The examiner stands behind the client and uses the elbow of the stabilising hand to ascertain whether any hitching occurs during testing. The testing hand is placed proximal to the wrist joint. Palpation of infraspinatus and teres minor muscles will assist in determining which muscle is implicated.

Resistance
Resist the client's rotation towards the ceiling in the direction of medial rotation.

MUSCLE TESTING
Infraspinatus

LENGTH BIAS TESTING

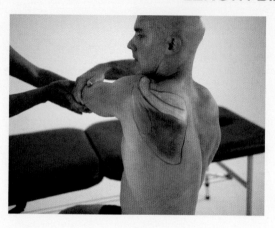

Client position

The client is seated in neutral lordosis and with the feet supported.

Instruction to client

Instruct the client to horizontally adduct the arm whilst keeping the elbow flexed to 90 degrees. Take the opposite hand to hold the elbow towards the body as the shoulder is internally rotated so that the hand turns to the floor.

Examiner position and notes

For this muscle, it is useful to palpate the resting tone of the muscle below the spine of the scapula or observe for wasting in this area. Palpation gives a more clear idea of whether the teres minor or infraspinatus is implicated.

4

KINESIO TAPING
Infraspinatus

STRENGTH TAPING

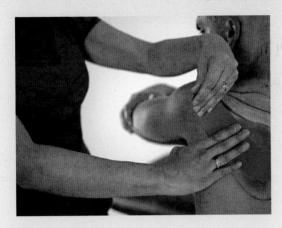

Client position

The client is seated in neutral lordosis and with the feet supported. Instruct the client to horizontally adduct the arm whilst keeping the elbow flexed to 90 degrees. Take the opposite hand to hold the elbow towards the body as the shoulder is internally rotated so that the hand turns to the floor.

Measurement of tape

Measure a length of tape from the medial border of the scapula to the greater tuberosity of the humerus. Cut the tape into a Y-strip to cover a broader area or maintain it as an I-strip to address particular fibres.

Tape application

For the I-strip: Apply the anchor with zero tension below the root of the spine of the scapula and apply the base with 25–35% tension over the infraspinous fossa below the spine of the scapula. Complete the taping by applying the anchor onto greater tuberosity of the humerus with zero tension. Rub the tape to activate the glue.

For Y application: Apply the common anchor at the greater tuberosity first and apply each tail along the muscle towards the medial border of the scapula with 25–35% tension. Complete the taping by applying the anchors with zero tension. Rub the tape to activate the glue.

STRENGTH TAPING

Reassessment

Reassess your client for changes in strength, tonal changes, functional changes and symptoms.

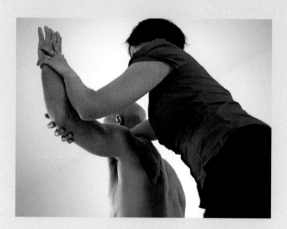

4

KINESIO TAPING
Infraspinatus

LENGTH TAPING

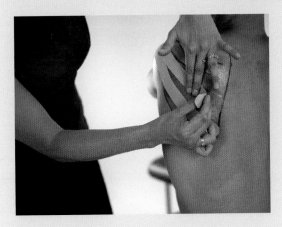

Client position

The client is seated in neutral lordosis and with the feet supported. Instruct the client to horizontally adduct the arm whilst keeping the elbow flexed to 90 degrees. Take the opposite hand to hold the elbow towards the body as the shoulder is internally rotated so that the hand turns to the floor.

Measurement of tape

Measure a length of tape from the medial border of the scapula to the greater tuberosity of the humerus. Cut the tape into a Y-strip to cover a broader area or maintain it as an I-strip to address particular fibres.

Tape application

For the I-strip: Apply the anchor with zero tension on the greater tuberosity of the humerus. With the tissue in the lengthened position, apply the base with 15–25% tension over the infraspinous fossa below the spine of the scapula. Complete the taping by applying the anchor onto the medial border of the scapula with zero tension. Rub the tape to activate the glue.

For Y application: Apply the common anchor at the greater tuberosity first and apply each tail along the muscle towards the medial border of the scapula with 15–25% tension. Complete the taping by applying the anchors with zero tension. Rub the tape to activate the glue.

LENGTH TAPING

Reassessment

Reassess your client for changes in length, strength, tonal changes, functional changes and symptoms.

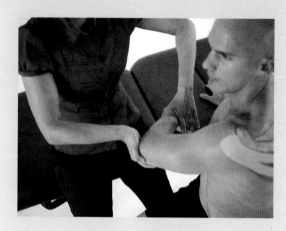

ANATOMY

Pectoralis major

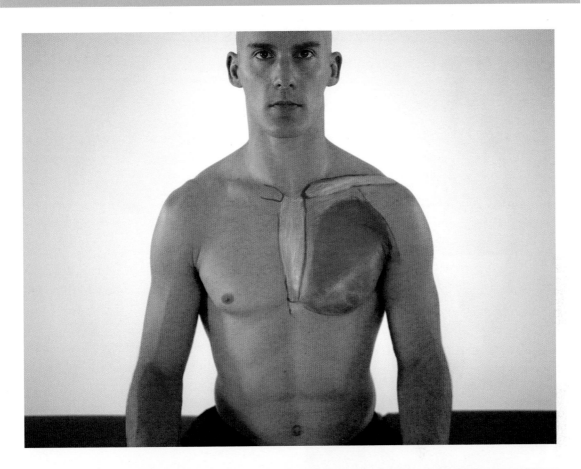

Pectoralis major

Origin:	Medial ½ of the clavicle, sternum and costal cartilages or ribs 1–7
Insertion:	Lateral lip of the bicipital groove of the humerus
Nerve supply:	Nerve root: C5–8, T1 Peripheral nerve: medial and lateral pectoral nerves
Function:	Adducts, medially rotates and horizontally flexes the upper arm at the glenohumeral joint. Functionally protracts the scapula at the scapulocostal joint
Clavicular head:	Flexes the upper arm at the glenohumeral joint
Sternocostal head:	Initiates extension when the upper arm is held in flexion

MUSCLE TESTING
Pectoralis major

STRENGTH BIAS TESTING

4

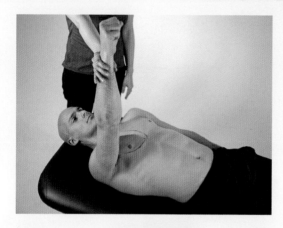

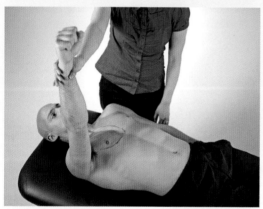

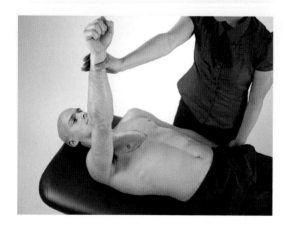

STRENGTH BIAS TESTING

Client position

The client is lying supine on the bed with the arm in 90 degrees flexion and 0 degree adduction and the elbow in 0 degree extension.

Instruction to client

For upper/clavicular fibres: Instruct the client to rotate the forearm as if turning a lever, so that the thumb is pointing diagonally towards the clavicle.

For middle fibres: Instruct the client to rotate the forearm as if turning a lever, so that the thumb is pointing horizontally.

For lower fibres: Instruct the client to rotate the forearm as if turning a lever, so that the thumb is pointing diagonally towards the opposite hip.

Examiner position and notes

The examiner stands to the opposite side of the bed so that the client's thumb is pointing towards the examiner for each range of testing. The examiner should use his/her body weight to assist with the testing rather than just using the upper body as resistance.

Resistance

The examiner applies a force on the distal radius in the direction opposite to where the thumb is pointing in the direction of the ulnar styloid.

MUSCLE TESTING
Pectoralis major

LENGTH BIAS TESTING

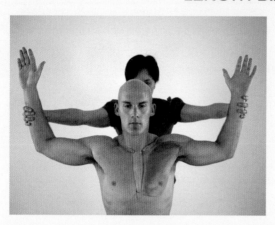

Client position

The client is seated in neutral lordosis and with the feet supported.

Instruction to client

The client is instructed to horizontally abduct the arm and rotate the hands up in a stop sign position for external rotation. To bias the clavicular head, the arm is abducted to 45 degrees instead of 90 degrees. The client should relax to allow the examiner to assess further into range.

Examiner position and notes

It is useful to do the seated test bilaterally to compare range and to also minimise compensatory trunk rotation. In this test the examiner is best placed standing behind the client to allow overpressure to be applied into the direction of horizontal abduction. The examiner may also choose to examine through an arc of movement for more specific deficits. The examiner should note any symptoms that are reproduced during the testing for re-evaluation after the intervention. Range should be compared to the non-affected side for a baseline of normal range when available.

LENGTH BIAS TESTING

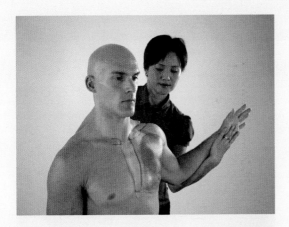

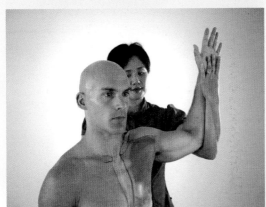

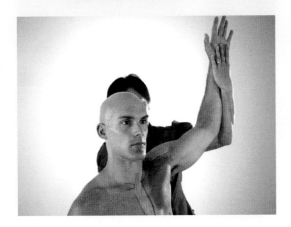

KINESIO TAPING
Pectoralis major

STRENGTH TAPING

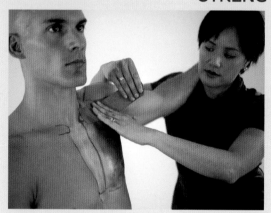

Upper fibres

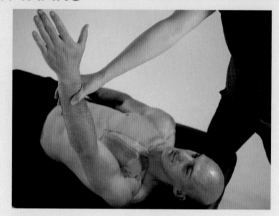

Upper fibres re-test

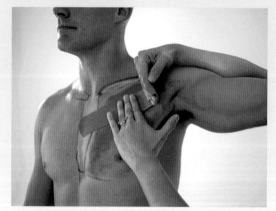

Middle fibres

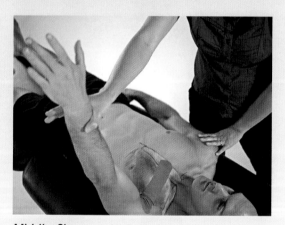

Middle fibres re-test

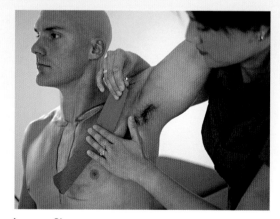

Lower fibres

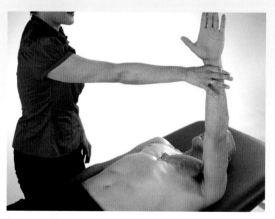

Lower fibres re-test

4

Client position

The client is seated with the arm held in abduction, external rotation and shoulder retraction.

Measurement of tape

Measure a length of tape from either the clavicular or sternal origin, as indicated by the testing. The tape can be cut into a thinner I-strip when treating a smaller-framed client or when having to treat multiple heads.

Tape application

Apply the anchor with zero tension over the clavicular or sternal head, as indicated by the testing. With the tissue in the lengthened position, apply the base with 25–35% tension towards the bicipital groove. Complete the taping by applying the final anchor with zero tension. Rub the tape to activate the glue.

Reassessment

Reassess your client for changes in strength, tonal changes, functional changes and symptoms.

KINESIO TAPING
Pectoralis major

LENGTH TAPING

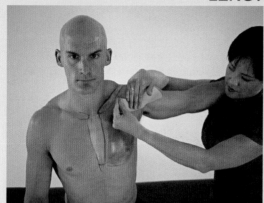

Upper fibres

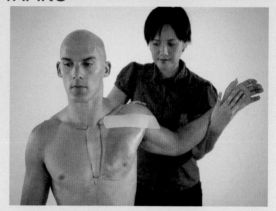

Upper fibres re-test

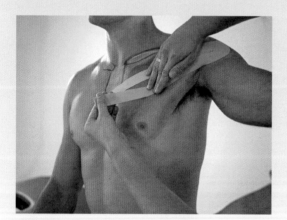

Middle fibres

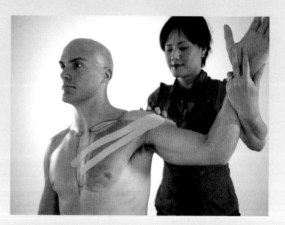

Middle fibres re-test

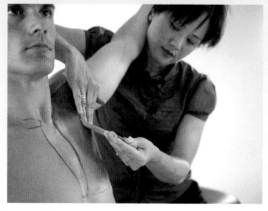

Lower fibres

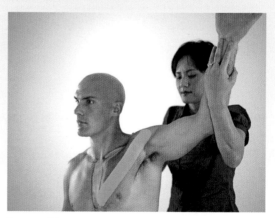

Lower fibres re-test

Client position

The client is seated with the arm held in abduction, external rotation and shoulder retraction.

Measurement of tape

Measure a length of tape from either the clavicular or sternal origin, as indicated by the testing. The tape can be cut into a Y-strip when addressing two different portions of the pectoralis major and for when treating a smaller-framed client.

Tape application

Apply the anchor over the bicipital grove with zero tension. With the tissue in a lengthened position, apply the base with 15–25% tension towards the clavicular or sternal head. Complete the taping by applying the final anchor with zero tension. Rub the tape to activate the glue.

For a Y-tape application, start the common anchor at the bicipital groove with zero tension. With each particular pectoral portion in a lengthened position, apply the tails separately towards the sternum or clavicle with 15–25% tension. Complete the taping by applying the final anchors with zero tension. Rub the tape to activate the glue.

Reassessment

Reassess your client for changes in length, strength, tonal changes, functional changes and symptoms.

4

ANATOMY
Pectoralis minor

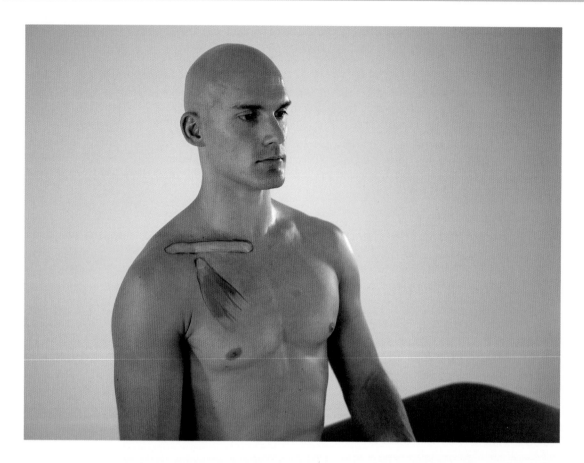

Pectoralis minor

Origin:	Anterior ribs 3–5
Insertion:	Coracoid process of the scapula
Nerve supply:	Nerve root: C8, T1 Peripheral nerve: medial pectoral nerve
Function:	Protracts, depresses and downwardly rotates the scapula at the scapulocostal joint

MUSCLE TESTING
Pectoralis minor

STRENGTH BIAS TESTING

Client position

The client is lying supine with the shoulder protracted and the elbow in 0 degree extension with the hand reaching towards the opposite hip with the thumb down.

Instruction to client

The client is instructed to maintain this position without resting the hand on the body.

Examiner position and notes

The examiner stands on the side to be tested and reaches across the body to resist above the wrist and also applies force on the ipsilateral shoulder towards retraction if needed. The shoulder placement is the opposite position to the strength test for lower trapezius and so in this way these muscles may be considered as antagonists during scapular movement.

Resistance

The examiner applies a force to lift the wrist and shoulder towards flexion and retraction (up towards the ceiling and then out).

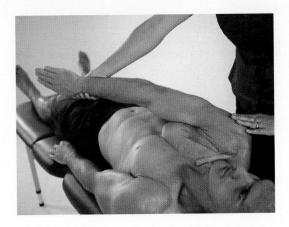

MUSCLE TESTING
Pectoralis minor

LENGTH BIAS TESTING

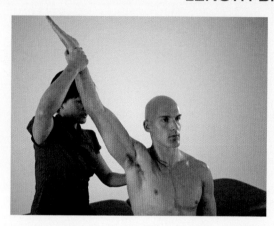

Client position

The client is seated in neutral lordosis and with the feet supported.

Alternatively, the client may be standing at a doorway.

Instruction to client

Instruct the client to consider the line between the shoulder and the contralateral hip, then instruct the client to take the arm out in a continuation of that line so that the arm is up and out at an angle with the thumb facing behind.

Alternative testing at the doorway: Instruct the client to abduct the upper limb to approximately 135 degrees at a doorway; then instruct the client to step forward with the ipsilateral leg or lean into the doorway.

Examiner position and notes

For the seated assessment, the examiner is positioned behind the client to stabilise the shoulder and to assess for resistance at end range. For the standing assessment, the examiner can be positioned in front of the client to palpate the shoulder. Palpation of the pectoralis minor at rest at the coracoid process will give a good indicator as to the resting tone and level of irritability of the tissue.

KINESIO TAPING
Pectoralis minor

STRENGTH TAPING

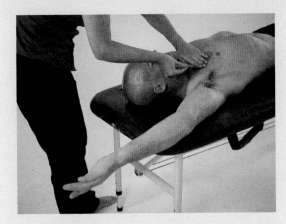

Client position
The client is lying supine with the shoulder abducted in a diagonal direction that continues the line from the contralateral hip to shoulder; the shoulder is resting in the overhead position.

Measurement of tape
Measure a length of tape from the coracoid process to the ribs 3–5. Fold the tape and cut as for a web cut. The web cut allows for movement of the pectoralis major whilst still facilitating normalisation of pectoralis minor function.

Tape application
Apply the anchor at rib 5 with zero tension. With the tissue in a lengthened position, apply the tape with 25–35% tension to the coracoid process. Complete the taping by applying the anchor with zero tension. Rub the tape to activate the glue.

Reassessment
Reassess your client for changes in strength, tonal changes, functional changes and symptoms.

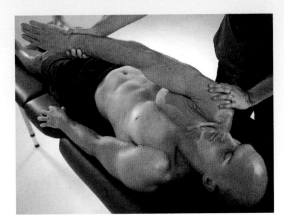

KINESIO TAPING
Pectoralis minor

LENGTH TAPING

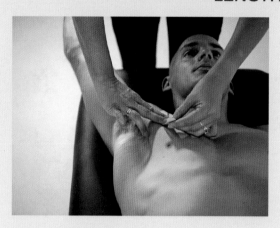

Client position

The client is lying supine with the shoulder abducted in a diagonal direction that continues the line from the contralateral hip to shoulder; the shoulder is resting in the overhead position.

Measurement of tape

Measure a length of tape from the coracoid process to the ribs 3–5. Cut the tape into a Y-strip or three fans.

Tape application

Apply the common anchor over the coracoid process with zero tension. With the tissue in the lengthened position, apply the base of each tail separately with 15–25% tension. Complete each tail by applying the anchor over the rib with zero tension. Rub the tape to activate the glue.

Reassessment

Reassess your client for changes in length, strength, tonal changes, functional changes and symptoms.

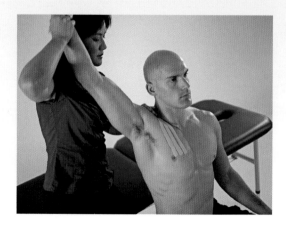

SHOULDER ASSESSMENT SHEET

Clinic: .... Date: ....

Client name: ....

Functional review

Functional limitation	Pre-test measure	Post-test measure

Muscle testing

Tested priority	Muscle	Strength		Length		Comments
		Right	Left	Right	Left	
	Upper trapezius					
	Middle trapezius					
	Lower trapezius					
	Coracobrachialis					
	Rhomboid					
	Levator scapula					
	Serratus anterior					
	Posterior deltoid					
	Middle deltoid					
	Anterior deltoid					
	Teres major					
	Latissimus dorsi					
	Supraspinatus					
	Infraspinatus					
	Pectoralis major					
	Pectoralis minor					

Treatment

Intervention	Re-test measures	Plan

Practitioner: .... Signature: ....

BIBLIOGRAPHY

Berryman Reese, N. M. (2012). *Muscle and sensory testing.* Missouri: Elsevier-Saunders.

Berryman Reese, N., & Bandy, W. D. (2010). *Joint range of motion and muscle length testing.* Missouri: Saunders Elsevier.

Calais-Germain, B. (1993). *Anatomy of movement* (12 ed.). Seattle: Eastland Press.

Comerford, M., & Mottram, S. (2012). *Kinetic control: the management of uncontrolled movement.* Sydney, Australia: Elsevier.

Kase, K., Hashimoto, T., & Okane, T. (1998). *Kinesio Taping perfect manual: amazing taping therapy to eliminate pain and muscle disorders.* Albuquerque: Kinesio Taping Association.

Kase, K., & Rock Stockheimer, K. (2006). *Kinesio Taping for lymphoedema and chronic swelling.* Albuquerque: Kinesio Taping Association.

Kase, K., Wallis, J., & Kase, T. (2003). *Clinical therapeutic applications of the Kinesio taping methods.* Albuquerque: Kinesio Taping Association.

Kendall, F. P., McCreary, E., Provance, P., Rodgers, M., & Romanic, W. (2005). *Muscles: testing and function with posture and pain.* Baltimore: Lippincott Williams Wilkins.

Standring, S., Borely, N., Collings, P., Crossman, A., Gatzoulis, M., Healy, J., … Wigley, C. (2008). *Gray's anatomy: the anatomical basis of clinical practice* (S. Susan Ed. 40 ed.). London, United Kingdom: Churchill Livingstone Elsevier.

4

Techniques for testing and taping the elbow

Biceps brachii and brachialis

Brachioradialis

Triceps brachii

ANATOMY

Biceps brachii and brachialis

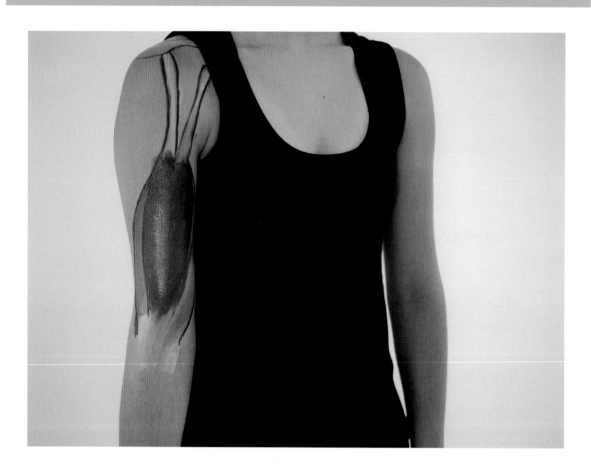

Biceps brachii

Origin:	Supraglenoid tubercle (long head) and coracoid process (short head) of the scapula
Insertion:	Radial tuberosity and deep fascia overlying the common flexor tendon
Nerve supply:	Nerve root: C5, C6 Peripheral nerve: musculocutaneous nerve
Function:	Flexes the forearm at the elbow joint, supinates the forearm at the radioulnar joint. Assists in the flexion of the shoulder. Long head abducts the arm at the glenohumeral joint; short head adducts the arm at the glenohumeral joint

Brachialis

Origin:	Distal ½ of anterior shaft of the humerus (distal to the deltoid tuberosity)
Insertion:	Tuberosity and coronoid process of the ulna
Nerve supply:	Nerve root: C5, C6, C7 Peripheral nerve: musculocutaneous nerve and radial nerve
Function:	Flexes the forearm at the elbow joint

MUSCLE TESTING
Biceps brachii and brachialis

STRENGTH BIAS TESTING

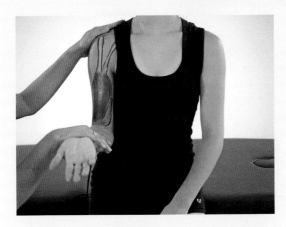

Client position
The client is seated with the feet supported. The shoulder is in a neutral position, the elbow flexed at 90 degrees and the forearm is supinated.

Instruction to client
The client is instructed to maintain the elbow at 90 degrees with the palm upwards as the examiner applies a downward force.

Examiner position and notes
The examiner is positioned in front of the client. The testing hand is placed proximal to the wrist and the stabilising hand on the shoulder to assess for compensatory shoulder hitching. Resist the client from flexing the forearm at the elbow joint and feel for a contraction of the biceps muscle and brachialis.

Resistance
The examiner applies force in the direction of the elbow extension.

MUSCLE TESTING
Biceps brachii and brachialis

LENGTH BIAS TESTING

Client position

The client is standing or seated in neutral lordosis and with the feet supported.

Instruction to client

The client is instructed to pronate the forearm with the elbow extended and take the shoulder into extension behind the back.

Examiner position and notes

The examiner is positioned standing behind and to the side of the client. The stabilising arm is applied to the posterior shoulder and the other hand at the wrist to maintain forearm pronation.

The examiner assesses for the range and quality of the movement. The examiner should note any symptoms that are reproduced during the testing for re-evaluation after the intervention. Range should be compared to the non-affected side for a baseline of normal range when available.

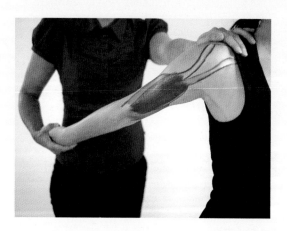

KINESIO TAPING
Biceps brachii and brachialis

STRENGTH TAPING

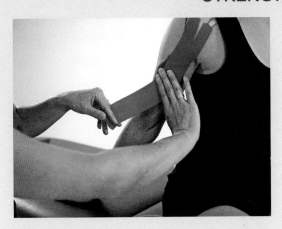

5

Client position
The client is seated with the shoulder in extension. Their arm is fully pronated and their elbow is in extension.

Measurement of tape
Measure a length of tape from the coracoid process of the scapula to the radial tuberosity.

Tape application
Apply the starting anchor with zero tension over the anterior acromion and in line with the bicipital groove. The second anchor is applied to the coracoid process with zero tension. With the tissue in a lengthened position, apply the base of the tape with 25–35% tension. Complete the taping with an anchor on the radial tuberosity with zero tension. Rub the tape to activate the glue.

Reassessment
Reassess your client for changes in strength, tonal changes, functional changes and symptoms.

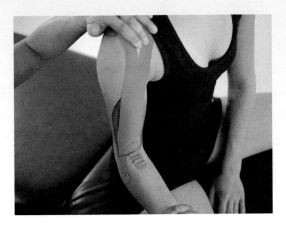

KINESIO TAPING
Biceps brachii and brachialis

LENGTH TAPING

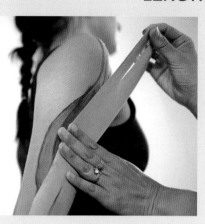

Client position

The client is seated with the shoulder in extension. The arm is fully pronated and the elbow is in extension.

Measurement of tape

Measure a length of tape from the coracoid process of the scapula to the radial tuberosity. Cut the tape into a Y-tape.

Tape application

Apply the common anchor onto the radial tuberosity with zero tension. With the tissue in the lengthened position, apply the lateral tail with 15–25% tension towards the acromion to approximate the superior labral attachment of the long head of biceps. Complete this tail application with zero tension on an anchor over the anterior acromion.

For the medial tail, take the arm into abduction in the extended position to apply the base with 15–25% tension. Complete this tail application with zero tension on the anchor over the coracoid process.

Reassessment

Reassess your client for changes in length, strength, tonal changes, functional changes and symptoms.

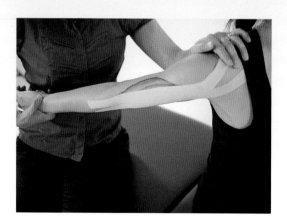

ANATOMY
Brachioradialis

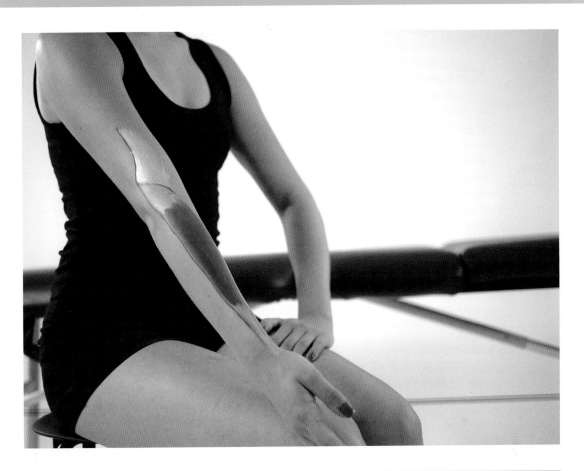

Brachioradialis

Origin:	Proximal ⅔ of the lateral supracondylar ridge of the humerus
Insertion:	Distal styloid process of the radius
Nerve Supply:	Nerve root: C5, C6, C7 Peripheral nerve: radial nerve
Function:	Flexes the forearm at the elbow joint

MUSCLE TESTING
Brachioradialis

STRENGTH BIAS TESTING

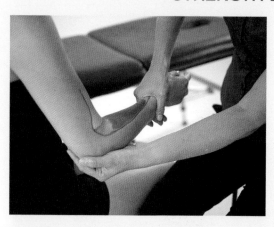

Client position

The client is seated with the arm relaxed and the forearm flexed at the elbow in a position halfway between full supination and full pronation. The thumb is facing up to the ceiling.

Instruction to client

The client is instructed to maintain the elbow and wrist position during the testing and attempts to prevent the examiner from extending the elbow.

Examiner position and notes

The examiner applies resistance to the anterior distal forearm just proximal to the wrist joint whilst the other hand stabilises the elbow.

Palpatory notes: The brachioradialis is superficial for the majority of its path except where the abductor pollicis longus and extensor pollicis brevis cross superficial to it at the distal forearm.

Resistance

The examiner applies a resistance in the direction of the elbow extension.

5

MUSCLE TESTING
Brachioradialis

LENGTH BIAS TESTING

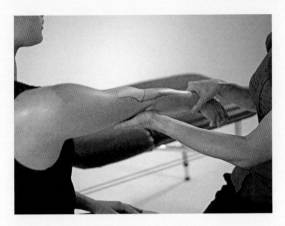

Client position
The client is seated in neutral lordosis and with the feet supported.

Instruction to client
The client is instructed to extend the elbow in front of the body. With the thumb facing the ceiling, the client is instructed to ulnar deviate by pointing the little finger towards the floor.

Examiner position and notes
The end range can be assessed by applying skin traction to the tissue before applying overpressure into the direction of the ulnar deviation. The other hand is used to support the elbow to maintain full extension. The overpressure can also be applied by the client so that the examiner is able to palpate the tissue. The examiner should note if there is a difference between the active and passive range of movement.

The examiner assesses for the range and quality of the movement. The examiner should note any symptoms that are reproduced during the testing for re-evaluation after the intervention. Range should be compared to the non-affected side for a baseline of normal range when available.

KINESIO TAPING
Brachioradialis

STRENGTH TAPING

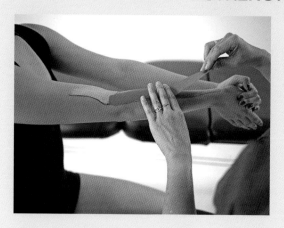

5

Client position

The client is seated with the elbow extended whilst the hand is in ulnar deviation. The client's other hand can assist to maintain the desired position.

Measurement of tape

Measure a length of tape from the supracondylar ridge of the humerus to the radial styloid. Cut the tape in half to create a 2.5 cm-wide strip. The remaining strip can be used for subsequent applications.

Tape application

Apply the anchor to the supracondylar ridge with zero tension. With the tissue in the lengthened position, apply the base of the tape with 25–35% tension towards the radial styloid. Complete the taping by applying the anchor on the radial styloid with zero tension. Rub the tape to activate the glue.

Reassessment

Reassess your client for changes in strength, tonal changes, functional changes and symptoms.

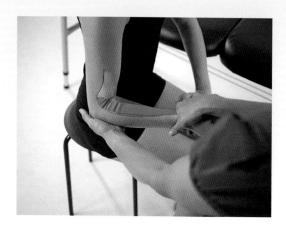

KINESIO TAPING
Brachioradialis

LENGTH TAPING

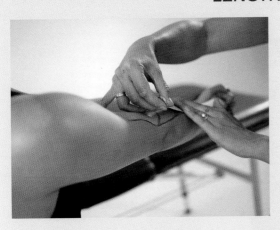

Client position
The client is seated with the elbow extended whilst the hand is in ulnar deviation. The client's other hand can assist to maintain the desired position.

Measurement of tape
With the tissue in the lengthened position, measure a length of tape from the supracondylar ridge of the humerus to the radial styloid. Cut the tape in half to create a 2.5 cm-wide strip. The remaining strip can be used for subsequent applications.

Tape application
Apply the anchor to the radial styloid with zero tension. With the tissue in the lengthened position, apply the base of the tape with 15–25% tension towards the lateral epicondyle. Complete the taping by applying the anchor on the supracondylar ridge with zero tension. Rub the tape to activate the glue.

Reassessment
Reassess your client for changes in length, strength, tonal changes, functional changes and symptoms.

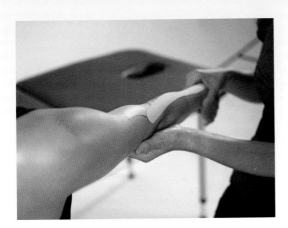

ANATOMY

Triceps brachii

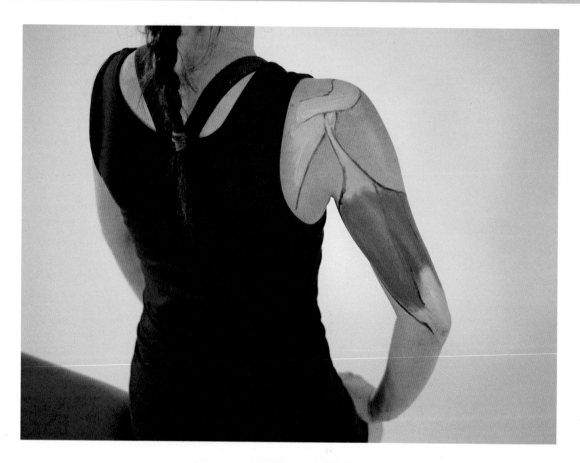

Triceps brachii	
Origin:	Infraglenoid tubercle of the scapula (long head) and the posterior shaft of the humerus (lateral and medial heads)
Insertion:	Olecranon process of the ulna
Nerve supply:	Nerve root C7, C8 Peripheral nerve: radial nerve
Function:	Entire muscle extends the forearm at the elbow joint. Long head adducts and extends the glenohumeral joint

MUSCLE TESTING
Triceps brachii

STRENGTH BIAS TESTING

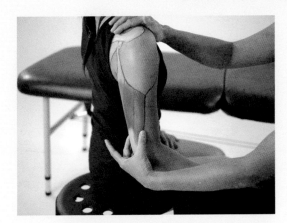 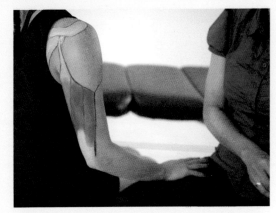

Client position

The client is seated with their arm relaxed and their forearm resting on the examiner's thigh. Alternatively, the client is lying prone with the arm abducted to 90 degrees and the elbow flexed to 90 degrees so that the hand is hanging off the table.

Instruction to client

The client is instructed to extend the forearm at the elbow joint by pressing the forearm against the thigh.

Alternative testing: Client is in supine. The client is instructed to extend the forearm at the elbow joint against resistance applied at the distal forearm.

Examiner position and notes

The examiner is seated anterior and to the side of the client and assesses for the amount of pressure applied on the thigh by the client, particularly when compared to the opposite side. The examiner is able to palpate the posterior surface of the upper arm during the testing and notes for any symptom reproduction or compensatory strategies noted. The shoulder may be stabilised during testing if necessary.

Alternative testing: The examiner is positioned standing to the side of the bed. Resistance is applied to the distal forearm by the examiner in the direction of elbow flexion as the client attempts to extend the elbow. The elbow is stable against the bed and so the available hand can be used to palpate the muscle during testing.

Resistance

No active resistance is applied by the examiner during the seated testing as the client controls the amount of force being applied to the examiner's thigh.

Alternative testing: Resistance is applied at the distal forearm in a direction towards the elbow flexion.

5

MUSCLE TESTING
Triceps brachii

LENGTH BIAS TESTING

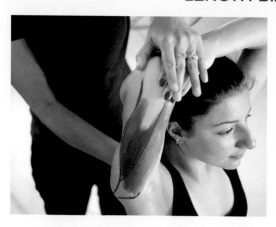

Client position

The client is seated in neutral lordosis and with the feet supported.

Instruction to client

The client is instructed to reach the hand behind the head and down the spine maximally. They may add further length by applying pressure into the elbow into a direction of shoulder flexion (elbow to ceiling).

Examiner position and notes

The examiner is positioned standing and observes any compensatory movement strategies as the client applies overpressure to the elbow. The examiner may stabilise the thorax or scapula as necessary and add overpressure at the elbow.

The examiner assesses for the range and quality of the movement. The examiner should note any symptoms that are reproduced during the testing for re-evaluation after the intervention. Range should be compared to the non-affected side for a baseline of normal range when available.

5

KINESIO TAPING
Triceps brachii

STRENGTH TAPING

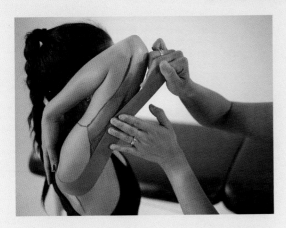

Client position
The client is seated with the hand placed behind the head; the hand is reaching maximally down the spine.

Measurement of tape
Measure a length of tape from posterior acromion process to the olecranon whilst in the lengthened position.

Tape application
Apply the starting anchor to the posterior acromion with zero tension. With the tissue in the lengthened position, apply the base of the tape with 25–35% tension. Complete the taping by applying the anchor to the olecranon and ulna with zero tension. Rub the tape to activate the glue.

Reassessment
Reassess your client for changes in strength, tonal changes, functional changes and symptoms.

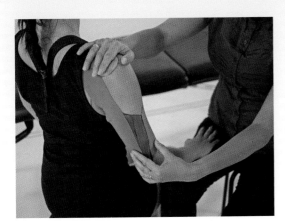

KINESIO TAPING
Triceps brachii

LENGTH TAPING

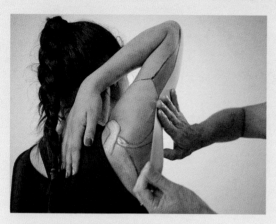

Client position

The client is seated with the hand placed behind the head; the hand is reaching maximally down the spine.

Measurement of tape

Measure a length of tape from the posterior acromion process to the olecranon whilst in the lengthened position.

Tape application

Apply the starting anchor to the ulna over the olecranon with zero tension. With the tissue in the lengthened position, apply the base of the tape with 15–25% tension over the muscle. Complete the taping by applying an anchor to the posterior acromion with zero tension. Rub the tape to activate the glue.

Reassessment

Reassess your client for changes in length, strength, tonal changes, functional changes and symptoms.

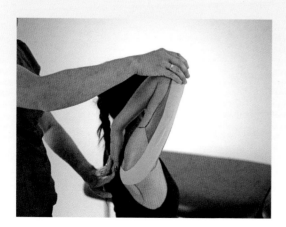

ELBOW ASSESSMENT SHEET

Clinic: .... Date: ....

Client name: ....

Functional review

Functional limitation	Pre-test measure	Post-test measure

Muscle testing

Tested priority	Muscle	Strength		Length		Comments
		Right	Left	Right	Left	
	Biceps brachii					
	Brachialis					
	Brachioradialis					
	Triceps brachii					

Treatment

Intervention	Re-test measures	Plan

Practitioner: .... Signature: ....

BIBLIOGRAPHY

Berryman Reese, N. M. (2012). *Muscle and sensory testing*. Missouri: Elsevier-Saunders.

Berryman Reese, N., & Bandy, W. D. (2010). *Joint range of motion and muscle length testing*. Missouri: Saunders Elsevier.

Calais-Germain, B. (1993). *Anatomy of movement* (12 ed.). Seattle: Eastland Press.

Comerford, M., & Mottram, S. (2012). *Kinetic control: the management of uncontrolled movement*. Sydney, Australia: Elsevier.

Kase, K., Hashimoto, T., & Okane, T. (1998). *Kinesio Taping perfect manual: amazing taping therapy to eliminate pain and muscle disorders*. Albuquerque: Kinesio Taping Association.

Kase, K., & Rock Stockheimer, K. (2006). *Kinesio Taping for lymphoedema and chronic swelling*. Albuquerque: Kinesio Taping Association.

Kase, K., Wallis, J., & Kase, T. (2003). *Clinical therapeutic applications of the Kinesio taping methods*. Albuquerque: Kinesio Taping Association.

Kendall, F. P., McCreary, E., Provance, P., Rodgers, M., & Romanic, W. (2005). *Muscles: testing and function with posture and pain*. Baltimore: Lippincott Williams Wilkins.

Standring, S., Borely, N., Collings, P., Crossman, A., Gatzoulis, M., Healy, J., … Wigley, C. (2008). *Gray's anatomy: the anatomical basis of clinical practice* (S. Susan Ed. 40 ed.). London, United Kingdom: Churchill Livingstone Elsevier.

5

Techniques for testing and taping the wrist and thumb

6

Brachioradialis

Pronator teres

Flexor carpi radialis

Flexor carpi ulnaris

Extensor carpi radialis longus and brevis

Pronator quadratus

Extensor carpi ulnaris

Supinator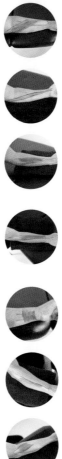

ANATOMY
Brachioradialis

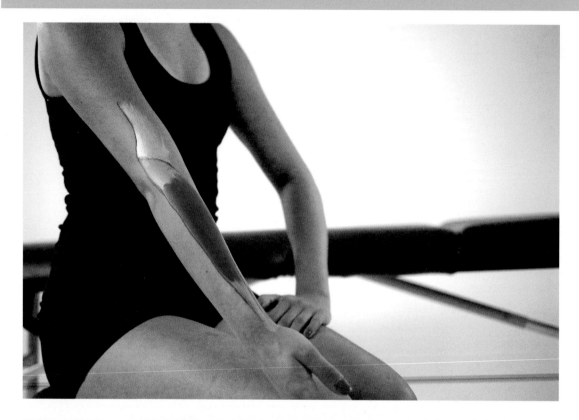

6

Brachioradialis

Origin:	Proximal ⅔ of the lateral supracondylar ridge of the humerus
Insertion:	Distal styloid process of the radius
Nerve supply:	Nerve root: C5, C6, C7 Peripheral nerve: radial nerve
Function:	Flexes the forearm at the elbow joint

MUSCLE TESTING
Brachioradialis

STRENGTH BIAS TESTING

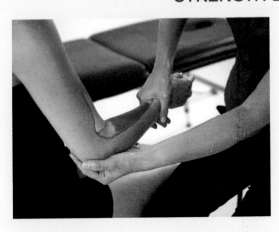

Client position

The client is seated with the arm relaxed and the forearm flexed at the elbow in a position halfway between full supination and full pronation. The thumb is up towards the ceiling.

Instruction to client

The client is instructed to maintain the elbow and wrist position during the testing and attempts to prevent the examiner from extending the elbow.

Examiner position and notes

The examiner applies resistance to the anterior distal forearm just proximal to the wrist joint whilst the other hand stabilises the elbow.

Palpatory notes: The brachioradialis is superficial for the majority of its path except where the abductor pollicis longus and extensor pollicis brevis cross superficial to it at the distal forearm. Keep this in mind when palpating the brachioradialis.

Resistance

The examiner applies a resistance in the direction of elbow extension.

MUSCLE TESTING
Brachioradialis

LENGTH BIAS TESTING

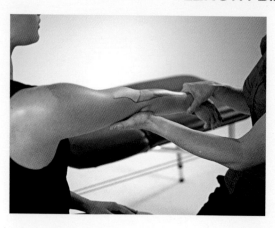

Client position

The client is seated in neutral lordosis and with the feet supported.

Instruction to client

The client is instructed to extend the elbow in front of the body. With the thumb facing the ceiling, the client is instructed to ulnar deviate by pointing the little finger towards the floor.

Examiner position and notes

The end range can be assessed by applying skin traction to the tissue before applying overpressure into the direction of ulnar deviation. The other hand is used to support the elbow to maintain full extension. The overpressure can also be applied by the client so that the examiner is able to palpate the tissue. The examiner should note if there is a difference between the active and passive range of movement.

The examiner assesses for the range and quality of the movement. The examiner should note any symptoms that are reproduced during the testing for re-evaluation after the intervention. Range should be compared to the non-affected side for a baseline of normal range when available.

KINESIO TAPING
Brachioradialis

STRENGTH TAPING

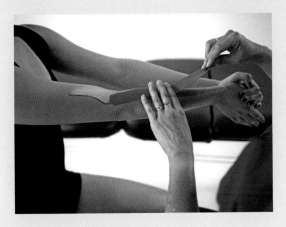

Client position

The client is seated with the elbow extended whilst the hand is in ulnar deviation. The client's other hand can assist to maintain the desired position.

Measurement of tape

Measure a length of tape from the supracondylar ridge of the humerus to the radial styloid. Cut the tape in half to create a 2.5 cm-wide strip. The remaining strip can be used for subsequent applications.

Tape application

Apply the anchor to the supracondylar ridge with zero tension. With the tissue in the lengthened position, apply the base of the tape with 25–35% tension towards the radial styloid. Complete the taping by applying the anchor on the radial styloid with zero tension. Rub the tape to activate the glue.

Reassessment

Reassess your client for changes in strength, tonal changes, functional changes and symptoms.

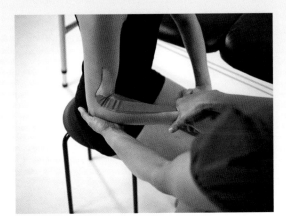

6

KINESIO TAPING
Brachioradialis

LENGTH TAPING

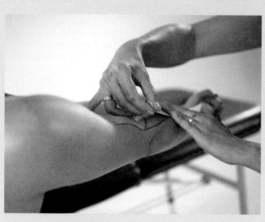

Client position

The client is seated with the elbow extended whilst the hand is in ulnar deviation. The client's other hand can assist to maintain the desired position.

Measurement of tape

With the tissue in the lengthened position, measure a length of tape from the supracondylar ridge of the humerus to the radial styloid. Cut the tape in half to create a 2.5 cm-wide strip. The remaining strip can be used for subsequent applications.

Tape application

Apply the anchor to the radial styloid with zero tension. With the tissue in the lengthened position, apply the base of the tape with 15–25% tension towards the lateral epicondyle. Complete the taping by applying the anchor on the supracondylar ridge with zero tension. Rub the tape to activate the glue.

Reassessment

Reassess your client for changes in length, strength, tonal changes, functional changes and symptoms.

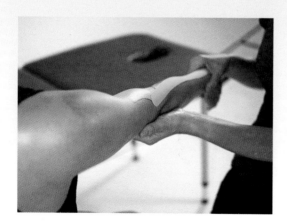

6

ANATOMY
Pronator teres

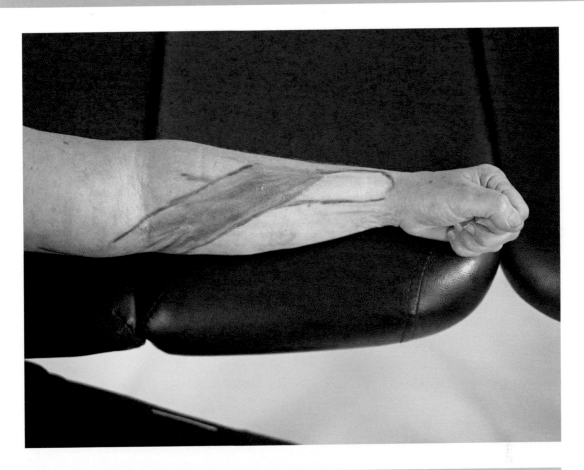

Pronator teres	
Origin:	Medial epicondyle of the humerus (via the common flexor tendon), medial supracondylar ridge of the humerus and the coronoid process of the ulna
Insertion:	Middle ⅓ of the lateral radius
Nerve supply:	Peripheral nerve: median nerve Nerve root: C6, C7
Function:	Pronates the forearm at the radioulnar joint and assists in flexing the forearm at the elbow joint

MUSCLE TESTING
Pronator teres

STRENGTH BIAS TESTING

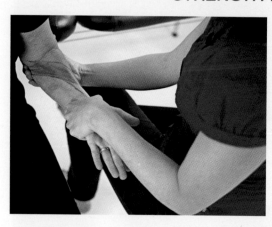

Client position

The client is seated with the shoulder in 0 degrees of abduction and the elbow partially flexed (90 degrees of elbow flexion is useful to help standardise the testing and re-testing) and full forearm supination. Alternatively, the client is lying supine with the elbow held against the side.

Instruction to client

The client is instructed to pronate the forearm whilst maintaining 90 degrees of elbow flexion and with the elbow maintained at the side of the body.

Examiner position and notes

The examiner is positioned in front of the client on the side being tested. The examiner stabilises the lateral elbow to prevent shoulder abduction whilst palpating the pronator teres with the thumb. With moderate force, resist the client from pronating the forearm at the radioulnar joint (proximal to the wrist). Performing a passive movement first allows determination of the client's available range of movement (ROM) whilst allowing for muscle palpation, and shows the client the movement desired. Avoid squeezing the radius and ulna together as this may be painful.

Resistance

Palpate the proximal anterior forearm with the thumb whilst applying resistance at the anterior distal forearm, proximal to the wrist joint.

MUSCLE TESTING
Pronator teres

LENGTH BIAS TESTING

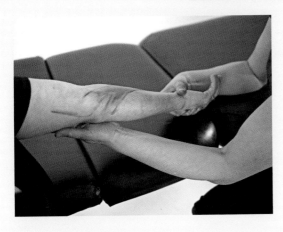

Client position
The client is seated with the feet supported.

Instruction to client
The client is instructed to extend the elbow and fully supinate the forearm by rotating the thumb away from the body and then continue the motion until the palm is facing away from the body; the thumb is pointing down or backwards.

Examiner position and notes
The examiner is positioned in front of the client, and observes any discomfort and alternative movement strategies as the client applies overpressure to the forearm. Palpate the muscle for tone and note any symptoms.

6

KINESIO TAPING
Pronator teres

STRENGTH TAPING

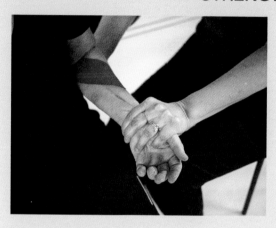

Client position

The client is seated with the elbow extended and the forearm supinated.

Measurement of tape

Measure a length of tape from the medial epicondyle obliquely down to the middle and lateral ⅓ of the radius. Cut the tape to the appropriate width for the client's musculature.

Tape application

Apply the starting anchor on the medial epicondyle with zero tension. With the tissue in the lengthened position, apply the base of the tape with 25–35% tension obliquely towards the mid-shaft of the lateral radius. Complete the taping by applying the final anchor with zero tension. Rub the tape to activate the glue.

Reassessment

Reassess your client for changes in strength, tonal changes, functional changes and symptoms.

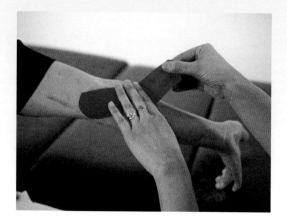

KINESIO TAPING
Pronator teres

LENGTH TAPING

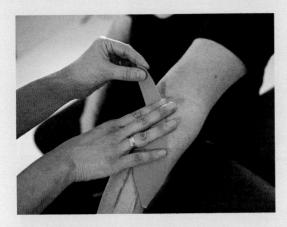

Client position

The client is seated with the elbow extended and the forearm supinated.

Measurement of tape

Measure a length of tape from the medial epicondyle obliquely down to the middle and lateral ⅓ of the radius. Cut this into a Y-strip with 2.5 cm-wide tails.

Tape application

Apply the starting anchor with zero tension at the middle ⅓ of the lateral radius. With the tissue in a lengthened position, apply the base of the tape with 15–25% tension towards the medial epicondyle. Complete the taping by applying the final anchor on the epicondyle with zero tension. Rub the tape to activate the glue.

Reassessment

Reassess your client for changes in length, strength, tonal changes, functional changes and symptoms.

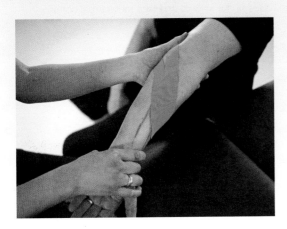

ANATOMY
Flexor carpi radialis

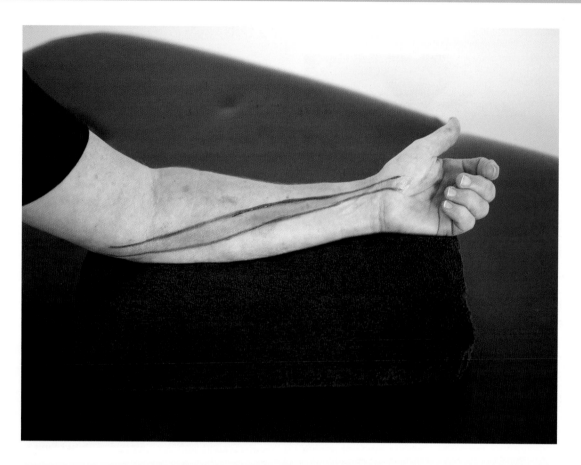

Flexor carpi radialis

Origin:	Medial epicondyle of the humerus via the common flexor tendon and deep antebrachial fascia
Insertion:	Radial side of the anterior hand at the bases of the second and third metacarpal bones
Nerve supply:	Peripheral nerve: median nerve Nerve root: C6, C7
Function:	Flexes and radially deviates (abducts) the hand at the wrist joint

MUSCLE TESTING
Flexor carpi radialis

STRENGTH BIAS TESTING

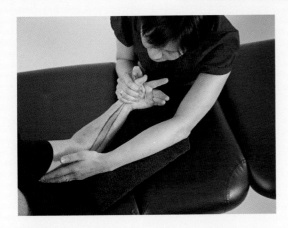

Client position
The client is seated with the arm relaxed and the forearm flexed at the elbow joint and fully supinated on a table or is supported by the examiner. Apply resistance proximal to the fingers against the wrist; the forearm rests in flexion. Bias the resistance to the second and third metacarpal heads.

Instruction to client
The examiner passively moves the wrist to show the client the desired movement as well as assessing for the range and quality of the movement. The client is instructed to flex the wrist towards the radial side by focusing on generating the flexion movement from the second and third fingers.

Examiner position and notes
The examiner is positioned in front of the client. Stabilise the posterior aspect of the distal humerus whilst palpating the tendon of the flexor carpi radialis at the base of the second metacarpal bone lateral to the midline of the forearm.

Note: This testing does not rule out palmaris longus. Care should also be taken to note if the fingers are flexing during testing as this indicates substitution by flexor digitorum superficialis or profundus.

Resistance
The examiner applies resistance over the thenar eminence along the volar aspect of the base of the first and second metacarpal bones in a direction of wrist extension and ulnar deviation.

6

MUSCLE TESTING
Flexor carpi radialis

LENGTH BIAS TESTING

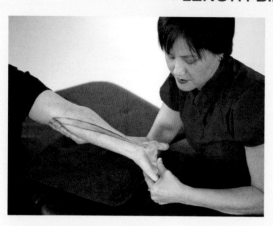

Client position
The client is seated with the feet supported.

Instruction to client
The client can assist with the length assessment by applying overpressure at the end of range. Instruct the client to extend the forearm fully and use the other hand to extend the wrist by holding the second and third digits; the palm will face away from the body. The client then adds ulnar deviation to stretch the tissue further by extending the fingers in the direction towards the little finger.

Examiner position and notes
The examiner is positioned in front of the client and observes any discomfort and alternative movement strategies as the client applies overpressure to the forearm. Palpate the muscle for tone and note any symptoms.

6

KINESIO TAPING
Flexor carpi radialis

STRENGTH TAPING

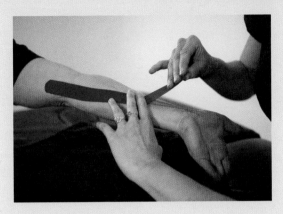

Client position
The client is seated with the forearm fully extended, and uses the other hand to extend the wrist holding the second and third digits, adding ulnar deviation to stretch the muscle further. Alternatively, the client can extend the fingers against the surface of the bed or table.

Measurement of tape
Measure a length of tape from the medial epicondyle to the base of the second metacarpal bone. Cut the tape into a 2.5 cm-wide strip.

Tape application
Apply the starting anchor with zero tension over the medial epicondyle. With the tissue in a lengthened position, apply the base of the tape with 25–35% tension on the volar forearm towards the second metacarpal bone. Complete the tape by applying the final anchor over the base of the second metacarpal bone with zero tension. The edge of the tape may also sit over the base of the third metacarpal. Rub the tape to activate the glue.

Reassessment
Reassess your client for changes in strength, tonal changes, functional changes and symptoms.

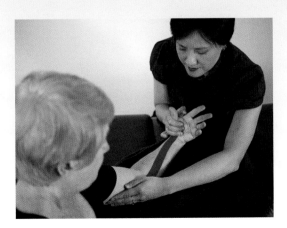

6

KINESIO TAPING
Flexor carpi radialis

LENGTH TAPING

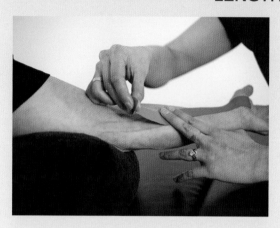

Client position

The client is seated with the forearm fully extended. They use the other hand to extend the wrist by holding the second and third digits, adding ulnar deviation to stretch the muscle further. Alternatively, the client can extend the fingers against the surface of the bed or table.

Measurement of tape

Measure a length of tape from the second and third metacarpal head up to the medial epicondyle. Cut the tape into a 2.5 cm-wide strip.

Tape application

Apply the starting anchor with zero tension over the base of the second metacarpal bone with the edge of the tape on the third metacarpal bone. With the tissue in a lengthened position, apply the base of the tape with 15–25% tension towards the common flexor origin. Complete the tape by applying the final anchor to the medial epicondyle with zero tension. Rub the tape to activate the glue.

Reassessment

Reassess your client for changes in length, strength, tonal changes, functional changes and symptoms.

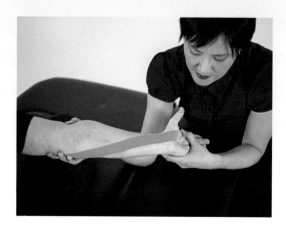

ANATOMY

Flexor carpi ulnaris

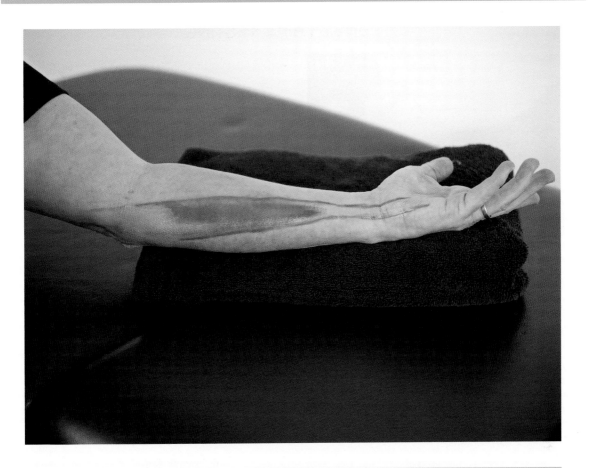

Flexor carpi ulnaris

Origin:	Medial epicondyle of the humerus via the common flexor tendon, proximal ⅔ of the ulna
Insertion:	The pisiform and via ligaments to the ulnar side of the anterior hand at the base of the fifth metacarpal bone and the hook of the hamate
Nerve supply:	Peripheral nerve: ulnar nerve Nerve root: C8, T1
Function:	Flexes and ulnar deviates (adducts) the hand at the wrist joint

6

MUSCLE TESTING
Flexor carpi ulnaris

STRENGTH BIAS TESTING

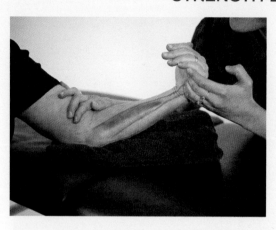

Client position

The client is seated with the arm relaxed and the forearm flexed at the elbow joint and fully supinated.

Instruction to client

The examiner passively moves the wrist towards flexion and ulnar deviation as the client is instructed to observe the desired movement. The client is instructed to maintain the position as a force is applied by the examiner to move the wrist and hand in the opposite direction.

Examiner position and notes

The examiner is positioned in front of the client. The examiner stabilises the upper limb whilst palpating the flexor carpi ulnaris.

Note: Care should also be taken to note if the fingers are flexing during testing as this indicates substitution by flexor digitorum superficialis or profundus.

Resistance

Apply resistance proximal to the fingers over the hypothenar eminence in a direction of extension towards the radial side.

6

MUSCLE TESTING
Flexor carpi ulnaris

LENGTH BIAS TESTING

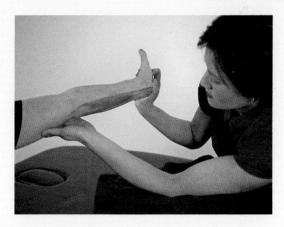

Client position

The client is seated with the feet supported.

Instruction to client

The client is instructed to extend the forearm fully and use the other hand to extend the wrist at the fingers. The client can add radial deviation to stretch the tissue further by applying force at the fifth and fourth digits in a direction of extension towards the thumb.

Examiner position and notes

The examiner is positioned in front of the client and observes any discomfort and alternative movement strategies as the client applies overpressure to the forearm.

Palpate the muscle for tone and note any symptoms. Alternatively, the overpressure may be applied by the examiner.

6

KINESIO TAPING
Flexor carpi ulnaris

STRENGTH TAPING

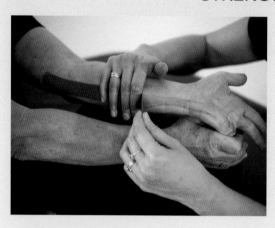

Client position

The client is seated with the forearm fully extended and the wrist held in extension by using the other hand to hold the fourth and fifth digit in extension towards the thumb.

Measurement of tape

Measure a length of tape from the medial epicondyle to the hypothenar eminence. Cut the tape into a 2.5 cm-wide strip.

Tape application

Apply the starting anchor with zero tension over the medial epicondyle. With the tissue in a lengthened position, apply the base of the tape with 25–35% tension on the volar forearm towards the hypothenar eminence. Complete the tape by applying the final anchor over the hyothenar eminence with zero tension. Rub the tape to activate the glue.

Reassessment

Reassess your client for changes in strength, tonal changes, functional changes and symptoms.

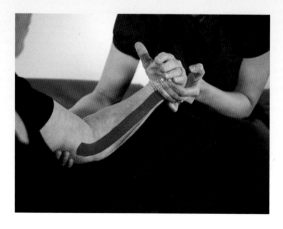

6

KINESIO TAPING
Flexor carpi ulnaris

LENGTH TAPING

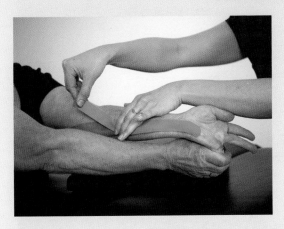

Client position

The client is seated with the forearm fully extended and the wrist held in extension by using the other hand to hold the fourth and fifth digit in extension towards the thumb.

Measurement of tape

Measure a length of tape from the hyponthenar eminence up to the medial epicondyle. Cut the tape into a 2.5 cm-wide strip.

Tape application

Apply the starting anchor with zero tension over the base of the fifth metacarpal bone. With the tissue in a lengthened position, apply the base of the tape with 15–25% tension towards the common flexor origin. Complete the tape by applying the final anchor to the medial epicondyle with zero tension. Rub the tape to activate the glue.

Reassessment

Reassess your client for changes in length, strength, tonal changes, functional changes and symptoms.

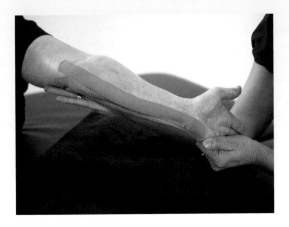

6

ANATOMY
Extensor carpi radialis longus and brevis

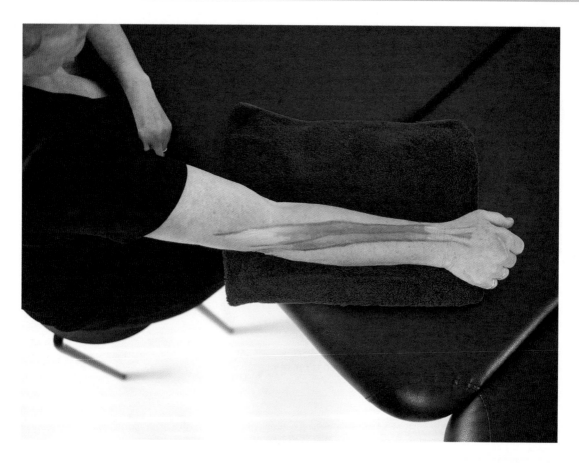

Extensor carpi radialis longus (ECRL)

Origin:	Distal ⅓ of the lateral supracondylar ridge of the humerus and lateral intermuscular septum
Insertion:	Radial side of the dorsal hand at the base of the second metacarpal bone
Nerve supply:	Peripheral nerve: radial nerve Nerve root: C6, C7
Function:	Radially deviates (abducts) and extends the hand at the wrist joint. Assists in flexing the forearm at the elbow joint

Extensor carpi radialis brevis (ECRB)

Origin:	Lateral epicondyle of the humerus via the common extensor tendon, radial collateral ligament of the elbow joint, and deep antebrachial fascia
Insertion:	Radial side of the dorsal hand at the base of the third metacarpal bone
Nerve supply:	Peripheral nerve: radial nerve Nerve root: C6, C7
Function:	Radially deviates (abducts) and extends the hand at the wrist joint

MUSCLE TESTING
Extensor carpi radialis longus and brevis

STRENGTH BIAS TESTING

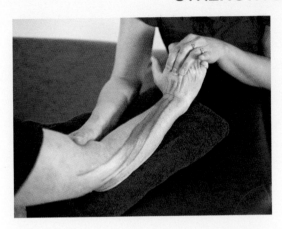 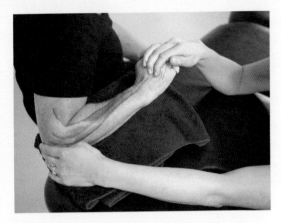

Client position
ECRL: The client is seated with the arm relaxed and the forearm slightly flexed at the elbow; the elbow is supported on a table.

ECRB: The client is seated with the elbow fully flexed; the forearm is supported and stabilised by the examiner's hand. Elbow flexion makes the extensor carpi radialis longus less effective by placing it in a shortened position.

Instruction to client
Instruct the client to radially deviate the wrist by bringing the thumb towards the elbow whilst extending the wrist.

Examiner position and notes
The examiner is positioned in front of the client whilst stabilising and supporting the tested forearm. Palpation notes: The ECRB is the most posterior of the radial group of muscles, brachioradialis is the most anterior and the ECRL is in the middle. The radial group of muscles can usually be pinched and separated from the rest of the muscles in the forearm.

Resistance
Resistance is applied against the dorsum of the hand along the second (ECRL) and third (ECRB) metacarpal bone in the direction of flexion and ulnar deviation.

6

MUSCLE TESTING
Extensor carpi radialis longus and brevis

LENGTH BIAS TESTING

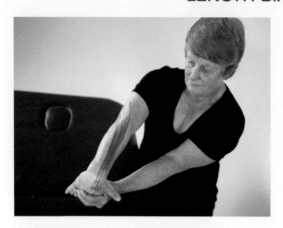

Client position
The client is seated with the feet supported.

Instruction to client
Self-administered testing: Instruct the client to extend the elbow with the wrist flexed, the client uses the other hand to give overpressure over the second and third metacarpal bones to flex and ulnar deviate the hand by pushing the dorsal hand back towards the body and out to the side of the little finger.

Therapist testing: With the client in elbow extension, the examiner applies a force over the dorsal second and third metacarpal bones in the direction of wrist flexion and ulnar deviation.

Examiner position and notes
The examiner is positioned to observe any discomfort and alternative movement strategies as the client applies overpressure to the forearm. A client-administered test allows the examiner to palpate the muscle for tone and note for any symptoms.

6

KINESIO TAPING
Extensor carpi radialis longus and brevis

STRENGTH TAPING

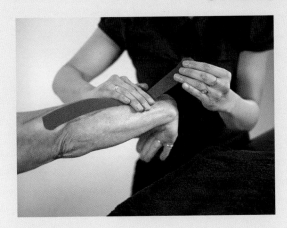

Client position
The client is seated with the elbow in extension, and uses the other hand to hold the second and third metacarpal bones into flexion and ulnar deviation of the wrist.

Measurement of tape
Measure a length of tape from the lateral epicondyle over the dorsal forearm to the base of the second metacarpal bone. Cut the tape into a 2.5 cm width to cover both ECRL and ECRB. Alternatively, use 1 cm-wide strips for individual muscle taping.

Tape application
Apply the starting anchor with zero tension over the lateral epicondyle. With the tissue in a lengthened position, apply the base of the tape with 25–35% tension on the dorsal forearm towards the second metacarpal bone. Complete the tape by applying the final anchor over the base of the second metacarpal bone with zero tension. Rub the tape to activate the glue.

Reassessment
Reassess your client for changes in strength, tonal changes, functional changes and symptoms.

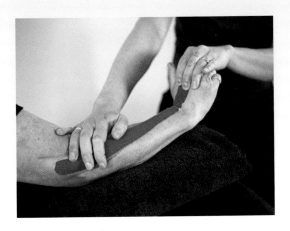
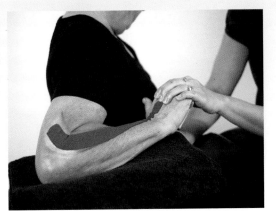

KINESIO TAPING
Extensor carpi radialis longus and brevis

LENGTH TAPING

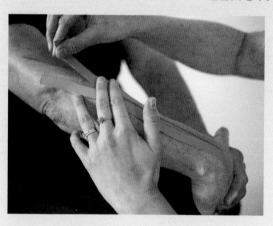

Client position

The client is seated with the elbow in extension, and uses the other hand to hold the second and third metacarpal bones into flexion and ulnar deviation of the wrist.

Measurement of tape

Measure a length of tape from the lateral epicondyle to the base of the second metacarpal bone. Cut the tape into a 2.5 cm-wide Y-strip. Alternatively use 1 cm-wide strips for individual muscle taping.

Tape application

Apply the starting anchor with zero tension over the base of the second metacarpal bone. With the tissue in a lengthened position, apply the base of the tape with 15–25% tension on the dorsal forearm towards the common extensor origin. Complete the tape by applying the final anchor to the lateral epicondyle with zero tension. Rub the tape to activate the glue.

Reassessment

Reassess your client for changes in length, strength, tonal changes, functional changes and symptoms.

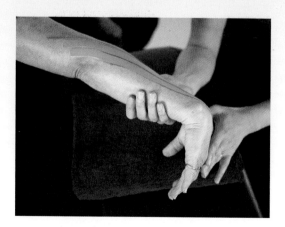

6

ANATOMY
Pronator quadratus

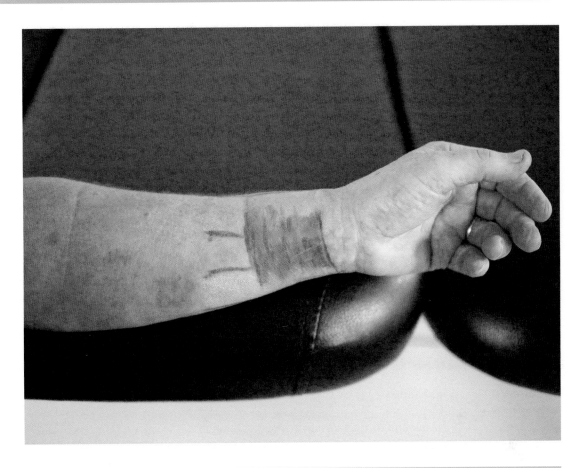

Pronator quadratus

Origin:	Anterior aspect of the distal ¼ of the ulna
Insertion:	Anterior aspect of the distal ¼ of the radius
Nerve supply:	Peripheral nerve: median nerve Nerve root: C8, T1
Function:	Pronates the forearm at the radioulnar joint

MUSCLE TESTING
Pronator quadratus

STRENGTH BIAS TESTING

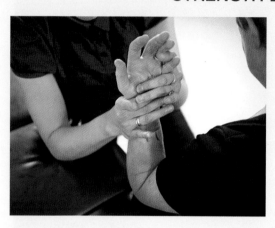

Client position

The client is seated with the upper limb in 0 degree abduction, full elbow flexion and full forearm supination. This makes the humeral head of pronator teres less effective due to its shortened position.

Instruction to client

The client is instructed to pronate the forearm whilst maintaining full elbow flexion.

Examiner position and notes

The examiner is positioned to the front or to the side being tested. With moderate force, resist the client from pronating the forearm at the radioulnar joint (proximal to the wrist). Performing a passive movement first allows determination of the client's available range of movement whilst allowing for muscle palpation, and shows the client the movement desired. Avoid squeezing the radius and ulna together because this may be painful.

Resistance

Palpate the distal anterior forearm whilst applying resistance at the anterior distal forearm, proximal to the wrist joint.

6

MUSCLE TESTING
Pronator quadratus

LENGTH BIAS TESTING

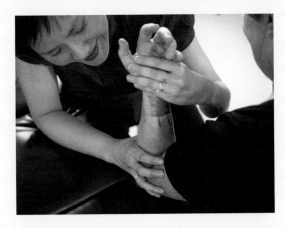

Client position

The client is seated with the upper limb in 0 degree abduction, full elbow flexion and full forearm supination. In this position, the humeral head of pronator teres is in a shortened position.

Instruction to client

The client is instructed to supinate the forearm by rotating the thumb away from the body and continue the motion until the palm is facing away from the body.

Examiner position and notes

The examiner is positioned in front of the client and observes any discomfort and alternative movement strategies as the client applies overpressure to the forearm. Pronator quadratus is deep and may be difficult to assess with palpation.

6

KINESIO TAPING
Pronator quadratus

STRENGTH TAPING

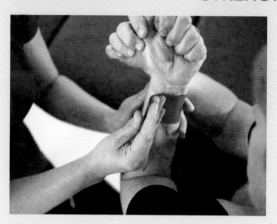

Client position

The client is seated and the elbow is flexed, the forearm is supinated and the position is held by the client.

Measurement of tape

Measure a length of tape from the lateral border of the radius, just above the styloid to the medial border of the ulna above the styloid.

Tape application

Apply the starting anchor with zero tension on the medial border of the ulna above the styloid process. With the tissue in a lengthened position, apply the base of the tape with 25–35% tension over the volar aspect of the forearm towards the lateral radius. Complete the taping by applying the final anchor to the distal and lateral radius with zero tension. Rub the tape to activate the glue.

Reassessment

Reassess your client for changes in strength, tonal changes, functional changes and symptoms.

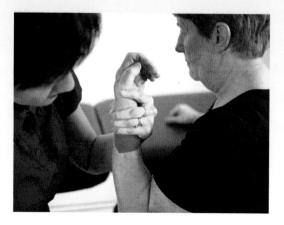

6

KINESIO TAPING
Pronator quadratus

LENGTH TAPING

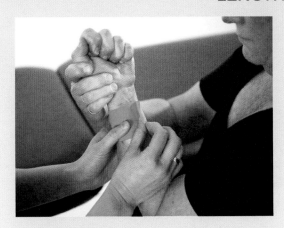

Client position
The client is seated and the elbow is flexed, the forearm is supinated and the position held by the client.

Measurement of tape
Measure a length of tape from the medial border of the ulna, just above the styloid to the lateral border of the radius above the styloid.

Tape application
Apply the starting anchor with zero tension, above the radial styloid on the lateral border of the radius. With the tissue in a lengthened position, apply the base of the tape with 15–25% tension on the volar forearm towards the medial border of the ulna above the styloid. Complete the tape by applying the final anchor over the ulna with zero tension. Rub the tape to activate the glue.

Reassessment
Reassess your client for changes in length, strength, tonal changes, functional changes and symptoms.

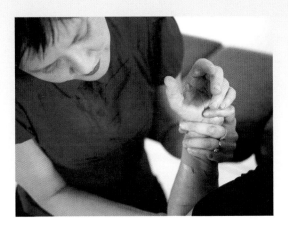

6

ANATOMY

Extensor carpi ulnaris

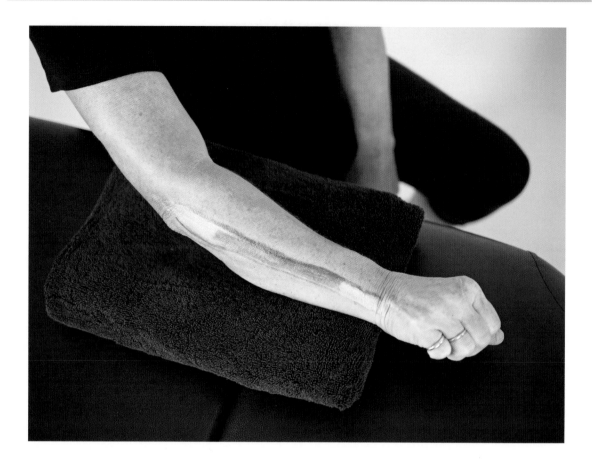

Extensor carpi ulnaris

Origin:	Lateral epicondyle of the humerus via the common extensor tendon, via the aponeurosis from the dorsal border of the ulna and deep antebrachial fascia
Insertion:	Ulnar side of the base of the fifth metacarpal bone
Nerve supply:	Peripheral nerve: radial nerve Nerve root: C6, C7, C8
Function:	Extends, and ulnar deviates (adducts) the wrist

6

MUSCLE TESTING
Extensor carpi ulnaris

STRENGTH BIAS TESTING

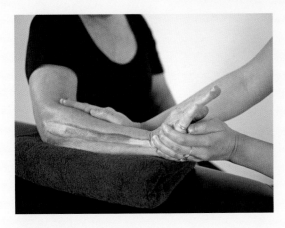

Client position
The client is seated with the feet supported. The elbow is flexed, and the forearm is pronated and supported on a flat surface.

Instruction to client
The client is instructed to extend the wrist and deviate to the ulnar side. Performing a passive movement first allows determination of the client's available range of movement and shows the client the movement desired.

Examiner position and notes
The examiner is positioned in front of the client. Stabilise and support the tested forearm. Palpate the tendon of the extensor carpi ulnaris distal to the ulnar styloid process.

Note: It is normal for the fingers to be in a position of passive flexion during testing. Active extension of the fingers as wrist extension is initiated suggests an attempt to substitute with the extensor digitorum, extensor indicis and extensor digiti minimi. To distinguish between the extensor digiti mimimi (EDM) and extensor carpi ulnaris (ECU), instruct the client to ulnar deviate the wrist joint. This engages the ECU but not the EDM. Alternatively, instruct the client to extend the fingers—this will engage the EDM but not the ECU.

Resistance
Apply resistance against the dorsum of the hand along the fifth metacarpal bone in a direction of flexion and towards the radial side.

6

MUSCLE TESTING
Extensor carpi ulnaris

LENGTH BIAS TESTING

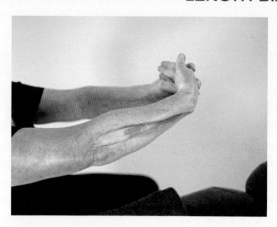

Client position

The client is seated with the feet supported.

Instruction to client

With the elbow in extension, the client is instructed to flex the wrist and use the other hand to give overpressure on the fifth digit to flex the wrist and radially deviate the hand by drawing the lateral border of the hand towards the direction of the thumb.

Examiner position and notes

The examiner is positioned in front of the client, and observes any discomfort and alternative movement strategies as the client applies overpressure to the forearm. Palpate proximally and at the middle ⅓ of the ulna, immediately posterior to the shaft of the ulna. Palpate the muscle for tone and note any symptoms.

6

KINESIO TAPING
Extensor carpi ulnaris

STRENGTH TAPING

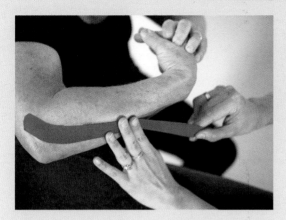

Client position

The client is seated with some elbow flexion, and uses the other hand to hold the fifth metacarpal bone into flexion and radial deviation of the wrist.

Note: Whilst the length testing is positioned with the elbow in extension, the taping process is with the elbow in flexion as this takes up tissue and skin 'slack' around the elbow and minimises skin irritation.

Measurement of tape

Measure a length of tape from the lateral epicondyle over the dorsal forearm to the base of the fifth metacarpal bone. Cut the tape into a 2.5 cm-wide strip.

Tape application

Apply the starting anchor with zero tension over the lateral epicondyle. With the tissue in a lengthened position, apply the base of the tape with 25–35% tension on the dorsal forearm towards the fifth metacarpal bone. Complete the taping by applying the final anchor over the ulnar side of the base of the fifth metacarpal bone with zero tension. Rub the tape to activate the glue.

Reassessment

Reassess your client for changes in strength, tonal changes, functional changes and symptoms.

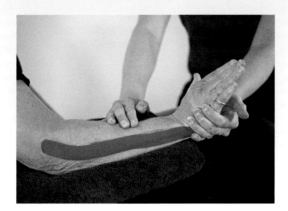

KINESIO TAPING
Extensor carpi ulnaris

LENGTH TAPING

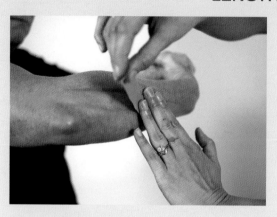

Client position

The client is seated with some elbow flexion, and uses the other hand to hold the fifth metacarpal bone into flexion and radial deviation of the wrist.

Note: Whilst the length testing is positioned with the elbow in extension, the taping process is with the elbow in flexion as this takes up tissue and skin 'slack' around the elbow and minimises skin irritation.

Measurement of tape

Measure a length of tape from the lateral epicondyle to the base of the fifth metacarpal bone. Cut the tape into a 2.5 cm-wide strip.

Tape application

Apply the starting anchor with zero tension over the ulnar side of the base of the fifth metacarpal bone. With the tissue in a lengthened position, apply the base of the tape with 15–25% tension on the dorsal forearm towards the common extensor origin. Complete the taping by applying the final anchor to the lateral epicondyle with zero tension. Rub the tape to activate the glue.

Reassessment

Reassess your client for changes in length, strength, tonal changes, functional changes and symptoms.

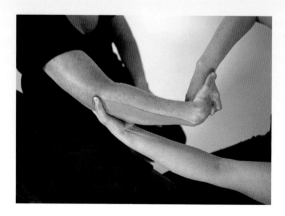

ANATOMY
Supinator

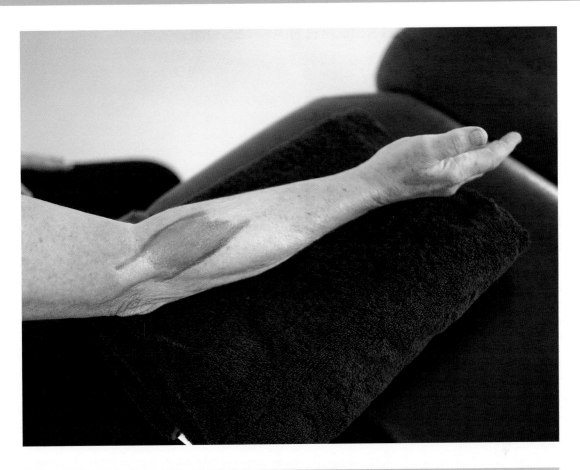

Supinator	
Origin:	Lateral epicondyle of the humerus and the supinator crest of the ulna, radial collateral ligament of the elbow, annular ligament of the radius
Insertion:	Tuberosity and oblique line of the radius; proximal ⅓ of the radius (posterior, lateral and anterior side)
Nerve supply:	Peripheral nerve: deep branch of the radial nerve Nerve root: C6
Function:	Supinates the forearm at the radioulnar joints

6

MUSCLE TESTING
Supinator

STRENGTH BIAS TESTING

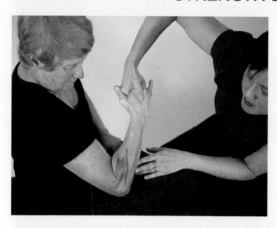

Client position

The client is seated with the shoulder in 0 degree abduction, full elbow flexion and full forearm pronation. Alternatively, the supinator can be tested in full elbow extension to decrease the mechanical leverage of biceps brachii and further implicate the supinator as the muscle to manage.

Instruction to client

The client is instructed to maintain supination of the forearm whilst the therapist is applying a force to rotate the forearm away from the body. The client attempts to do this whilst maintaining the starting position of full elbow flexion or elbow extension (testing at the inner or outer range of biceps brachii).

Examiner position and notes

The examiner is positioned in front or laterally to access the side being tested. If the elbow is not fixed on a stable surface, the therapist stabilises the lateral elbow to prevent shoulder abduction.

The examiner applies resistance at the distal forearm, proximal to the wrist in the direction of pronation.

Performing a passive movement first allows determination of the client's available range of movement and shows the client the movement desired. In the absence of distal wrist pathology, and for ease of handling and better examiner grip, the examiner may hold the client's hand as if to do a handshake to apply resistance. To palpate, push the brachioradialis muscle laterally and palpate deep toward the head and shaft of the radius to find the supinator.

Resistance

The examiner grips the distal wrist and applies resistance in the direction of pronation. The client attempts to maintain the starting test position.

6

MUSCLE TESTING
Supinator

LENGTH BIAS TESTING

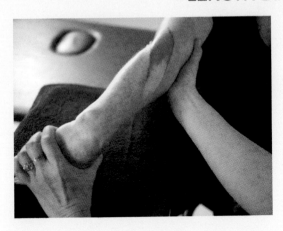

Client position
The client is seated with the feet supported.

Instruction to client
The client is instructed to maintain the elbow in extension as they rotate the palm inwards. They continue to rotate the wrist and forearm in this direction until the maximal available active range is reached. At the end position, it is usual for the wrist to be in flexion with the fingers pointing away from the body.

Examiner position and notes
The examiner is positioned in front of the client, and observes any discomfort and alternative movement strategies. Either the examiner or the client can apply overpressure to the forearm. Palpate the muscle for tone and note any symptoms.

6

KINESIO TAPING
Supinator

STRENGTH TAPING

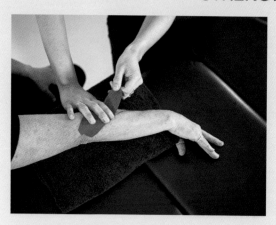

Client position

The client is seated with the elbow extended and the forearm fully pronated.

Measurement of tape

Measure a length of tape from the anterior (volar) superior ⅓ of the radius to the lateral epicondyle. Cut this into a web cut for coverage of larger forearms.

Tape application

Apply the starting anchor with zero tension at the lateral epicondyle and dorsal surface of the radius. With the tissue in a lengthened position, apply the base of the tape with 25–35% tension obliquely towards volar surface of the proximal ⅓ of the radius. Complete the taping by applying the final anchor with zero tension. Rub the tape to activate the glue.

Reassessment

Reassess your client for changes in strength, tonal changes, functional changes and symptoms.

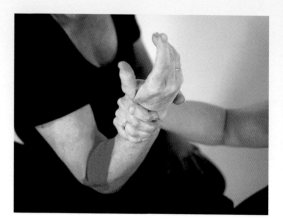
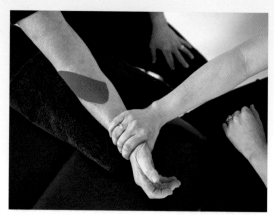

KINESIO TAPING
Supinator

LENGTH TAPING

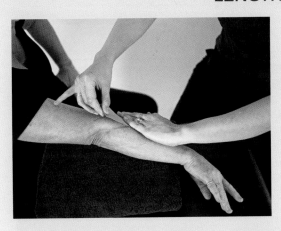

Client position
The client is seated with the elbow extended and the forearm fully pronated.

Measurement of tape
Measure a length of tape from the anterior (volar) superior ⅓ of the radius to the lateral epicondyle. Cut this into a web cut for coverage of larger forearms.

Tape application
Apply the starting anchor with zero tension at the anterior proximal ⅓ of the radius. With the tissue in a lengthened position, apply the base of the tape with 15–25% tension obliquely towards the lateral epicondyle. Complete the taping by applying the final anchor on the lateral epicondyle with zero tension. Rub the tape to activate the glue.

Reassessment
Reassess your client for changes in length, strength, tonal changes, functional changes and symptoms.

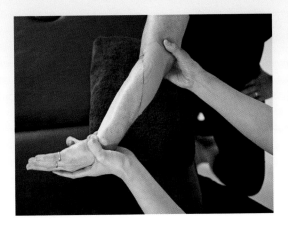

6

WRIST ASSESSMENT SHEET

Clinic: .... Date: ....

Client name: ....

Functional review

Functional limitation	Pre-test measure	Post-test measure

Muscle testing

Tested priority	Muscle	Strength		Length		Comments
		Right	Left	Right	Left	
	Brachioradialis					
	Pronator teres					
	Flexor carpi radialis					
	Flexor carpi ulnaris					
	Extensor carpi radialis longus and brevis					
	Pronator quadratus					
	Extensor carpi ulnaris					
	Supinator					

Treatment

Intervention	Re-test measures	Plan

Practitioner: .... Signature: ....

6

BIBLIOGRAPHY

Berryman Reese, N. M. (2012). *Muscle and sensory testing*. Missouri: Elsevier-Saunders.

Berryman Reese, N., & Bandy, W. D. (2010). *Joint range of motion and muscle length testing*. Missouri: Saunders Elsevier.

Calais-Germain, B. (1993). *Anatomy of movement* (12 ed.). Seattle: Eastland Press.

Comerford, M., & Mottram, S. (2012). *Kinetic control: the management of uncontrolled movement*. Sydney, Australia: Elsevier.

Kase, K., Hashimoto, T., & Okane, T. (1998). *Kinesio Taping perfect manual: amazing taping therapy to eliminate pain and muscle disorders*. Albuquerque: Kinesio Taping Association.

Kase, K., & Rock Stockheimer, K. (2006). *Kinesio Taping for lymphoedema and chronic swelling*. Albuquerque: Kinesio Taping Association.

Kase, K., Wallis, J., & Kase, T. (2003). *Clinical therapeutic applications of the Kinesio taping methods*. Albuquerque: Kinesio Taping Association.

Kendall, F. P., McCreary, E., Provance, P., Rodgers, M., & Romanic, W. (2005). *Muscles: testing and function with posture and pain*. Baltimore: Lippincott Williams Wilkins.

Standring, S., Borely, N., Collings, P., Crossman, A., Gatzoulis, M., Healy, J., … Wigley, C. (2008). *Gray's anatomy: the anatomical basis of clinical practice* (S. Susan Ed. 40 ed.). London, United Kingdom: Churchill Livingstone Elsevier.

6

Latissimus dorsi

Quadratus lumborum

Erector spinae (iliocostalis lumborum)

Erector spinae (iliocostalis thoracis)

Multifidus (transversospinales group)

Rectus abdominis

Internal and external obliques

Psoas major

Transversus abdominis

ANATOMY
Latissimus dorsi

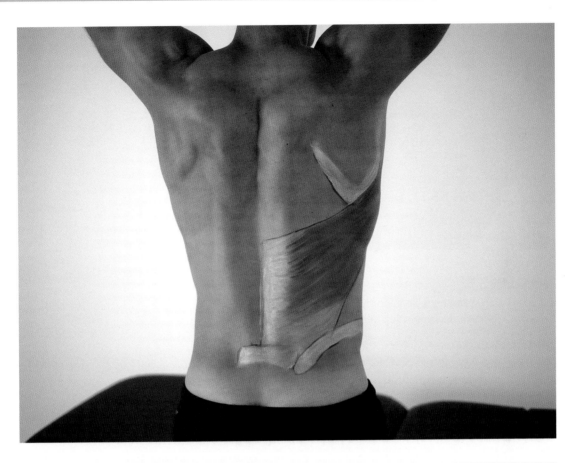

Latissimus dorsi

Origin:	Via the thoracolumbar fascia; spinous process T7–L5, posterior sacrum, posterior iliac crest, lowest three to four ribs and the inferior angle of the scapula
Insertion:	Medial lip of the bicipital groove of the humerus
Nerve supply:	Nerve root: C6–8 Peripheral nerve: thoracodorsal nerve
Function:	With the origin fixed, the latissimus dorsi extends, adducts and medially rotates the arm at the shoulder joint. Additionally depresses the shoulder girdle and assists in lateral flexion of the trunk. With the insertion fixed, the latissimus dorsi assists in tilting the pelvis both anteriorly and laterally. Acting bilaterally, assists in hyper-extending the spine and anteriorly tilting the pelvis or in flexing the spine. Acting with the contralateral gluteal muscles the latissimus dorsi has a role in assisting load transfer across the pelvic girdle by providing stability

7

MUSCLE TESTING
Latissimus dorsi

STRENGTH BIAS TESTING

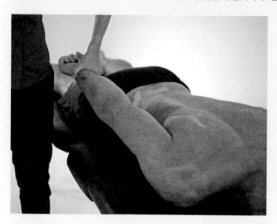

Client position

The client is prone with the shoulder held in internal rotation with the palm facing upwards. The shoulder is also in extension and adduction behind the back but without resting on the body.

Instruction to client

The client is instructed to resist the force applied by the examiner by maintaining the shoulder and upper limb position in internal rotation, extension and adduction without trying to hold against the back or buttocks during the testing.

Examiner position and notes

The examiner is positioned to the side of the client. The testing hand is placed proximal to the wrist (proximal to the elbow in the case of elbow pathology). The examiner should note for a compromised strategy which can be indicated with trunk rotation, alternative leg lifting and shoulder hitching.

Resistance

The examiner applies resistance in the direction of shoulder flexion and abduction to clear the trunk.

7

MUSCLE TESTING
Latissimus dorsi

LENGTH BIAS TESTING

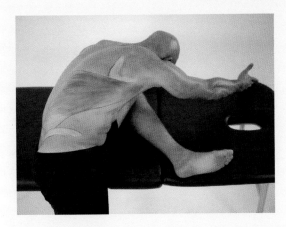

Client position

The client is sitting sideways on a plinth, the opposite hip is abducted and the trunk flexed and laterally flexed away from the side being tested. The arm is reaching forward diagonally across the body with the forearm supinated.

Instruction to client

The client is instructed to take the arm into lateral rotation, flexion and adduction in the overhead position in front of the body whilst also performing trunk flexion, lateral flexion and rotation away from the side being tested

Examiner position and notes

The examiner is positioned to assess for the range and quality of the movement. The examiner should note any symptoms that are reproduced during the testing for re-evaluation after the intervention. Range should be compared to the non-affected side for a baseline of normal range when available.

7

KINESIO TAPING
Latissimus dorsi

STRENGTH TAPING

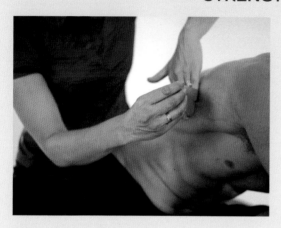

Client position

The client is sitting sideways on a plinth, the opposite hip is abducted, and the trunk flexed and laterally flexed away from the side being tested. The arm is reaching forward diagonally across the body with the forearm supinated.

Measurement of tape

Measure a length to tape from the sacrum to the medial aspect of the axilla. Fold the tape in two and cut down as for a web cut leaving a 5 cm anchor at both ends.

Tape application

Apply the starting anchor at the sacrum with zero tension. With the tissue in the lengthened position, lightly apply the base of the tape with 25–35% tension towards the axilla. Apply the anchor onto the axilla with zero tension and then lift the base of the tape and apply at appropriate angles to cover the muscle, its rib attachments and its scapular attachments. Rub the tape to activate the glue.

Reassessment

Reassess your client for changes in strength, tonal changes, functional changes and symptoms.

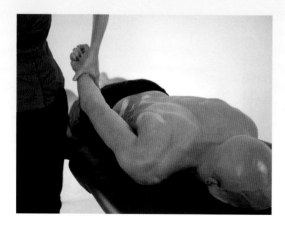

7

KINESIO TAPING
Latissimus dorsi

LENGTH TAPING

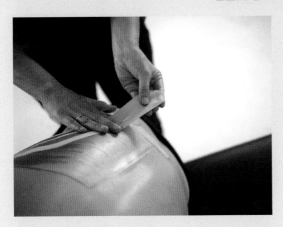

Client position
The client is sitting sideways on a plinth, the opposite hip is abducted, and the trunk flexed and laterally flexed away from the side being tested. The arm is reaching forward diagonally across the body with the forearm supinated.

Measurement of tape
Measure a length to tape from the sacrum to the medial aspect of the axilla. Fold the tape in two and cut down as for a web cut leaving a 5 cm anchor at both ends.

Tape application
Apply the starting anchor adjacent to the axilla with zero tension. With the tissue in the lengthened position, lightly lay the base of the tape with 15–25% tension towards the sacrum. Apply the anchor onto the sacrum with zero tension and then lift the base of the tape and apply at appropriate angles to cover the muscle, its rib attachments and its scapular attachments. Rub the tape to activate the glue.

Reassessment
Reassess your client for changes in length, strength, tonal changes, functional changes and symptoms.

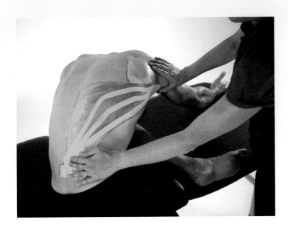

7

ANATOMY
Quadratus lumborum

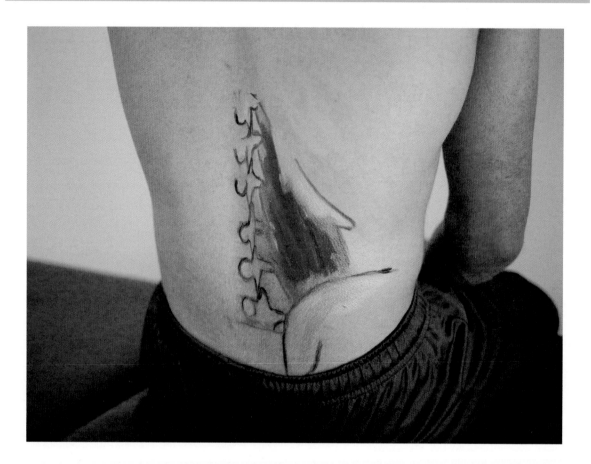

Quadratus lumborum

Origin:	Iliolumbar ligament, iliac crest
Insertion:	Inferior border of the last rib and transverse processes of the upper four lumbar vertebrae
Nerve supply:	T12, L1, 2, 3 Peripheral nerve: lumbar plexus
Function:	Anteriorly tilts the pelvis at the lumbosacral joint via its attachment to the iliac crest. Has a role in elevating the pelvis in the upright position and during gait. Acts with other muscles during lateral trunk flexion

MUSCLE TESTING
Quadratus lumborum

STRENGTH BIAS TESTING

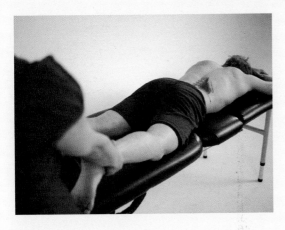

Client position
The client is in prone position with the leg abducted in a line that follows the orientation of the quadratus lumborum fibres.

Instruction to client
The client is instructed to hitch the hip being tested towards the same shoulder; the hip should be in slight extension so that the leg is not resting on the bed. The client should attempt to hold the hip hitch position during the test.

Examiner position and notes
The examiner is positioned at the foot of the bed opposite to the line of pull of the muscle fibres. The ankle is held above the malleolus as this position best provides the examiner with a mechanical advantage and a better grip and ability to use their own body weight to apply resistance during the test.

For the testing of a client with the presence of weak hip muscles or hip pathology, pressure may be given over the posterolateral iliac crest in a direction that opposes the line of the muscle pull. However, in the presence of a hip weakness, the examiner should determine whether the hip muscles may indeed need to be prioritised over management of quadratus lumborum with taping.

The quadratus lumborum acts with other muscles in lateral trunk flexion and lateral trunk stability. Whilst functional testing may implicate the muscle in standing, the elevation of the pelvis in standing or during gait is also a function of the contralateral adductors as well as the ipsilateral lateral abdominal muscles. The testing position in prone allows for a distinction between these other synergists for lateral stability. However the test does require that there is no underlying hip or knee pathology.

Resistance
The examiner offers resistance to the movement by placing a traction force on the leg above the ankle in a direction of extension and abduction.

7

MUSCLE TESTING
Quadratus lumborum

LENGTH BIAS TESTING

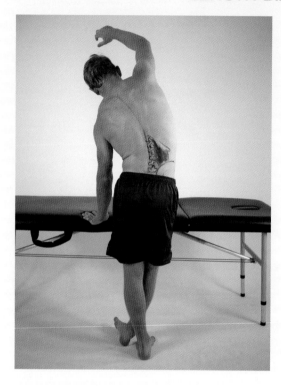

Client position

The client stands next to a wall or bed for support if necessary. The side being tested is furthest from the support structure, the ipsilateral foot is placed in front of the other, and the feet are inverted and rest on the floor. The upper body is stabilised by the contralateral hand holding the wall or the bed.

Instruction to client

The client is instructed to reach above the head with the ipsilateral arm in order to laterally flex the trunk. The hip may move laterally during the testing.

Examiner position and notes

The examiner is positioned behind the client to assess for range, the quality of the movement and for any anomalies in the spinal alignment during testing.

7

KINESIO TAPING
Quadratus lumborum

STRENGTH TAPING

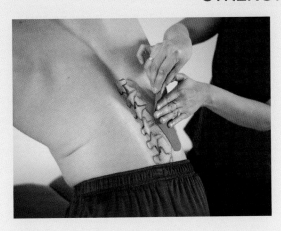

Client position
The client is in standing and instructed to laterally flex and reach over to the contralateral side. The pelvis is tucked under to create a slight lumbar flexion.

Measurement of tape
A length of tape is measured from the medial posterior iliac crest to the last rib adjacent to the lumbar spine transverse processes.

Tape application
The tape may be cut into an X-strip or Y-strip to cover a larger surface area or be maintained as an I-strip. Apply the starting anchor with zero tension on the posterior iliac crest. Apply the base of the tape with 25–35% tension up towards the last rib and the adjacent lumbar spine transverse processes. Apply the final anchor with zero tension. Rub the tape to activate the glue.

Reassessment
Reassess your client for change in strength, tonal changes, functional changes and symptoms.

7

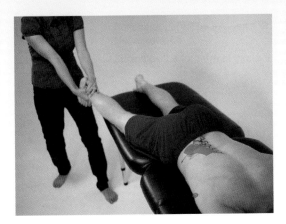

KINESIO TAPING
Quadratus lumborum

LENGTH TAPING

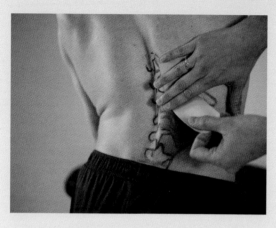

Client position

The client stands and is instructed to laterally flex and reach over to the contralateral side. The pelvis is tucked under to create a slight lumbar flexion.

Measurement of tape

A length of tape is measured from the medial posterior iliac crest to the last rib adjacent to the lumbar spine transverse processes.

Tape application

The tape may be cut into an X-strip or Y-strip to cover a larger surface area or be maintained as an I-strip. Apply the starting anchor with zero tension on the last rib adjacent to the transverse process of the upper lumbar spine. Apply the base of the tape down towards the posterior iliac crest with 15–25% tension. Apply the anchor on the iliac crest with zero tension. Rub the tape to activate the glue.

7

LENGTH TAPING

Reassessment

The client is reassessed for the range of movement, symptoms and palpated for changes in tone. A restoration of length may also yield strength improvements where a strength deficit was detected prior to the taping. In these circumstances, the strength should also be reassessed. Any functional deficits can also be reassessed for changes.

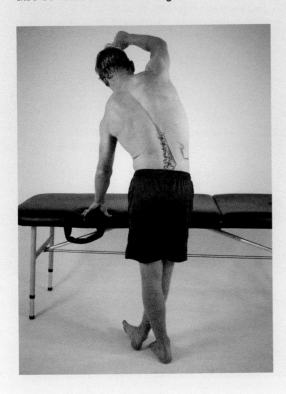

ANATOMY
Erector spinae (iliocostalis lumborum)

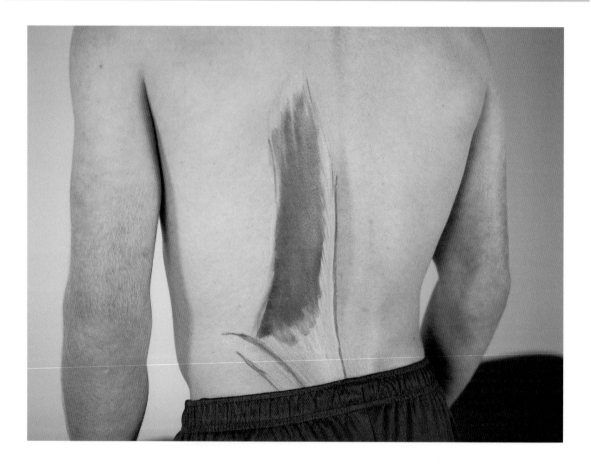

Erector spinae (iliocostalis lumborum)

Origin:	Medial crest of the sacrum, spinous processes of L1–5, T11–12, posterior medial lip of the iliac crest, supraspinous ligament
Insertion:	Via tendons into the inferior borders of the angles of the lower six or seven ribs. In the cervical and thoracic region, most of the erector spinae is located lateral to the laminar groove (lower portion of muscle shown)
Nerve supply:	T12, L1, 2, 3 Peripheral nerve: lumbar plexus
Function:	Bilaterally extends the vertebral column and the lower thoracic area, draws the ribs downward. Anteriorly tilts and elevates the pelvis at the lumbosacral joint Acting unilaterally, extends, rotates and laterally flexes the trunk to the ipsilateral side. Eccentrically acts to allow trunk flexion when in an upright position

MUSCLE TESTING
Erector spinae (iliocostalis lumborum)

STRENGTH BIAS TESTING

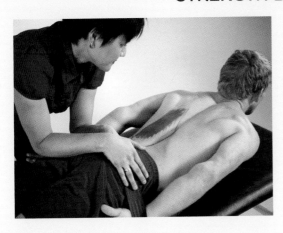

Client position

Client is lying prone on a bed with a pillow underneath the pelvis.

Instruction to client

The client is instructed to extend the trunk off the bed and hold this position. A slight testing bias can be created by rotating the ipsilateral trunk and shoulder up during the extension movement on the side being tested.

Examiner position and notes

The examiner stands to the side of the client to assess for directional bias, muscle activity and imbalances. The pelvis and lower limb are stabilised on the plinth with belts over the pelvis and lower limb.

Additional support to stabilise the pelvis may be offered by the examiner during the testing.

Resistance

It is not necessary for the examiner to apply force on the trunk as the examination requires extension against the resistance of gravity. The application of undue force may exacerbate conditions. Applying light force on one side of the trunk compared to the other may show a weakness in one side's capacity to hold the position. This should only be attempted when the examiner is sure this test will not irritate the client's condition.

7

MUSCLE TESTING
Erector spinae (iliocostalis lumborum)

LENGTH BIAS TESTING

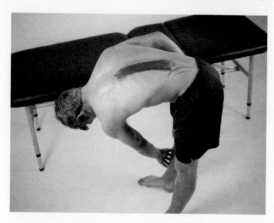

Client position

The client sits or stands with the feet firmly supported.

Instruction to client

The client is instructed to slowly flex the trunk by rounding out the trunk whilst reaching towards the opposite leg and sliding the hand down towards the floor.

Examiner position and notes

Observation of where the flexion movement of the trunk is or is not occurring shows the muscle's ability to lengthen. Once it is clear a component of the erector spinae groups is involved in the presenting problem then palpate the area. Palpation of the muscle tone and muscle fibres helps to specify the direction of tape application and over which fibres the tape should be applied to yield maximal effects.

7

KINESIO TAPING
Erector spinae (iliocostalis lumborum)

STRENGTH TAPING

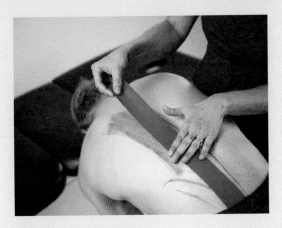

Client position
The client is seated or standing. The client is instructed to slowly flex the trunk by rounding out the trunk whilst reaching towards the opposite leg and floor.

Measurement of tape
A length of tape is measured from the sacrum to the spinal level above the level of deficit.

Tape application
Apply the starting anchor to the lower segment of the spine (typically at the ilium or sacrum) with zero tension. With the tissue in the lengthened position, apply the base of the tape with 25–35% tension over the identified muscle fibres. Apply the final anchor with zero tension at the segment above those in deficit. Rub the tape to activate the glue.

Reassessment
Reassess your client for changes in strength, tonal changes, functional changes and symptoms.

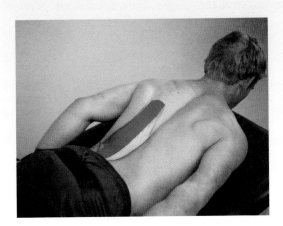

7

KINESIO TAPING
Erector spinae (iliocostalis lumborum)

LENGTH TAPING

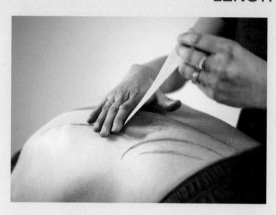

Client position

The client is seated or standing. The client is instructed to slowly flex the trunk by rounding out the trunk whilst reaching towards the opposite leg and floor.

Measurement of tape

A length of tape is measured from the sacrum to the spinal level above the level of deficit.

Tape application

Apply the starting anchor with zero tension above the upper spinal segment. With the tissue in a lengthened position, apply the base of the tape over the pathway of the identified fibres down towards the ilium and sacrum with 15-25% tension. Apply the final anchor with zero tension over the sacrum or ilium. Rub the tape to activate the glue.

Reassessment

The client is reassessed for range of movement, symptoms and palpated for changes in tone. A restoration of length may also yield strength improvements where a strength deficit was detected prior to the taping, in these circumstances, the strength should also be reassessed. Any functional deficits can also be reassessed for changes.

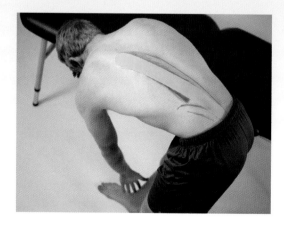

7

ANATOMY

Erector spinae (iliocostalis thoracis)

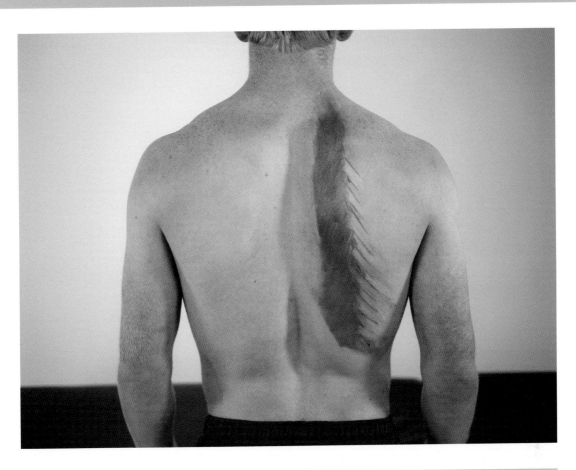

Erector spinae (iliocostalis thoracis)

Origin:	Via tendons from the upper borders of angles of lower six ribs
Insertion:	Cranial borders of angles of the upper six ribs and transverse process of the seventh cervical vertebrae
Nerve supply:	Posterior branch of the spinal nerve
Function:	Bilaterally extends the vertebral column. Acting unilaterally, extends, rotates and laterally flexes the upper trunk to the ipsilateral side, may draw the ribs downwards. Eccentrically acts to allow upper trunk flexion when in an upright position

7

MUSCLE TESTING
Erector spinae (iliocostalis thoracis)

STRENGTH BIAS TESTING

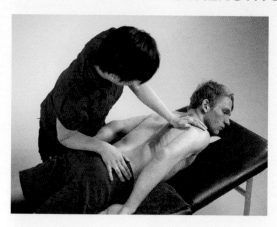

Client position
The client is instructed to lie prone on the bed.

Instruction to client
The thoracic area is placed in ipsilateral rotation, extension; lateral flexion will occur as a coupling movement with this activity.

Examiner position and notes
The examiner is standing on the contralateral side to the one being tested. The level to be tested is placed in ipsilateral rotation, extension; lateral flexion will occur as a coupling movement with this activity.

Resistance
The resistance is applied via the heel of the hand placed between the spine and the scapula. Resistance is applied over the muscle in the direction down towards a neutral position on the bed.

7

MUSCLE TESTING
Erector spinae (iliocostalis thoracis)

LENGTH BIAS TESTING

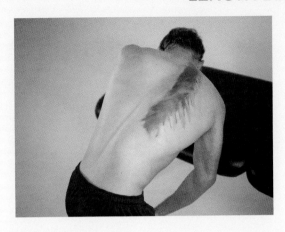

Client position

The client is seated or standing (whichever is more comfortable for the client). The spine is flexed with the trunk curling over and the upper limb reaching towards the opposite foot. The neck is also flexed.

Instruction to client

The client is instructed to slowly flex the trunk by flexing the neck and rounding out the trunk whilst reaching towards the floor. Length testing for one side can be enhanced by adding some lateral flexion towards the opposite side as well as rotation.

Examiner position and notes

Observation of where the flexion movement of the trunk is or is not occurring shows the muscle's ability to lengthen. Once it is clear that a component of the erector spinae groups is involved in the presenting problem then palpate the area. Palpation of the muscle tone and muscle fibres helps to specify the direction of tape application and over which fibres the tape should be applied to yield maximal effects.

7

KINESIO TAPING
Erector spinae (iliocostalis thoracis)

STRENGTH TAPING

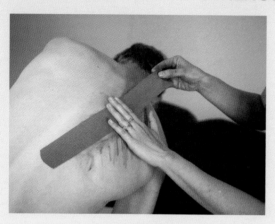

Client position

The client is seated or standing (whichever is more comfortable for the client). The spine is flexed with the trunk curling over and the upper limb reaching towards the opposite foot. The neck is also flexed.

Measurement of tape

A length of tape is measured from the sacrum to the spinal level above the level of deficit.

Tape application

Apply the starting anchor with zero tension to the lower segment of the thorax. With the tissue in a lengthened position, apply the base of the tape with 25–35% tension over the identified muscle fibres. Apply the final anchor with zero tension at the segment above those in deficit. Rub the tape to activate the glue.

Reassessment

Reassess your client for change in strength, tonal changes, functional changes and symptoms.

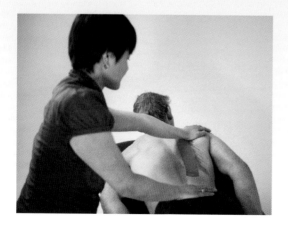

7

KINESIO TAPING
Erector spinae (iliocostalis thoracis)

LENGTH TAPING

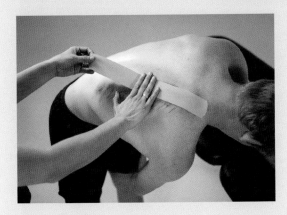

Client position
The client is seated or standing (whichever is more comfortable for the client). The spine is flexed with the trunk curling over and the upper limb reaching towards the opposite foot. The neck is also flexed.

Measurement of tape
A length of tape is measured from the lower thorax to the spinal level above the level of deficit.

Tape application
Apply the starting anchor with zero tension above the upper spinal segment. With the tissue in a lengthened position, apply the base of the tape over the identified fibres and pathway down towards the ilium and sacrum with 15–25% tension. Apply the final anchor with zero tension over the lower thorax. Rub the tape to activate the glue.

Reassessment
The client is reassessed for range of movement, symptoms and palpated for changes in tone. A restoration of length may also yield strength improvements where a strength deficit was detected prior to the taping—in these circumstances, the strength should also be reassessed. Any functional deficits can also be reassessed for changes.

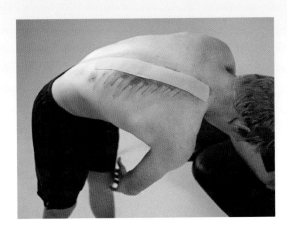

7

ANATOMY
Multifidus (transversospinales group)

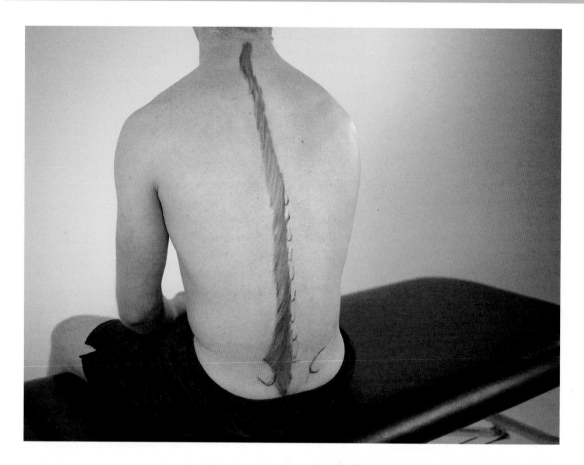

Multifidus (transversospinales group)

Origin:	Posterior surface of the sacrum
Insertion:	Located within the laminar groove (the area between the spinous process and transverse process)
Nerve supply:	Dorsal rami of the spinal nerves
Function:	Deep fibres assist in stabilising the spinal segments. Superficial fibres assist in spinal segmental extension. By orientation of the fibres, they provide contralateral rotation to vertebrae for appropriate stacking of spinal segments

7

MUSCLE TESTING
Multifidus (transversospinales group)

STRENGTH BIAS TESTING

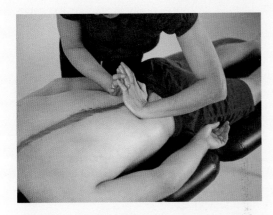

Handling for testing shown in prone which can be used for both prone or supine testing

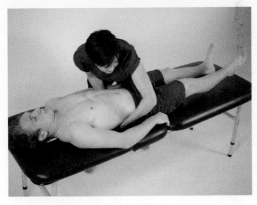

Lying on back with leg lift

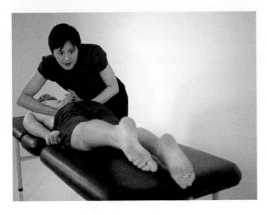

Prone leg extension (face down)

Client position

The client is lying supine for the active straight leg raise (ASLR) test or prone for the prone leg extension (PLE) test.

STRENGTH BIAS TESTING

Instruction to client

The client is instructed to lift the leg with the knee extended, to a height of 10 cm. The client is instructed to rate the perceived effort in lifting the leg; 0/5 for no effort, 5/5 for maximal effort.

The ASLR test score is taken as a baseline measure of the client's functional ability to stabilise the pelvis in order to transfer load as the leg is lifted, whilst strategy and symptoms are noted by the examiner. The client is reminded that this is a test of perceived effort and that they should score on the effort experienced with the task and not the symptoms.

The examiner then asks the client to repeat the test, this time with the tensional forces of the muscle contraction supplemented by the examiner. The client is asked to re-rate the perceived effort. The baseline effort is then compared to the effort experienced during examiner-supplemented testing. If there are no changes in perceived effort during the supplemented testing, then taping of multifidus is not indicated.

Clients with an extension provocation bias to their function may demonstrate more meaningful scores with a PLE test. For a PLE test, the client is instructed to extend the leg off the bed by extending the hip and maintaining knee extension. The ankle is only required to lift above the bed by 10 cm. A baseline measure of effort is taken and compared to the supplemented testing.

Examiner position and notes

For the baseline testing, the examiner is positioned at the foot or head of the bed to best assess for the movement quality.

For the supplemented muscle testing, the examiner is positioned to the side of the client and places the heels of the hands either side of the multifidus muscles (lateral to the bulk of the muscles) in the lumbar spine. The examiner applies a compressive force medially towards the spine to supplement the tensional vector that would otherwise be generated if the muscle was contracted. The examiner should only apply gentle forces which could be created by the muscle activation and replicated by the tape to create change.

The examiner is reminded that the role of the deep multifidus is described in the literature as a stabilising muscle, whilst the superficial multifidus has a role in extension. In acute low back pain, the deep multifidus may be inhibited in its function. However, in chronic low back pain the superficial multifidus may be overactive. As the taping process will overlay both components of the multifidus, the primary taping technique used will be decided based on the length and strength assessments and which test is more significant with respect to the history and the presenting symptoms of the client.

The testing described distinctly relates to the use of Kinesio Tape and the value that it would give to an individual's function when applied to this part of the body. The intention of this resource is to provide useful testing procedures that would be available to any practitioner without the need for additional equipment. Of course, the everyday practitioner with access to additional testing equipment is encouraged to use these tools.

The use of the active straight leg raise (ASLR) during the testing of the multifidus is intentional. The ASLR test has been proven in literature to be a reliable test to measure the capacity of the active muscle system to generate sufficient tension to allow for the transfer of load across the pelvis. It can be an extremely useful clinical test to ascertain the effectiveness of treatment.

The testing shown here interprets the role of multifidus in stabilising the pelvis for the client being tested.

For the baseline testing: If the client is aware of an increase in perceived effort with the ASLR (particularly when compared to the contralateral side), then the test will be valuable.

The examiner should assess for the quality of the movement independently of the client when assessing the baseline as well as during the supplemented test.

STRENGTH BIAS TESTING

Once the baseline ASLR is established, the examiner attempts to supplement the forces otherwise created by an active muscle contraction of the lower multifidus as it stabilises the lumbar spine. This is done by gathering tension in the low back by taking up tissue slack across the lumbosacral junction and approximating it towards the centre.

An improvement in perceived effort during the ASLR with an examiner-supplemented force in the region implies that taping to replicate the handling forces of the examiner would be appropriate.

If the baseline test is positive for perceived effort but the test is unchanged with the supplemented support over multifidus, then the test remains positive but taping over the multifidus is not indicated and unlikely to yield improvements to the ASLR tests. That is, the source of this increased effort is not from this muscle, and testing of other muscles is warranted.

If the client is not aware of any perceived effort during the baseline ASLR and the execution of the test is normal, then this test may be inappropriate for them as it has no meaning to their individual experience or symptoms. Testing in the prone position may have more meaning for the client and this is recommended instead; their condition may have an extension provocation bias which has more meaning to their personal experience with extension provocation testing.

If the client reports no perceived effort with the testing and yet the examiner is aware of compromised strategies such as breath holding, trunk twisting, abdominal bulging, upper limb activity and others, then the test is valuable to the examiner. However, the client is likely to be compromised in proprioceptive awareness and may have a chronic condition which has altered their perception of what would be considered normal. The examiner should apply the supplemented test to the client and ascertain if this improves their perceived effort beyond what they thought would be 'normal'. This would indicate taping for the multifidus. The examiner should also independently assess whether there is an improvement in movement during the test that the client may not yet be aware of. This would also indicate that taping of the multifidus may be appropriate for improving function. If there is no improvement in movement with the assisted test and the client is not aware of any changes, then the test may still be valuable to the examiner but taping of the multifidus is not indicated.

Resistance

No resistance is applied by the examiner; rather, the examiner adds a force across the segment from one hand to the other to supplement the stabilising vector otherwise created by the multifidus muscle. An improvement in the perceived effort of the ASLR in the absence of a length restriction indicates strength taping may be beneficial. It is important to assess the tone and length of the multifidus. It is not uncommon for chronic conditions to have short or overactive superficial multifidus. In these situations, the testing may improve perceived effort but the taping indicated would be a lengthening tape in order to restore function.

MUSCLE TESTING
Multifidus (transversospinales group)

LENGTH BIAS TESTING

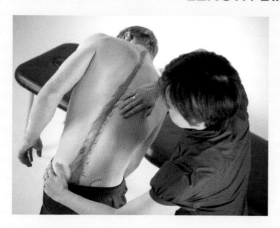

Client position

The client is seated or standing (whichever is more comfortable for the client). The spine is flexed with the trunk curling over towards the knees. The right shoulder is rotated to the left knee, right elbow to the left knee, for taping the left multifidus and vice versa for the right side.

Instruction to client

The client is instructed to reach towards the ipsilateral knee (to the side of the multifidus to be tested) with the opposite upper limb. The client is then instructed to slide the hand down the leg. Rather than reaching down the leg as far as possible, the client should attempt to round out the back during the movement.

Examiner position and notes

The examiner assesses for even contribution to flexion of the spine at the spinal segments. A flattening of the spine with increased flexion above and below the segment suggests that the segment is not moving and may be limited by the length of soft tissue and muscles. An overactive or short multifidus may induce a 'weakness' in segmental control and respond to the strength testing. In this case, a length application should be applied as the first intervention.

7

KINESIO TAPING
Multifidus (transversospinales group)

STRENGTH TAPING

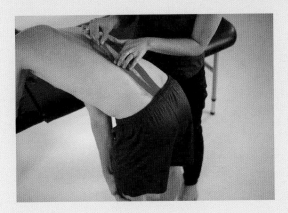

Client position

The client is seated or standing (whichever is more comfortable for the client). The spine is flexed with the trunk curling over towards the knees. The right shoulder is rotated to the left knee, right elbow to left knee, for taping the left multifidus and vice versa for the right mulitifidus.

Measurement of tape

With the client in a lengthened position, measure a length of tape from the apex of the sacrum to one inch above the segments indicated. Cut the tape in a Y-strip with each tail 2.5 cm wide.

Tape application

Apply the common anchor with zero tension on the sacrum starting above the apex. With the tissue in a lengthened position, apply the base of one tail with 25–35%, tension just lateral to the spinous process. Complete the tape by applying the final anchor with zero tension. In the same manner, apply the other tail, remembering to reach to the other side to lengthen the tissue. Rub the tape to activate the glue.

Reassessment

Reassess your client for changes in length, strength, tonal changes, functional changes and symptoms. The perceived effort in the active straight leg raise or prone extension test should improve to approximate or equal the quality of movement achieved with the supplemented test.

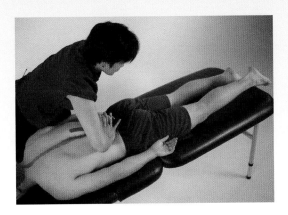

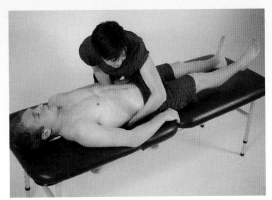

KINESIO TAPING
Multifidus (transversospinales group)

LENGTH TAPING

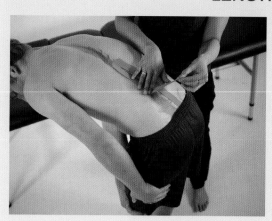

Client position

The client is seated or standing (whichever is more comfortable for the client). The spine is flexed with the trunk curling over towards the knees. The right shoulder is rotated to the left knee, right elbow to the left knee, for taping the left multifidus and vice versa for the right multifidus.

Measurement of tape

With the client in a lengthened position, measure a length of tape from the apex of the sacrum to one inch above the segments indicated. Cut the tape in a Y-strip with each tail 2.5 cm wide.

Tape application

Apply the starting anchor with zero tension above the segments indicated in testing. Apply the base of one tail with 15–25% tension just lateral to the spinous process and down onto the sacrum, ending above the apex of the sacrum with the final anchor with zero tension. In the same manner, apply the other tail and remember to reach to the other side to lengthen the tissue. Rub the tape to activate the glue.

7

LENGTH TAPING

Reassessment

Reassess your client for changes in length, strength, tonal changes, functional changes and symptoms. The segment of interest should have convolutions when in a neutral position but may have less convolutions than more mobile segments. The active straight leg raise (ASLR) test or prone leg extension (PLE) test should yield improvements in perceived effort.

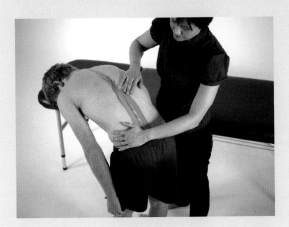

ANATOMY
Rectus abdominis

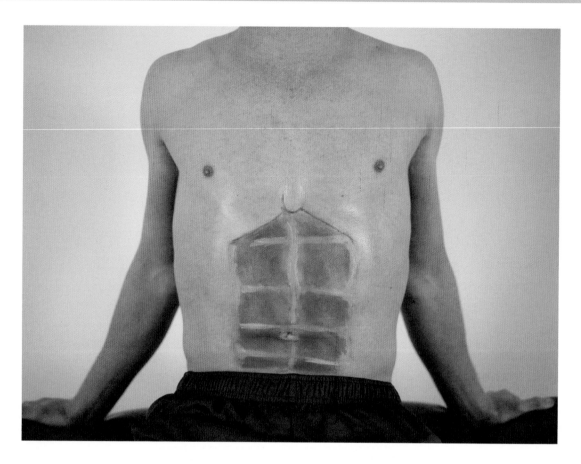

Rectus abdominis

Origin:	Pubic crest and pubic symphysis
Insertion:	Costal cartilages of ribs 5–7 and xiphoid process of the sternum
Nerve supply:	Nerve root: T5–12 Peripheral nerve: ventral rami
Function:	Flexes the vertebral column. In supine position, it tilts the pelvis posteriorly or approximates the thorax towards the pelvis

MUSCLE TESTING
Rectus abdominis

STRENGTH BIAS TESTING

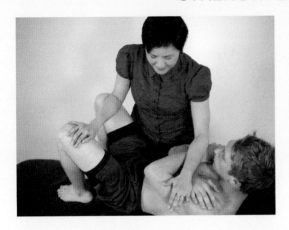 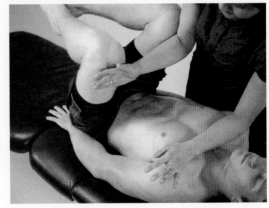

Client position

The client is lying supine with the hips and knees in flexion as for a sit-up. The arms are placed across the chest.

Instruction to client

Upper abdominals: The client is instructed to perform an abdominal curl up by bringing the chest towards the knees.

Lower abdominals: The client is instructed to raise the knees so that they point to the ceiling, hips and knees are held in a table-top position (shins horizontal) whilst the client is lying supine. The arms are resting by the side of the body. The client is instructed to raised their pelvis off the floor and reach the pelvis towards the ceiling whilst bringing the knees towards the chest.

Examiner position and notes

The examiner is positioned to the side of the client and notes if there is compensatory overactivity at the neck or chest, or whether the strategy requires breath holding. The examiner should note for symmetry and symptom reproduction as well as loss of range. Resistance need only be applied if the antigravity testing is non-significant.

Resistance

Upper abdominals: If the testing is not significant on contraction against gravity alone, the examiner may add resistance by applying a force over the arms of the client (crossed over the chest) in the direction that would return the trunk to the bed. The examiner's other arm is used to stabilise the legs.

Lower abdominals: Resistance may be applied to the thigh in the direction that would return the feet to the bed. The upper body should be stabilised with the forearm resting over the upper chest.

MUSCLE TESTING
Rectus abdominis

LENGTH BIAS TESTING

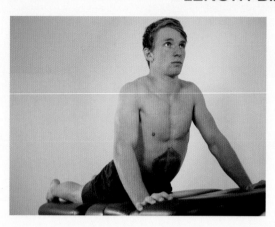

Client position

The client is in a lunge position supported by their extended arms on a bed.

With shoulder complications, the client can extend over a therapy ball with the legs extended and arms flexed to maximal available range or in horizontal abduction.

Instruction to client

The client is instructed to place the hands adjacent to the shoulders. The client is then instructed to push through the hands so that the upper body moves away from the bed whilst maintaining the pelvis on the bed.

Examiner position and notes

The examiner is positioned to the side of the client. A sensation of tension, increased resting tone and lack of range indicates that length taping may be beneficial.

7

KINESIO TAPING
Rectus abdominis

STRENGTH TAPING

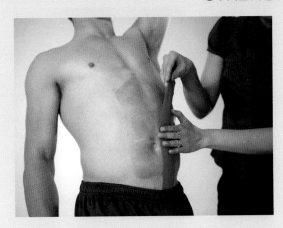

Client position

The client is in a standing lunge position with the arms reaching overhead or in a lunge position supported by their extended arms. With shoulder complications, the client can extend over a therapy ball with the legs extended and arms flexed to maximal available range or in horizontal abduction.

For clients who have difficulty repositioning or have poor mobility, instruct the client to reach the arms overhead whilst in a supine position.

In addition to each test position, the client is instructed to take a deep breath to blow out their abdominal wall when the base of the tape is applied.

Measurement of tape

With the client in the lengthened position, measure two lengths of tape from the costal cartilages adjacent to the sternum down to the pubic bone (direct application of tape onto the pubic bone may be limited depending on the client).

Tape application

For upper abdominal deficits the pubic bone is considered to be the origin. Apply the starting anchor as close to the pubic bone as possible with zero tension. With the tissue in the lengthened position, apply the base of the tape with 25–35% tension towards the costal cartilages on the same side. Complete the taping by applying the final anchor with zero tension on the costal cartilages. Repeat the application on the other side if indicated by the testing. Rub the tape to activate the glue.

For lower abdominal deficits the pubic bone is considered to be the insertion. Apply the starting anchor at the costal cartilages with zero tension. With the tissue in a lengthened position, apply the base of the tape with 25–35% tension towards the pubic bone. Complete the taping by applying the final anchor with zero tension as close to the pubic bone as possible. Repeat the application on the other side if indicated by the testing. Rub the tape to activate the glue.

7

STRENGTH TAPING

Reassessment

Reassess your client for changes in strength, tonal changes, functional changes and symptoms.

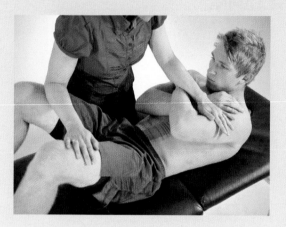 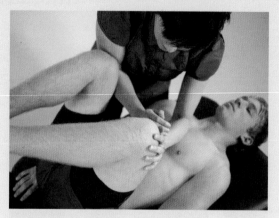

KINESIO TAPING
Rectus abdominis

LENGTH TAPING

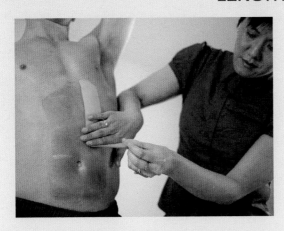

Client position

The client is in a standing lunge position with the arms reaching overhead or in a lunge position supported by their extended arms.

With shoulder complications, the client can extend over a therapy ball with the legs extended and arms flexed to maximal available range or in horizontal abduction.

For clients who have difficulty repositioning or poor mobility, instruct the client to reach the arms overhead in the supine position.

In addition to each test position, the client is instructed to take a deep breath to blow out their abdominal wall when the base of the tape is applied.

Measurement of tape

With the client in the lengthened position, measure two lengths of tape from the costal cartilages adjacent to the sternum down to the pubic bone (direct application of tape onto the pubic bone may be limited depending on the client).

Tape application

For upper abdominal deficits: the pubic bone is considered to be the origin. Apply the starting anchor with zero tension to the costal cartilage. With the tissue in the lengthened position, apply the base with 15–25% tension down to the pubic symphysis on one side of the umbilicus. Complete the taping by applying the final anchor with zero tension to an area as close to the pubic bone as possible. Repeat the application on the other side if indicated by testing. Rub the tape to activate the glue.

For lower abdominal deficits: the pubic bone is considered to be the insertion. Start the beginning anchor as close to the pubic bone as possible with zero tension. With the tissue in the lengthened position, apply the base of the tape over on one side of the umbilicus with 15–25% tension up towards the 'origin' at the costal cartilage/sternum on the same side. Complete the taping by applying the final anchor on the 'origin' at the costal cartilage with zero tension. Repeat the application on the other side if indicated by testing. Rub the tape to activate the glue.

LENGTH TAPING

Reassessment

Reassess your client for changes in length, strength, tonal changes, functional changes and symptoms.

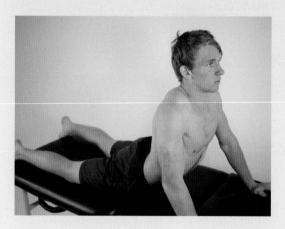

7

ANATOMY
Internal and external obliques

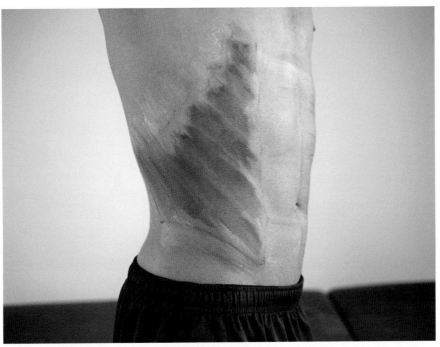

External Oblique shown on client's right side

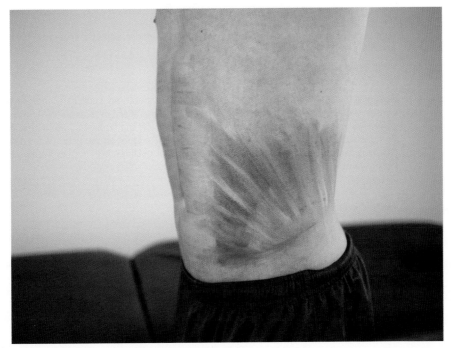

Internal Oblique shown on client's left side

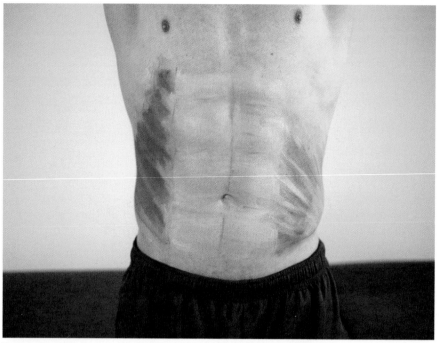

External and Internal Obliques (one on each side of client)

External obliques

Origin:	Anterior fibres: external surfaces of ribs 5–8 interdigitating with the serratus anterior Lateral fibres: external surfaces of rib 9 interdigitating with the serratus anterior, external surfaces of ribs 10–12 interdigitating with latissimus dorsi
Insertion:	Via a broad aponeurosis to the linea alba Lateral fibres; ipsilateral inguinal ligament into the anterior-superior spine and pubic tubercle and the external lip of the anterior ½ of the iliac crest
Nerve supply:	Peripheral nerve: ventral rami Nerve root: T5–12
Function:	Acting bilaterally, the anterior fibres flex the vertebral column, support, compress and contain the abdominal viscera, depress the thorax and assist in respiration. Acting unilaterally, the anterior fibres work synergistically with the contralateral internal obliques to flex and rotate the thorax towards the contralateral side when the pelvis is fixed. When the thorax is fixed, the unilateral activity of the external obliques with the contralateral internal obliques rotates the contralateral pelvis posteriorly

Internal obliques

Origin:	Anterior and middle ⅓ of the iliac crest
Insertion:	Via a broad aponeurosis to the linea alba
Nerve supply:	Nerve root: T7–12, L1 Peripheral nerve: Iliohypogastric and ilioinguinal, ventral rami
Function:	Acting bilaterally, the lateral fibres flex the vertebral column and depress the thorax. Acting unilaterally, the anterior superior fibres act synergistically with the ipsilateral external oblique to laterally flex the vertebral column to the same side. These fibres also work with the contralateral external obliques to flex and rotate the trunk

7

MUSCLE TESTING
Internal and external obliques

STRENGTH BIAS TESTING

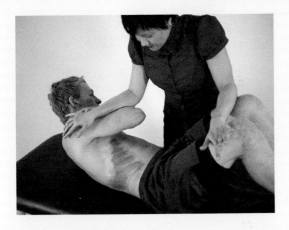

Client position

The client is lying supine with the hips and knees flexed so that the feet are resting on the bed. The arms are placed across the chest with the hands resting on the opposite shoulder.

Instruction to client

The client is instructed to curl up and bring the contralateral lower rib cage over towards the ipsilateral knee (towards the examiner). Right external obliques and left internal obliques testing is shown.

Examiner position and notes

The examiner stands to the ipsilateral side of the internal obliques being tested and stabilises the thigh and hips. The examining hand is placed over the contralateral shoulder and upper arm.

Resistance

The examiner applies a force onto the shoulder and upper arm in the direction that would return the trunk to a neutral position. It is important for the examiner to use their own body weight to apply the resistance rather than exert force through only the upper limb. The testing should be directed towards returning the trunk to the bed rather than just testing the anterior shoulder.

7

MUSCLE TESTING
Internal and external obliques

LENGTH BIAS TESTING

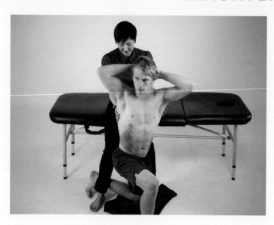

Client position

The client is in a kneeling lung position with the hands clasped behind the head. The external oblique muscle being tested is on the side with the knee in front and the internal oblique being tested on the side with the knee in the kneeling position. Clients with knee problems may be assessed in alternative positions such as a standing lunge position. Clients with shoulder problems may be assessed with the hands across the chest or behind the back.

Instruction to client

The client is instructed to rotate the upper body towards the side with the knee in front whilst maintaining the pelvic position.

Examiner position and notes

The examiner assesses for the quality of movement, range and symptom reproduction. Overpressure may be applied if it does not irritate the client's condition and the examiner may attempt to feel for where the resistance to movement may be coming from. Palpation may show more specific muscle tone areas requiring management or further assessment.

7

KINESIO TAPING
Internal and external obliques

STRENGTH TAPING

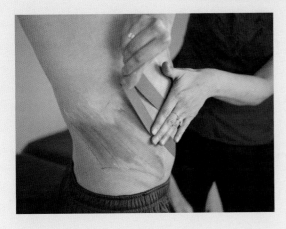

Client position
The client is in a kneeling lunge position as per the length testing position with the hands clasped behind the head or back, and rotated.

Measurement of tape
Measure a length of tape from the lateral midline of the ribs to the contralateral anterior superior iliac spine (ASIS). Fold the tape in half, cut down the centre as for a web cut or a basket weave to cover a larger surface area.

Tape application
For the purpose of function, the origin for the external oblique is considered to be the contralateral ASIS via its fascial connections to the contralateral internal oblique. The client is instructed to hold a deep breath during the taping so as to increase abdominal distension and rib cage excursion. Apply the starting anchor with zero tension over the contralateral ASIS. Apply the base of the tape with 25–35% tension towards the lateral midline of the ribs (the tape should point towards the scapula). Complete the taping by applying the final anchor on the lateral ribs with zero tension. Rub the tape to activate the glue.

7

STRENGTH TAPING

Reassessment

Reassess your client for change in strength, tonal changes, functional changes and symptoms.

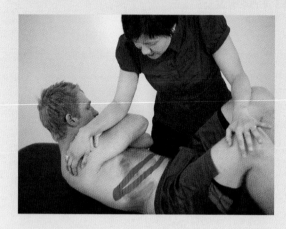

KINESIO TAPING
Internal and external obliques

LENGTH TAPING

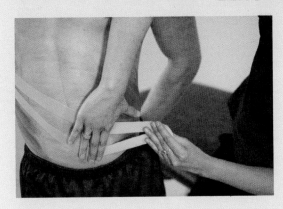

Client position
The client is in a kneeling lunge position as per the length testing position with the hands clasped behind the head or back, and rotated.

Measurement of tape
Measure a length of tape from the lateral midline of the ribs to the contralateral ASIS. Fold the tape in half, cut down the centre as for a web cut or a basket weave cut to cover a larger surface area.

Tape application
For the purpose of function, the origin for the external oblique is considered to be the contralateral ASIS via its fascial connections to the contralateral internal oblique. The client is instructed to hold a deep breath during the taping so as to increase abdominal distension and rib cage excursion. Apply the starting anchor with zero tension over the lateral midline of the ribs (the tape should point towards the scapula). Apply the base of the tape with 15–25% tension towards the contralateral ASIS whilst avoiding the umbilicus. Complete the taping by applying the final anchor on the ASIS with zero tension. Rub the tape to activate the glue.

Reassessment
Reassess your client for changes in length, strength, tonal changes, functional changes and symptoms.

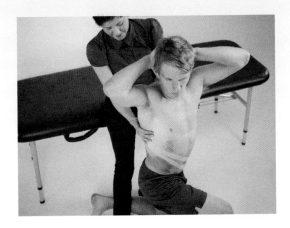

7

ANATOMY
Psoas major

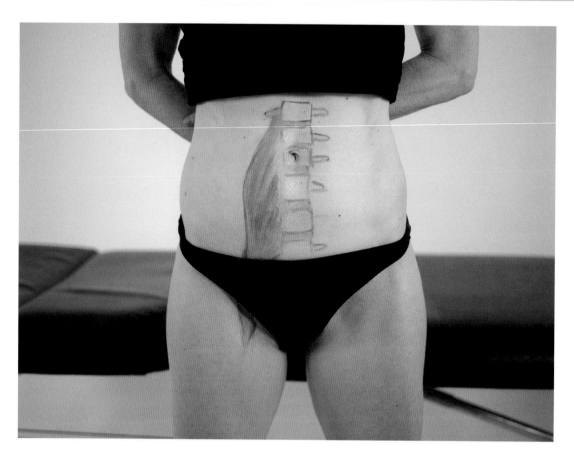

7

Psoas major	
Origin:	Anterior surfaces of the transverse processes of the T12 and the lumbar vertebrae, sides of the bodies and corresponding intervertebral discs of the last thoracic and all lumbar vertebrae. These include membranous arches that extend over the sides of the bodies of the lumbar vertebrae
Insertion:	Lesser trochanter of the femur
Nerve supply:	Nerve root: L1, 2, 3, 4 Peripheral nerve: lumbar plexus
Function:	With the origin fixed, iliopsoas flexes the hip joint by flexing the femur on the trunk. They may assist in lateral rotation of the hip joint. When acting bilaterally, they flex the hip joint by flexing the trunk on the femur. The lower fibres of psoas major will act to increase lumbar lordosis with the insertion fixed whilst the upper fibres will act to assist lumbar flexion, and lateral flexion when acting unilaterally

MUSCLE TESTING
Psoas major

STRENGTH BIAS TESTING

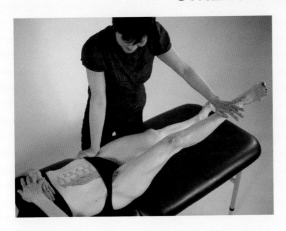

Client position
The client is lying supine with the legs in extension.

Instruction to client
The client is instructed to maintain knee extension whilst performing hip flexion in a position of slight lateral rotation.

Examiner position and notes
The examiner stands to the side of the limb being tested and stabilises the opposite pelvis. The examining hand is placed proximal to the ankle joint.

Resistance
Resistance is applied at the anterior medial aspect of the distal tibia in a direction of hip extension and slight abduction in a direction opposite to the line of pull of the muscle.

7

MUSCLE TESTING
Psoas major

LENGTH BIAS TESTING

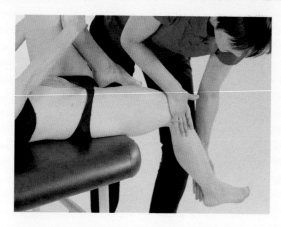 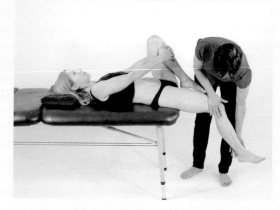

Client position
The client is instructed to sit at the end of a plinth.

Instruction to client
The client is instructed to hold the contralateral knee to the chest and is assisted by the examiner into the supine position whilst maintaining the knee-to-chest position.

Examiner position and notes
The examiner is positioned to the side of the bed in order to assist the client into the supine position. Once in the testing position, the examiner may assess for hip extension range off the edge of the bed. Psoas and iliacus tension is indicated when the hip is held in some flexion and/or external rotation. For symptomatic clients, the decision to tape iliacus or psoas may also be assisted by the client; if the examiner rotates the hip internally or externally whilst in extension, the client is often able to confirm in which area the resistance is mainly experienced.

7

KINESIO TAPING
Psoas major

STRENGTH TAPING

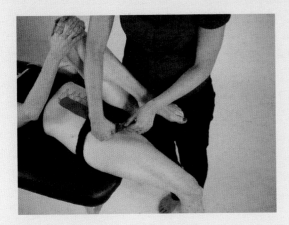

Client position

The client is lying supine with one hip in extension over the side or end of the bed. Alternatively, if a bed is not available, the client may be in the kneeling lunge position. In the lunge position, the ipsilateral arm is reaching above the head when the client is able to do so.

Measurement of tape

Measure a length of tape from the umbilicus to the inner thigh. It is more practical to have a length of tape that is too long rather than one that is not long enough.

Tape application

The application for the psoas muscle is completed in two stages in order to work around underwear. The hip is resting in extension and internal rotation over the edge of the bed. The starting anchor is placed with zero tension above the level of the umbilicus and adjacent to the midline. The client is instructed to further lengthen the abdominal tissue by taking a deep breath and blowing out the abdominal wall to create abdominal distension whilst the base of the tape is applied with 25–35% tension towards the underwear. When the practitioner reaches the top of the underwear, the client is allowed to breathe normally again whilst the practitioner folds the tape up and slides the tape (and the remainder of the backing) under the underwear. The client is instructed to again take a deep breath and blow out their abdominal wall whilst the rest of the tape base is applied with 25–35% tension. The final anchor is applied with zero tension distal to the lesser trochanter. Rub the tape to activate the glue or instruct the client to activate the glue.

7

STRENGTH TAPING

Reassessment

Reassess your patient for changes in length, strength, tonal changes, functional changes and symptoms.

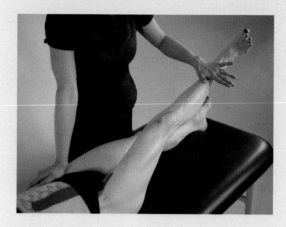

KINESIO TAPING
Psoas major

LENGTH TAPING

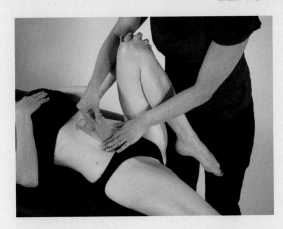

Client position

The client is lying supine with one hip in extension over the side or end of the bed. Alternatively, if a bed is not available, the client may be in the kneeling lunge position. In the lunge position, the ipsilateral arm is reaching above the head when the client is able to do so.

Measurement of tape

Measure a length of tape from the umbilicus to the inner thigh. It is more practical to have a length of tape that is too long rather than one that is not long enough.

Tape application

The application for the psoas muscle is completed in two stages in order to work around underwear. The hip is resting in extension and internal rotation over the edge of the bed. The starting anchor is placed with zero tension distal to the lesser trochanter. With the tissue in the lengthened position, the base of the tape is applied with 15–25% tension towards the underwear. When the practitioner reaches the bottom of the underwear, the practitioner folds the tape up and slides the tape (and the remainder of the backing) under the underwear. The client is instructed to take a deep breath and blow out their abdominal wall to maximise tissue stretch via abdominal distension, whilst the rest of the tape base is applied with 15–25% tension. The final anchor is applied with zero tension adjacent to the midline. Rub the tape to activate the glue or instruct the client to activate the glue.

7

LENGTH TAPING

Reassessment

Reassess the client for changes in length, strength, tonal changes, functional changes and symptoms. For testing where strength was also in deficit, re-test for a normalisation of strength bias testing.

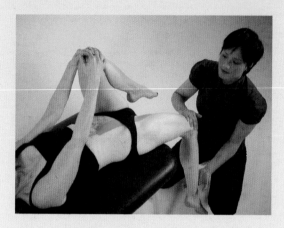

ANATOMY
Transversus abdominis

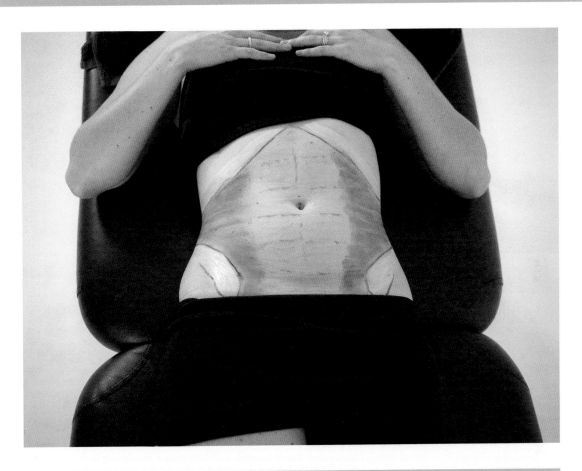

Transversus abdominis

Origin:	Inner surface of the cartilages of the lower six ribs interdigitating with the diaphragm, thoracolumbar fascia, anterior lip of the iliac crest and lateral ⅓ of the inguinal ligament
Insertion:	Linea alba via a broad aponeurosis, pubic crest
Nerve supply:	Nerve root: T7–12, L1 Peripheral nerve: ventral divisions of iliohypogastric and ilioinguinal
Function:	Acts as a girdle to flatten the abdominal wall, support the abdominal viscera, and provide a more stable platform for limb movements and load transfer to occur. Upper fibres act to decrease the infrasternal angle (expiration), and the lower fibres act to support pelvic stability

7

MUSCLE TESTING
Transversus abdominis

STRENGTH BIAS TESTING

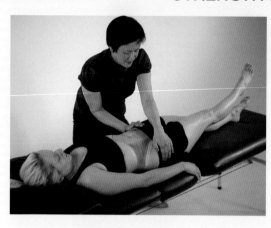

Client position

The client is lying supine on a bed in preparation for the supine active straight leg raise (ASLR) test.

Instruction to client

The client is instructed to lift the leg with the knee extended, to a height of 10 cm. The client is instructed to rate the perceived effort in lifting the leg; 0/5 for no effort, 5/5 for maximal effort.

The ASLR test score is taken as a baseline measure of the client's functional ability to stabilise the pelvis in order to transfer load as the leg is lifted. Strategy and symptoms are noted by the examiner. The client is reminded that this is a test of perceived effort and that they should score on the effort experienced with the task and not the symptoms.

The examiner then asks the client to repeat the test, this time with the tensional forces of the muscle contraction supplemented by the examiner. The client is asked to re-rate the perceived effort. The baseline effort is then compared to the effort experienced during examiner supplemented testing. If there are no changes in perceived effort during the supplemented testing, then taping of transversus abdominis is not indicated.

Clients with an extension provocation bias to their functional ability may demonstrate more meaningful scores with a prone leg extension (PLE) test. For a PLE test, the client is instructed to extend the leg off the bed by extending the hip and maintaining the knee extension. The ankle is only required to lift above the bed by 10 cm. A baseline measure of effort is taken and compared to the supplemented testing.

Examiner position and notes

The examiner is positioned to the side of the client and places the heels of the hands on the anterior iliac crests, then gathers the tissue either side and approximates this to the midline. Note that this is *not* a compression of the iliac spine. The examiner should only apply gentle forces that could be replicated by the tape (and gentle muscle contractions) to create change.

The use of the ASLR during the testing of transversus abdominis is intentional. The ASLR test has been proven in literature to be a reliable test to measure the capacity of the active muscle system to generate sufficient tension to allow for the transfer of load across the pelvis. It can be an extremely useful clinical test to ascertain the effectiveness of treatment.

The testing described distinctly relates to the use of Kinesio Tape and the value that it would give to an individual's function when applied to this part of the body. The intention of this resource is to provide useful testing procedures that would be available to any practitioner without the need for additional equipment. Of course, the everyday practitioner with access to additional testing equipment is encouraged to use these tools.

The testing shown here interprets the role of transversus abdominis in stabilising the pelvis for the client being tested.

For the baseline testing: If the client is aware of an increase in perceived effort with the ASLR (particularly when compared to the contralateral side), then the test will be a valuable test.

The examiner should assess for the quality of the movement independently of the client when assessing the baseline as well as during the supplemented test.

Once the baseline ASLR is established, the examiner attempts to supplement the forces otherwise created by an active muscle contraction of the lower transversus abdominis as it stabilises the anterior pelvic wall. This is done by gathering tension in the anterior abdominal wall by taking up tissue slack across the anterior lower pelvis and approximating it towards the centre.

An improvement in perceived effort during the ASLR with an examiner-supplemented force in the region implies that taping to replicate the handling forces of the examiner would be appropriate.

If the baseline test is positive for perceived effort but the test is unchanged with the supplemented support over transversus abdominis, then the test remains positive. However taping over the transversus abdominis is not indicated and unlikely to yield improvements to the ASLR tests. That is, the source of this increased effort is not from this muscle, and testing of other muscles is warranted.

If the client is not aware of any perceived effort during the baseline ASLR and the execution of the test is normal, then this test may be inappropriate for them as it has no meaning to their individual experience or symptoms. Testing in the prone position may have more meaning for the client and this is recommended instead; their condition may have an extension bias which has more meaning to their personal experience with extension provocation testing.

If the client reports no perceived effort with the testing and yet the examiner is aware of compromised strategies such as breath holding, trunk twisting, abdominal bulging, upper limb activity and others, then the test is valuable but the client is likely to be compromised in proprioceptive awareness and may have a chronic condition which has altered their perception of what would be considered normal. The examiner should apply the supplemented test to the client and ascertain if this improves their perceived effort beyond what they thought would be 'normal'. This would indicate taping for the TA. The examiner should also independently assess whether there is an improvement in movement of the test that the client may not yet be aware of. This would also indicate that taping of the TA may be appropriate for improving function. If there is no improvement in movement with the assisted test and the client is not aware of any changes, then the test may still be valuable to the examiner but taping of the TA is not indicated.

Resistance

No resistance is applied by the practitioner, rather, the practitioner adds a force across the segment from one hand to the other to supplement the stabilising vector otherwise created by the lower TA muscle. The force applied attempts to replicate a gentle gathering of tension as would be generated by an appropriate muscle contraction. An improvement in the perceived effort of the ASLR or PLE in the absence of a length restriction or abdominal discomfort indicates strength taping may be appropriate.

MUSCLE TESTING
Transversus abdominis

LENGTH BIAS TESTING

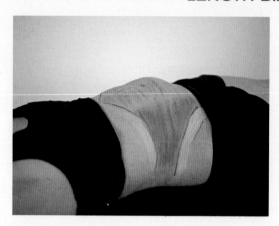
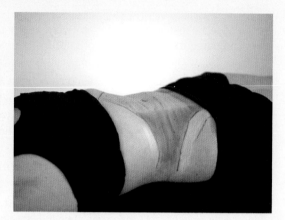

Client position

The client is lying supine on a bed.

Instruction to client

The client is instructed to take a deep breath in to blow out the abdominal wall (abdominal distension) and note if there is any discomfort or restriction in the abdominal region before relaxing again.

Examiner position and notes

The examiner is positioned at either end of the bed to assess if there is an imbalance in the abdominal wall movement during the breathing. A restriction may also indicate other muscles and structures in the abdominal region that warrant further assessment. The examiner is reminded that a cluster of tests may be used to better confirm or rule out other structures.

The examiner should further palpate the abdomen, noting for any discomfort.

The examiner is reminded that the testing serves to indicate a location for the delivery of the tape with specific tension in order to increase or decrease tone of a muscle in an area. A positive test for discomfort and tension implies that taping to relax the muscle may be warranted.

Whilst the taping shown on the following pages focuses on the lower transversus abdominis, it would be more appropriate to apply the tape over the site of tension vectors in clients who demonstrate findings in other locations of the anterior abdominal wall.

KINESIO TAPING
Transversus abdominis

STRENGTH TAPING

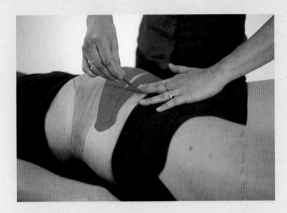

Client position

The client is lying supine on the bed. For additional length in the tissue, the hips may be abducted.

Measurement of tape

Two lengths of tape are measured from one ASIS to the other and cut into a Y-strip.

Tape application

The common anchor is applied to one ASIS with no tension. The client is instructed to take a deep breath in order to distend the abdomen. For those with larger bodies, it may be appropriate to have them assist by holding the abdomen up and away from the pubis during the application. Then each tail is applied underneath the umbilicus at the level of the ASIS with 25–35% tension. The final anchors are applied over the opposite ASIS with zero tension. The second tape is applied in the same fashion with the initial anchor on the opposite ASIS to the first, with each tail interdigitating with the first. Rub the tape to activate the glue.

Reassessment

Reassess your patient for changes in length, strength, tonal changes, functional changes and symptoms. The perceived effort in the active straight leg raise or prone extension test should improve to approximate or equal the quality of movement achieved with the supplemented test.

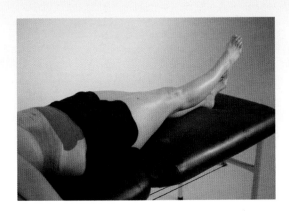

KINESIO TAPING
Transversus abdominis

LENGTH TAPING

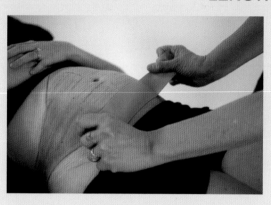

Client position

The client is lying supine on the bed. For additional length in the tissue, the hips may be abducted.

Measurement of tape

A length of tape is measured from one ASIS to the other. The tape can be maintained as an I-strip or cut into basket weave to cover a larger surface area. Additional tape strips may be required for larger clientele.

Tape application

The tape is folded in half and the backing torn in the middle to expose the glue. The tape backing is removed to either anchor and the tape stretched to 15–25% tension in the middle of the tape. The client is instructed to take a deep breath in order to distend the abdomen. For those with larger bodies, it may be appropriate to have them assist by holding the abdomen up and away from the pubis during the application. The tape is applied underneath the umbilicus at the level of the ASIS with the 15–25% tension. The client is allowed to breathe normally whilst the practitioner applies each anchor over the ASIS with zero tension. Rub the tape to activate the glue.

Reassessment

Reassess your patient for changes in length, strength, tonal changes, functional changes and symptoms. The active straight leg raise test or prone leg extension test should yield improvements in perceived effort.

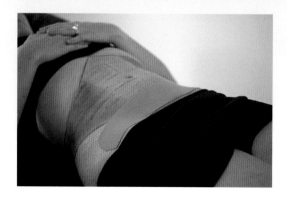

TRUNK ASSESSMENT SHEET

Clinic: .... Date: ....

Client name: ....

Functional review

Functional limitation	Pre-test measure	Post-test measure

Muscle testing

Tested priority	Muscle	Strength		Length		Comments
		Right	Left	Right	Left	
	Latissimus dorsi					
	Quadratus lumborum					
	Erector spinae (iliocostalis lumborum)					
	Erector spinae (iliocostalis thoracis)					
	Multifidus (transversospinales group)					
	Rectus abdominis					
	Internal and external oblique					
	Psoas major					
	Transversus abdominis					

Treatment

Intervention	Re-test measures	Plan

Practitioner: .... Signature: ....

BIBLIOGRAPHY

Berryman Reese, N., & Bandy, W. D. (2010). *Joint range of motion and muscle length testing*. Missouri: Saunders Elsevier.

Berryman Reese, N. M. (2012). *Muscle and sensory testing*. Missouri: Elsevier-Saunders.

Bridges, T. (2013a). *Can load transfer through the pelvis (as measured by the active straight leg raise) be improved through the use of Kinesio taping?* Paper presented at the 8th Interdisciplinary World Congress on Low Back and Pelvic Pain, Dubai.

Bridges, T. (2013b). *Hip intervention crosses the pelvic girdle: a thought provoking case study*. Paper presented at the 8th Interdisciplinary World Congress on Low Back and Pelvic Pain, Dubai.

Calais-Germain, B. (1993). *Anatomy of movement* (12th ed.). Seattle: Eastland Press.

Comerford, M., & Mottram, S. (2012). *Kinetic control: the management of uncontrolled Movement*. Sydney, Australia: Elsevier.

Hides, J., Richardson, C., & Jull, G. (1996). Multifidus muscle recovery is not automatic following an acute, first episode of low back pain. *Spine, 21*(23), 2763–2769.

Kase, K., Hashimoto, T., & Okane, T. (1998). *Kinesio Taping perfect manual: amazing taping therapy to eliminate pain and muscle disorders*. Albuquerque: Kinesio Taping Association.

Kase, K., & Rock Stockheimer, K. (2006). *Kinesio Taping for lymphoedema and chronic swelling*. Albuquerque: Kinesio Taping Association.

Kase, K., Wallis, J., & Kase, T. (2003). *Clinical therapeutic applications of the Kinesio taping methods*. Albuquerque: Kinesio Taping Association.

Kendall, F. P., McCreary, E., Provance, P., Rodgers, M., & Romanic, W. (2005). *Muscles: testing and function with posture and pain*. Baltimore: Lippincott Williams Wilkins.

Mens, J. M. A., Vleeming, A., & C.J., S. (2007). Straight leg raising: a clinical approach to the load transfer functions across the pelvic girdle. *The Journal of Manual & Manipulative Therapy, 15*, 133–141.

Mens, J. M. A., Vleeming, A., C.J., S., Koes, B. W., & Stam, H. J. (2001). Reliability and validity of the active straight leg raise test in posterior pelvic pain since pregnancy. *Spine, 26*, 1167–1171.

Mens, J. M. A., Vleeming, A., C.J., S., Koes, B. W., & Stam, H. J. (2002). Validity of the active straight-leg-raise test for measuring disease severity in patients with posterior pelvic pain since pregnancy. *Spine, 27*(2), 196.

Mens, J. M. A., Vleeming, A., Schnidjers, C. J., & Stam, H. J. (1997). Active straight-leg-raise test: a clinical approach to load transfer function of the pelvic girdle. In A. Vleeming, V. Mooney, C. Schnidjers, T. Dorman, & R. Stoeckart (Eds.), *Movement, stability and low back pain: the essential role of the pelvis* (pp. 425–431). Edinburgh: Churchill Livingstone.

O'Sullivan, P. B., Beales, D. J., Beetham, J. A., Cripps, J., Graf, F., Lin, T. B., . . . Avery, A. (2002). Altered motor control strategies in subjects with sacroiliac joint pain during the active straight-leg-raise test. *Spine, 27*(1), E1–E8.

Richardson, C., Jull, G., Hodges, P., & Hides, J. (1999). *Therapeutic exercises for spinal segmental stabilization in low back pain: scientific basis and clinical approach*. Edinburgh: Churchill Livingstone.

Standring, S., Borely, N., Collings, P., Crossman, A., Gatzoulis, M., Healy, J., . . . Wigley, C. (2008). *Gray's anatomy: the anatomical basis of clinical practice* (S. Susan Ed. 40 ed.). London, United Kingdom: Churchill Livingstone Elsevier.

7

Techniques for testing and taping the pelvic girdle and hip

Pectineus and adductor brevis

Adductor longus

Gracilis

Adductor magnus

Psoas major and minor

Iliacus

Tensor fasciae latae

Gluteus medius and gluteus minimus

Gluteus maximus

Piriformis

Quadratus femoris and obturator externus

Gemellus superior, gemellus inferior and obturator internus

ANATOMY
Pectineus and adductor brevis

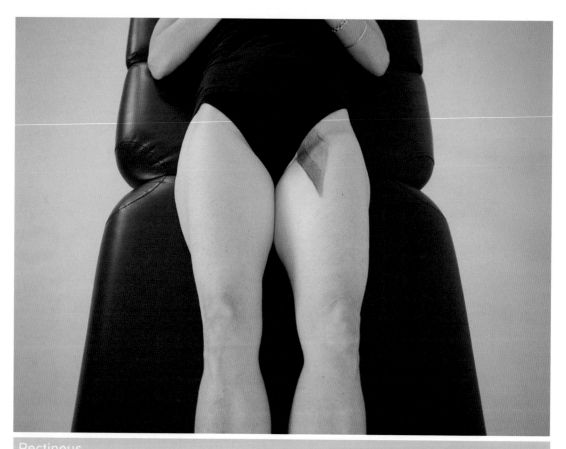

Pectineus

Origin:	Surface of the superior ramus of the pubis
Insertion:	Pectineal line of the femur
Nerve supply:	Nerve root: L2, 3, 4 Peripheral nerve: femoral and obturator
Function:	Adducts and flexes the hip joint

Adductor brevis

Origin:	Outer surface of the inferior ramus of the pubis
Insertion:	Distal ⅔ of the pectineal line and proximal half of the of the medial lip of the linea aspera
Nerve Supply:	Nerve root: L2, 3, 4 Peripheral nerve: obturator
Function:	Adducts and flexes the hip joint

8

MUSCLE TESTING
Pectineus and adductor brevis

STRENGTH BIAS TESTING

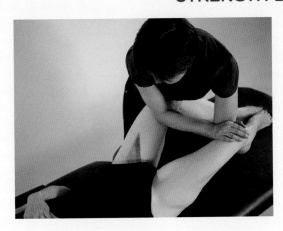

Client position

The client is lying supine with both knees flexed to 90 degrees and with the feet resting on the bed.

Instruction to client

The client is instructed to maintain hip adduction by holding the knees together against the resistance of the examiner.

Examiner position and notes

For bilateral testing, the examiner is positioned to the side of the bed and places the heels of the hand on the inside of the thigh. For the safety of the examiner, the forearm line should be relatively perpendicular to the client's lower leg and the examiner's humerus may rest on the inside of the client's thigh and knee. Overzealous or particularly strong clients may overpower the examiner during testing. Therefore the placement of the forearms between the knees and one arm perpendicular to the client's movement ensures an end range for the client's adduction as it is stopped by the forearm bones. This testing of the adductor group has the hip in some flexion to bias more anterior fibres and to direct the taping. Additional information can be gathered from palpation and a thorough history.

Resistance

The examiner applies a force along the shaft of their forearm in a direction which moves the knees apart and the hip towards abduction. The client is instructed to match the force to avoid the leg being moved.

8

MUSCLE TESTING
Pectineus and adductor brevis

LENGTH BIAS TESTING

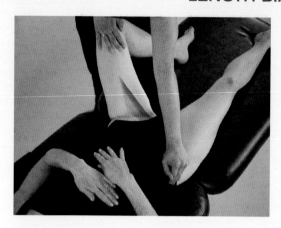

Client position

The client is lying supine with the hip and knee flexed and the foot adjacent to the contralateral knee and in line with the hip.

Instruction to client

The client is instructed to let their knee fall to the side (abduction).

Examiner position and notes

The examiner is positioned to the side of the client and supports the client at end range if irritable; if not irritable, the examiner assesses for the passive range with gentle overpressure. The opposite pelvis is stabilised during the testing. Additional palpation may give clarity as to the direction of the fibres to be managed.

8

KINESIO TAPING
Pectineus and adductor brevis

STRENGTH TAPING

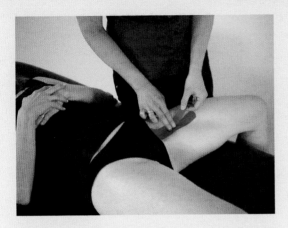

Client position
The client is lying in supine with the hip abducted and the knee flexed whilst resting over the edge of the bed.

Measurement of tape
A length of tape is measured from the pubis to the proximal ⅓ of the femur. The direction and length of the tape is best appreciated when the client is instructed to lightly contract the muscle whilst held in the lengthened position.

Tape application
The starting anchor is applied with zero tension over the pubic bone or as close to the pubic bone as possible. With the tissue in the lengthened position, the base of the tape is applied towards the proximal ⅓ of the medial femur with 25–35% tension. The final anchor is applied on the proximal femur with zero tension. Rub the tape to activate the glue or instruct the client to activate the glue.

Reassessment
Reassess your client for changes in strength, tonal changes, functional changes and symptoms.

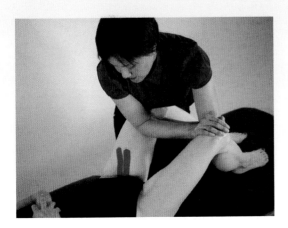

8

KINESIO TAPING
Pectineus and adductor brevis

LENGTH TAPING

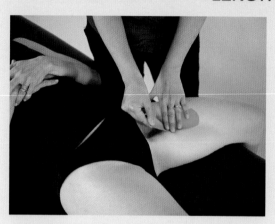

Client position

The client is positioned in supine with the hip and knee flexed so that the foot is resting next to the contralateral knee. The knee is then taken laterally to induce abduction of the hips.

Measurement of tape

A length of tape is measured from the pubis to the proximal ⅓ of the femur. The direction and length of the tape is best appreciated when the client is instructed to lightly contract the muscle whilst held in the lengthened position.

Tape application

The starting anchor is applied with zero tension over the proximal ⅓ of the femoral shaft behind the border of the sartorius. With the tissue in the lengthened position, the base of the tape is applied with 15–25% tension towards the pubis. The final anchor is applied as close to the pubis as permissible with zero tension. Rub the tape to activate the glue or instruct the client to activate the glue.

Reassessment

Reassess your client for changes in length, strength, tonal changes, functional changes and symptoms.

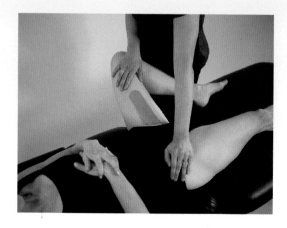

ANATOMY

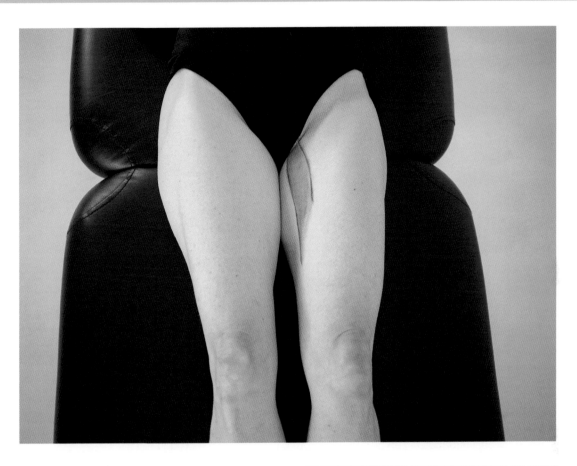

Adductor longus

Origin:	Anterior surface of the pubis at the junction of the crest and symphysis
Insertion:	Middle ⅓ of the medial lip of the linea aspera
Nerve supply:	Nerve root: L2, 3, 4 Peripheral nerve: obturator
Function:	Adducts and flexes the hip joint

MUSCLE TESTING
Adductor longus

STRENGTH BIAS TESTING

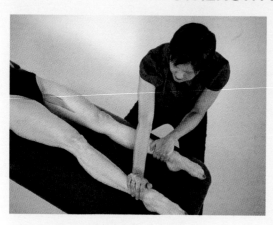

Client position

The client is lying supine with both hips in a neutral position and the knees extended.

Instruction to client

The client is instructed to maintain hip adduction by holding the ankles together against the resistance of the examiner.

Examiner position and notes

For bilateral testing, the examiner is positioned to the side of the bed and holds each leg above the ankle. This testing of the adductor group has the hip in a neutral position to bias more midline fibres and to direct taping. Additional information can be gathered from palpation and a thorough history.

The examiner should be positioned in the squat or lunge position to better stabilise themselves to apply force during the test. Resistance applied above the ankle offers the examiner better grip and mechanical leverage but requires the absence of knee pathologies in the client.

Resistance

The examiner applies a force above the ankles in a direction that separates them and abducts the hip from the midline.

8

MUSCLE TESTING
Adductor longus

LENGTH BIAS TESTING

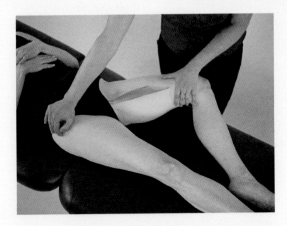

Client position

The client is lying supine, the side to be examined has the hip flexed so that the foot is resting adjacent to the contralateral calf and the big toe is adjacent to the contralateral medial malleolus.

Instruction to client

The client is instructed to allow the hip to abduct by letting the knee fall away from the midline.

Examiner position and notes

The examiner is positioned to the side of the client and supports the leg during the testing. The opposite hip is stabilised with the upper hand during the abduction movement and end range can be assessed with overpressure if the client is not irritable. Additional palpation may give clarity as to the direction of the fibres to be managed.

8

KINESIO TAPING
Adductor longus

STRENGTH TAPING

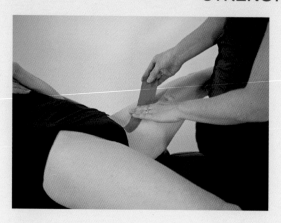

Client position

The client is lying supine with the knee extended. The practitioner takes the hip into abduction and supports the leg at the end of range. Alternatively the leg can be held at end range by the client using a strap around the foot.

Measurement of tape

A length of tape is measured from the pubis to the middle ⅓ of the femur. The direction and length of the tape is best appreciated when the client is instructed to lightly contract the muscle whilst held in the lengthened position.

Tape application

The starting anchor is applied with zero tension over the pubic bone or as close to the pubic bone as possible. With the tissue in the lengthened position, the base of the tape is applied towards the middle ⅓ of the medial femur with 25–35% tension. The final anchor is applied on the middle of the femur with zero tension. Rub the tape to activate the glue or instruct the client to activate the glue.

Reassessment

Reassess your client for change in strength, tonal changes, functional changes and symptoms.

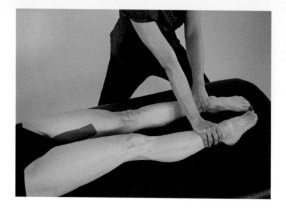

8

KINESIO TAPING
Adductor longus

LENGTH TAPING

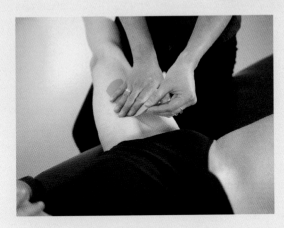

Client position
The client is lying supine with the knee extended. The practitioner takes the hip into abduction and supports the leg at the end of range. Alternatively, the leg can be held at end range by the client using a strap around the foot.

Measurement of tape
A length of tape is measured from the pubis to the middle ⅓ of the femur. The direction and length of the tape is best appreciated when the client is instructed to lightly contract the muscle whilst held in the lengthened position.

Tape application
The starting anchor is applied with zero tension over the middle ⅓ of the femoral shaft behind the border of the sartorius. With the tissue in the lengthened position, the base of the tape is applied with 15–25% tension towards the pubis. The final anchor is applied as close to the pubis as permissible with zero tension. Rub the tape to activate the glue or instruct the client to activate the glue.

8

LENGTH TAPING

Reassessment

The client is reassessed for range of movement and symptoms, and palpated for changes in tone. A restoration of length may also yield strength improvements where a strength deficit was detected prior to the taping; in these circumstances, the strength should also be reassessed. Any functional deficits can also be reassessed for changes.

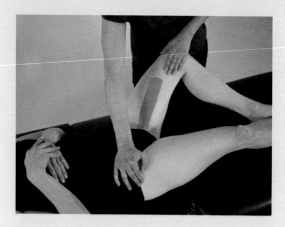

ANATOMY
Gracilis

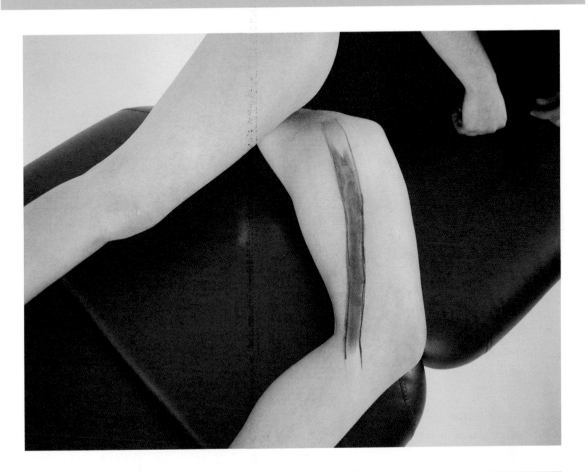

Gracilis

Origin:	Ischiopubic ramus
Insertion:	Medial tibia distal to the condyle (pes anserinus)
Nerve supply:	Peripheral nerve: Nerve root: L2, 3, 4 Anterior branch of obturator nerve
Function:	Adducts, flexes and medially rotates the knee; adducts the hip

8

MUSCLE TESTING
Gracilis

STRENGTH BIAS TESTING

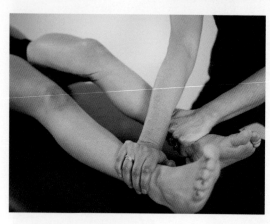

Client position

The client is lying supine with the leg to be tested in slight knee flexion and internal rotation of the tibia. The ankle is then taken towards the midline adjacent to the contralateral ankle.

Instruction to client

The client is instructed to keep the legs together whilst the examiner applies a force to attempt to separate the legs.

Examiner position and notes

The examiner stands to the side of the client and holds the legs above the ankle whilst standing in a stable lunge or squat position.

Resistance

The examiner applies a force at the ankle in the direction of abduction away from the opposite ankle.

8

MUSCLE TESTING
Gracilis

LENGTH BIAS TESTING

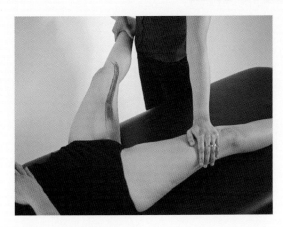

Client position

The client is lying supine with the hip and pelvis in neutral and the knee extended with lateral tibial rotation.

Instruction to client

The client is instructed to allow their leg to be taken out to the side as far as possible whilst keeping the knee extended and the pelvic position maintained.

Examiner position and notes

The examiner supports the leg in the horizontal plane and facilitates the abduction of the leg. The other hand may be used to stabilise the opposite lower limb. The leg is placed in lateral tibial rotation prior to the abduction. The examiner stops when a compensatory movement in the hip is noted or a countermovement in the opposite leg.

8

KINESIO TAPING
Gracilis

STRENGTH TAPING

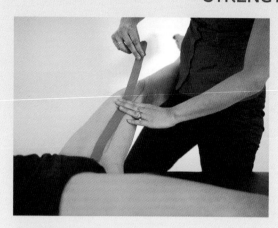

Client position

The client lies supine with the hip in abduction, lateral rotation and flexion resting against a wall, the examiner's side or with the assistance of a belt.

Measurement of tape

Measure a length of tape from the ischiopubic ramus to the medial proximal tibia. Depending on the size of the muscle, the tape may be cut down its length to create a 2.5 cm-wide strip.

Tape application

Apply the starting anchor with zero tension as close to the ischiopubic ramus as possible. Apply the base of the tape with 25–35% tension towards the pes anserine on the proximal medial tibia. Complete the tape by applying the final anchor on the tibia with zero tension. Rub the tape to activate the glue or instruct the client to activate the glue.

Reassessment

Reassess your client for changes in strength, tonal changes, functional changes and symptoms.

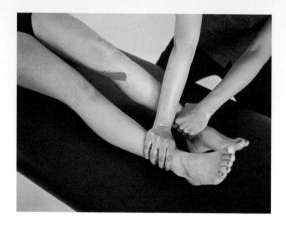

8

KINESIO TAPING
Gracilis

LENGTH TAPING

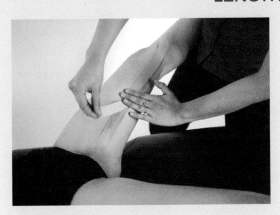

Client position

The client is lying supine with the hip in abduction, lateral rotation and flexion resting against a wall, the examiner's side or with the assistance of a belt.

Measurement of tape

Measure a length of tape from the ischiopubic ramus to the medial proximal tibia. Cut the tape into a 2.5 cm-wide strip if the client is smaller in size.

Tape application

Apply the starting anchor with zero tension over the pes anserine at the medial tibia. With the tissue in the lengthened position, apply the base of the tape with 15–25% tension towards the ischiopubic ramus. Complete the tape by applying the final anchor as close as possible to the ischiopubic ramus with zero tension. Rub the tape to activate the glue or instruct the client to activate the glue.

Reassessment

The client is reassessed for range of movement, symptoms and palpated for changes in tone. A restoration of length may also yield strength improvements where a strength deficit was detected prior to the taping; in these circumstances, the strength should also be reassessed. Any functional deficits can also be reassessed for changes.

8

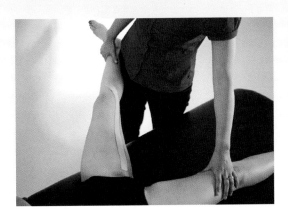

ANATOMY
Adductor magnus

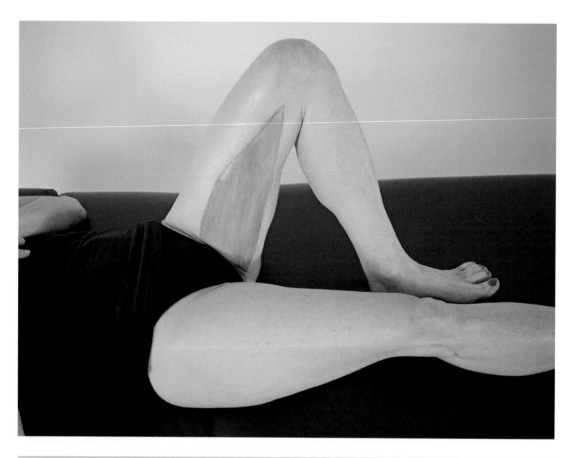

Adductor magnus

Origin:	Inferior pubic ramus, ramus of the ischium, and ischial tuberosity
Insertion:	Medial to the gluteal tuberosity, middle of the linea aspera, medial supracondylar line and the adductor tubercle on the medial condyle of the femur
Nerve supply:	Nerve root L2, 3, 4 and L4, 5, S1 Peripheral nerves: obturator and sciatic
Function:	Adducts the hip joint. Anterior fibres arising from the pubic ramus flex the hip whilst posterior fibres arising from the ischial tuberosity assist in hip extension

8

MUSCLE TESTING
Adductor magnus

STRENGTH BIAS TESTING

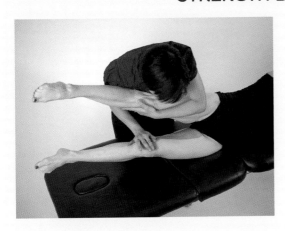

Client position
The client is in a sidelying position with the tested hip on the bed.

Instruction to client
The client is instructed to lift the lower leg to meet the one supported by the examiner. The leg and hip should remain in a neutral position or slight hip extension.

Examiner position and notes
The examiner is positioned behind the client and supports the upper leg in the abducted position. Depending on the weight and ability of the client, this support can be done with the knee flexed or extended. This testing of the adductor group has the hip in some extension and against gravity to bias more posterior fibres and the larger muscle belly of the adductor magnus to direct taping. Additional information can be gathered from palpation and a thorough history.

Resistance
Testing is positive if the client is unable to lift the lower leg against gravity or deviates from the neutral position. Additional resistance by applying a downward force on the lower limb can be used if testing against gravity is not significant.

8

MUSCLE TESTING
Adductor magnus

LENGTH BIAS TESTING

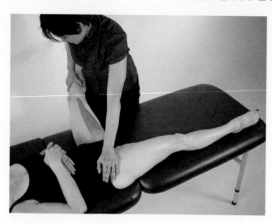

Client position

The client is lying supine with the hip and knee in a neutral position.

Instruction to client

The client is instructed to relax as the examiner abducts the leg.

Examiner position and notes

The examiner is positioned to the side of the client and supports the leg during the testing. The client's hip is taken into abduction range with the leg extended. The examiner may rest the client's leg against the examiner's outer hip or thigh for support. To bias the ischial component of the adductor length test, the hip is taken into further flexion range. Additional palpation may give clarity as to the direction of the fibres to be managed.

8

KINESIO TAPING
Adductor magnus

STRENGTH TAPING

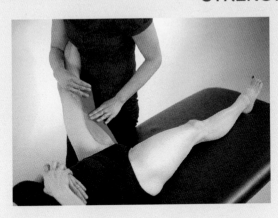

Client position

The client is positioned in supine with the knee extended. The practitioner takes the hip into abduction and supports the leg at the end of range. Alternatively the leg can be held at end range by the client using a strap.

Measurement of tape

A length of tape is measured from the pubis to the distal ⅓ of the femur above the medial femoral condyle. The direction and length of the tape is best appreciated when the client is instructed to lightly contract the muscle whilst held in the lengthened position. For particularly 'weak' muscles, two strips of tape may be appropriate to provide more stimulation by covering a larger surface area.

Tape application

The starting anchor is applied with zero tension over the pubic bone or as close to the pubic bone as is practically possible. With the tissue in the lengthened position, the base of the tape is applied towards the distal ⅓ of the femur above the medial condyle with 25–35% tension. The final anchor is applied on the distal femur with zero tension. Rub the tape to activate the glue or instruct the client to activate the glue.

Reassessment

Reassess your client for changes in strength, tonal changes, functional changes and symptoms.

8

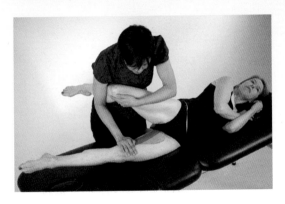

KINESIO TAPING
Adductor magnus

LENGTH TAPING

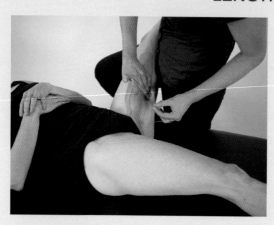

Client position

The client is positioned in supine with the knee extended. The practitioner takes the hip into abduction and supports the leg at the end of range. Alternatively, the leg can be held at end range by the client using a strap.

Measurement of tape

A length of tape is measured from the pubis to the distal ⅓ of the femur above the medial femoral condyle. The direction and length of the tape is best appreciated when the client is instructed to lightly contract the muscle whilst held in the lengthened position. The tape may be cut into a Y-strip (as shown in the picture) to create a larger region or influence or may be kept as an I-strip to specifically address a local region of tension.

Tape application

The starting anchor is applied with zero tension over the distal ⅓ of the femoral shaft behind the border created by the sartorius. With the tissue in the lengthened position, the base of the tape is applied with 15–25% tension towards the pubis. The final anchor is applied as close to the pubis as permissible with zero tension. Rub the tape to activate the glue or instruct the client to activate the glue.

8

LENGTH TAPING

Reassessment

Reassess the client for changes in length, strength, tonal changes, functional changes and symptoms. For testing where strength was also in deficit, re-test for a normalisation of strength bias testing.

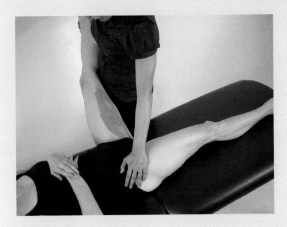

ANATOMY

Psoas major and minor

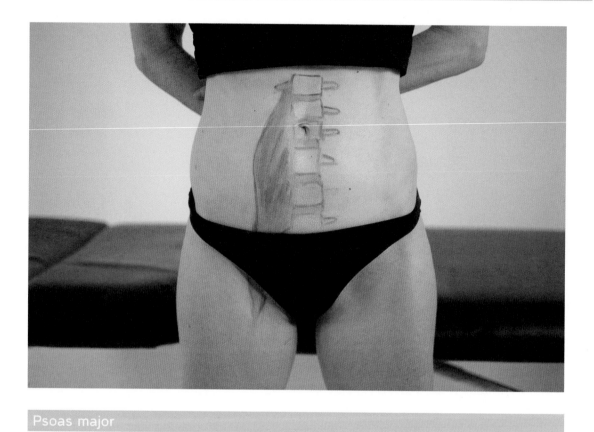

Psoas major

Origin:	Anterior surfaces of the transverse processes of the T12 and the lumbar vertebrae, sides of the bodies and corresponding intervertebral discs of the last thoracic and all lumbar vertebrae including membranous arches that extend over the sides of the bodies of the lumbar vertebrae
Insertion:	Lesser trochanter of the femur
Nerve supply:	Nerve root: L1, 2, 3, 4 Peripheral nerve: lumbar plexus
Function:	With the origin fixed, iliopsoas flexes the hip joint by flexing the femur on the trunk. They may assist in lateral rotation of the hip joint. When acting bilaterally, they flex the hip joint by flexing the trunk on the femur. The lower fibres of psoas major will act to increase lumbar lordosis with the insertion fixed whilst the upper fibres will act to assist lumbar flexion, and lateral flexion when acting unilaterally

Psoas minor

Origin:	Sides of the bodies of the 12th thoracic and first lumbar vertebra and the intervertebral disc between them
Insertion:	Iliopectineal eminence, arcuate line of the ilium and the iliac fascia
Nerve supply:	Nerve root: L1, 2 Peripheral nerve: lumbar plexus
Function:	Creates tension, assists in lumbar spine on a stable pelvis or pelvic flexion when the spine is fixed

8

MUSCLE TESTING
Psoas major

STRENGTH BIAS TESTING

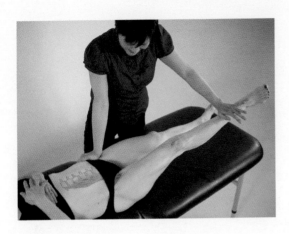

Client position

The client is lying supine with the legs in extension.

Instruction to client

The client is instructed to maintain the knee extension whilst performing a hip flexion in a position of slight lateral rotation.

Examiner position and notes

The examiner stands to the side of the limb being tested and stabilises the opposite pelvis. The examining hand is placed proximal to the ankle joint.

Resistance

Resistance is applied at the anterior medial aspect of the distal tibia in a direction of hip extension and slight abduction in a direction opposite to the line of pull of the muscle.

8

MUSCLE TESTING
Psoas major

LENGTH BIAS TESTING

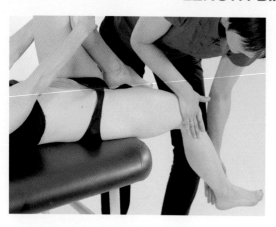 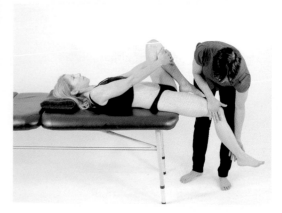

Client position
The client is instructed to sit at the end of a plinth.

Instruction to client
The client is instructed to hold the contralateral knee to the chest and is assisted by the examiner into the supine position whilst maintaining the knee-to-chest position. The hip being tested is allowed to rest into extension off the edge of the bed. The thigh should not be resting on the bed.

Examiner position and notes
The examiner is positioned to the side of the bed in order to assist the client into the supine position. Once in the testing position, the examiner may assess for hip extension range off the edge of the bed. Psoas and iliacus tension is indicated when the hip is held in some flexion and/or external rotation. For symptomatic clients, the decision to tape iliacus or psoas may also be assisted by the client; if the examiner rotates the hip internally or externally whilst in extension, the client is often able to confirm which area the resistance is mainly experienced in and can direct the placement of the tape to address the angle of either to psoas major or the iliacus.

8

KINESIO TAPING
Psoas major

STRENGTH TAPING

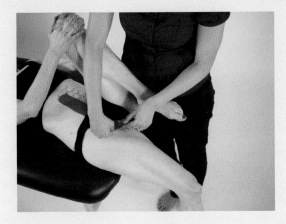

Client position

The client is positioned in supine with one hip in extension over the side or end of the bed. Alternatively, if a bed is not available, the client may be in the kneeling lunge position. The ipsilateral arm is reaching above the head when able in the lunge position.

Measurement of tape

Measure a length of tape from the umbilicus to the inner thigh. It is more practical to have a length of tape that is too long rather than one that is not long enough.

Tape application

The application for the psoas muscle is completed in two stages in order to work around underwear. The hip is resting in extension and internal rotation over the edge of the bed. The starting anchor is placed with zero tension above the level of the umbilicus and adjacent to the midline. The client is instructed to further lengthen the abdominal tissue by taking a deep breath and blowing out the belly to create abdominal wall distension whilst the base of the tape is applied with 25–35% tension towards the underwear. When the practitioner reaches the top of the underwear, the client is allowed to breathe normally again whilst the practitioner folds the tape up and slides the tape (and the remaining backing) under the underwear. The client is instructed to again take a deep breath and blow out their stomach whilst the rest of the tape base is applied with 25–35% tension. The final anchor is applied with zero tension distal to the lesser trochanter. Rub the tape to activate the glue or instruct the client to activate the glue.

8

STRENGTH TAPING

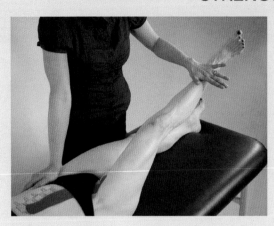

Reassessment

Reassess your patient for changes in length, strength, tonal changes, functional changes and symptoms.

8

KINESIO TAPING
Psoas major

LENGTH TAPING

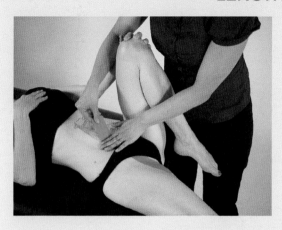

Client position

The client is positioned in supine with one hip in extension over the side or end of the bed. Alternatively, if a bed is not available, the client may be in the kneeling lunge position. The ipsilateral arm is reaching above the head when able when in the lunge position.

Measurement of tape

Measure a length of tape from the umbilicus to the inner thigh. It is more practical to have a length of tape that is too long rather than one that is not long enough.

Tape application

The application for the psoas muscle is completed in two stages in order to work around underwear. The hip is resting in extension and internal rotation over the edge of the bed. The starting anchor is placed with zero tension distal to the lesser trochanter. With the tissue in the lengthened position, the base of the tape is applied with 15–25% tension towards the underwear. When the practitioner reaches the bottom of the underwear the practitioner folds the tape up and slides the tape (and the remaining backing) under the underwear. The client is then instructed to take a deep breath and blow out their stomach to maximise tissue stretch via abdominal wall distension, whilst the rest of the tape base is applied with 15–25% tension. The final anchor is applied with zero tension adjacent to the midline. Rub the tape to activate the glue or instruct the client to activate the glue.

8

LENGTH TAPING

Reassessment

Reassess the client for changes in length, strength, tonal changes, functional changes and symptoms. For testing where strength was also in deficit, re-test for a normalisation of strength bias testing.

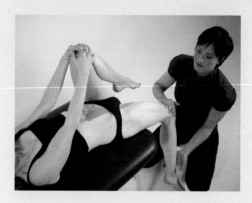

ANATOMY
Iliacus

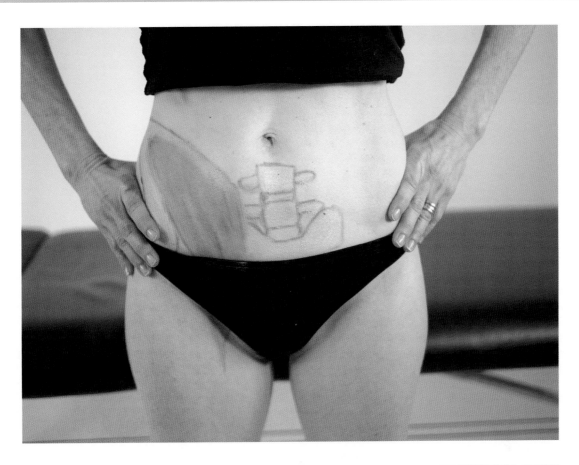

Iliacus	
Origin:	Superior ⅔ of the iliac fossa, internal lip of the iliac crest, iliolumbar ligament, ventral sacroiliac ligament, ala of the sacrum
Insertion:	Lateral side of the tendon of the psoas major just distal to the lesser trochanter
Nerve supply:	Nerve root: L1, 2, 3, 4 Peripheral nerve: femoral
Function:	Flexes and laterally rotates the hip

8

MUSCLE TESTING
Iliacus

STRENGTH BIAS TESTING

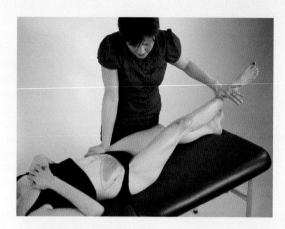

Client position

The client is in supine with the hip and knee in neutral.

Instruction to client

The client is instructed to maintain knee extension whilst performing hip flexion in a position of slight lateral rotation.

Examiner position and notes

The examiner stands to the side of the limb being tested and stabilises the opposite pelvis. The examining hand is placed proximal to the ankle joint.

Resistance

Resistance is applied at the anterior medial aspect of the distal tibia in a direction of hip extension and slight abduction in a direction opposite to the line of pull of the muscle.

8

MUSCLE TESTING
Iliacus

LENGTH BIAS TESTING

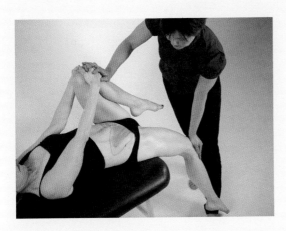

Client position
The client is instructed to sit at the end of a plinth.

Instruction to client
The client is instructed to hold the contralateral knee to the chest and is assisted by the examiner into the supine position whilst maintaining the knee-to-chest position. The hip being tested is allowed to rest into extension off the edge of the bed. The thigh should not be resting on the bed.

Examiner position and notes
The examiner is positioned to the side of the bed in order to assist the client into the supine position. Once in the testing position, the examiner may assess for hip extension range off the edge of the bed. Psoas and iliacus tension is indicated when the hip is held in some flexion and/or external rotation. For symptomatic clients, the decision to tape iliacus or psoas may also be assisted by the client; if the examiner rotates the hip internally or externally whilst in extension, the client is often able to confirm which area the resistance is mainly experienced in and can direct the placement of the tape to address the angle of either psoas major or the iliacus.

8

KINESIO TAPING
Iliacus

STRENGTH TAPING

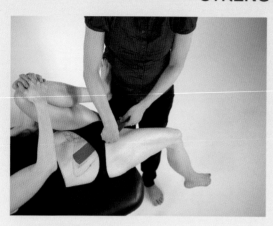

Client position

The client is lying supine with one hip in extension over the side or end of the bed. Alternatively, if a bed is not available, the client may be in the kneeling lunge position. When in the lunge position, the ipsilateral arm is reaching above the head if the client is able to do so.

Measurement of tape

Measure a length of tape from the lateral iliac crest to the inner thigh. It is more practical to have a length of tape that is too long rather than one that is not long enough.

Tape application

The application for the iliacus muscle is completed in two stages in order to work around underwear. The hip is resting in extension and internal rotation over the edge of the bed. The starting anchor is placed with zero tension adjacent to the iliac crest laterally. The client is instructed to further lengthen the abdominal tissue by taking a deep breath and blowing out the belly to create abdominal distension whilst the base of the tape is applied with 25–35% tension towards the underwear. When the practitioner reaches the top of the underwear, the client is allowed to breathe normally again whilst the practitioner folds the tape up and slides the tape (and the remaining backing) under the underwear. The client is instructed to again take a deep breath and blow out their stomach whilst the rest of the tape base is applied with 25–35% tension. The final anchor is applied with zero tension distal to the lesser trochanter. Rub the tape to activate the glue or instruct the client to activate the glue.

8

STRENGTH TAPING

Reassessment

Reassess your patient for changes in length, strength, tonal changes, functional changes and symptoms.

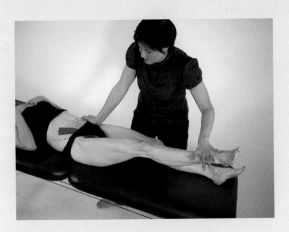

8

KINESIO TAPING
Iliacus

LENGTH TAPING

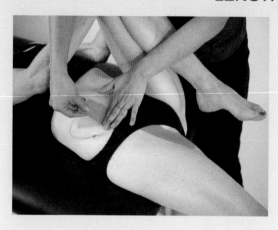

Client position

The client is lying supine with one hip in extension over the side or end of the bed. Alternatively, if a bed is not available, the client may be in the kneeling lunge position. When in the lunge position, the ipsilateral arm is reaching above the head if the client is able to do so.

Measurement of tape

Measure a length of tape from the lateral iliac crest to the inner thigh. It is more practical to have tape that is too long rather than one that is not long enough.

Tape application

The application for the iliacus muscle is completed in two stages in order to work around underwear. The hip is resting in extension and internal rotation over the edge of the bed. The starting anchor is placed with zero tension distal to the lesser trochanter. With the tissue in the lengthened position, the base of the tape is applied with 15–25% tension towards the underwear. When the practitioner reaches the bottom of the underwear, the practitioner folds the tape up and slides the tape (and the remaining backing) under the underwear. The client is instructed to take a deep breath and blow out their stomach; to maximise tissue stretch via abdominal distension, whilst the rest of the tape base is applied with 15–25% tension. The final anchor is applied with zero tension adjacent to iliac crest laterally. Rub the tape to activate the glue or instruct the client to activate the glue.

8

LENGTH TAPING

Reassessment

Reassess the client for changes in length, strength, tonal changes, functional changes and symptoms. For testing where strength was also in deficit, re-test for a normalisation of strength bias testing.

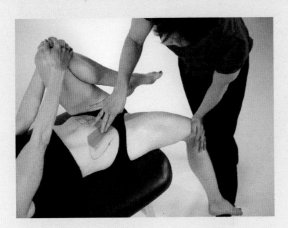

ANATOMY
Tensor fasciae latae

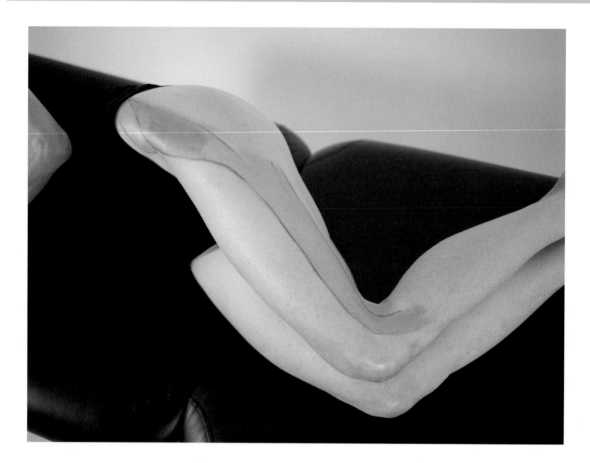

Tensor fasciae latae

Origin:	Anterior part of the external lip of the iliac crest, outer surface of the anterior superior iliac spine
Insertion:	Iliotibial tract of the fascia latae at the junction of the proximal and middle third of the thigh
Nerve supply:	Nerve root: L4, 5, S1 Peripheral nerve: superior gluteal
Function:	Flexes, medially rotates and abducts the hip joint, tensions the fascia latae and may assist in knee extension via the illiotibial tract

MUSCLE TESTING
Tensor fasciae latae

STRENGTH BIAS TESTING

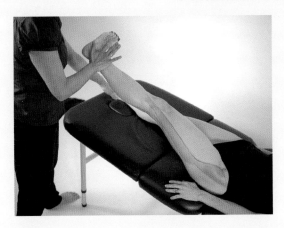

Client position
The client is lying supine with the knee in extension and with the hip internally rotated.

Instruction to client
The client is instructed firstly to internally rotate the hip by turning the foot inwards towards the opposite foot. They are then instructed to maintain knee extension and the foot position whilst performing hip flexion in a position of slight abduction.

Examiner position and notes
The examiner stands to the side of the leg being tested and applies a force above the ankle joint.

Resistance
Resistance is applied at the anterior lateral aspect of the distal tibia in a direction of hip extension and slight adduction to return the leg towards the bed. It is not necessary to apply resistance to the rotatory component.

8

MUSCLE TESTING
Tensor fasciae latae

LENGTH BIAS TESTING

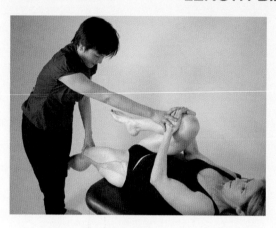

Client position

The client is lying supine at the end of a bed.

Instruction to client

The client is instructed to stand and rest the ischium at the end of a plinth. The client is then instructed to hold the contralateral knee to the chest and is assisted by the examiner into the supine position whilst maintaining the knee-to-chest position. The hip to be tested should be allowed to rest into extension and the thigh should not be supported by the bed.

Examiner position and notes

The examiner is positioned to the side of the bed in order to assist the client into the supine position. Once the client is in the testing position, the examiner may assess for hip extension range off the edge of the bed. Tensor fasciae latae (TFL) shortness may be indicated when the hip is held in some flexion, abduction and/or internal rotation. The knee may also be limited in flexion as TFL extends the knee through its connection via the iliotibial tract. The examiner may test for the resistance to the various elements of movement by applying overpressure at the end range. Further information gained with a thorough history and assessment with palpation is valuable in order to confirm findings.

8

KINESIO TAPING
Tensor fasciae latae

STRENGTH TAPING

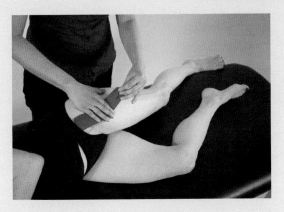

Client position

The client is in a sidelying position. The non-taped leg is below with the hip flexed. This lower knee may be held by the client in order to assist with support. The hip to be taped is on top with the hip in extension, external rotation and hip adduction towards the floor behind the bed.

Measurement of tape

A length of tape is measured from the anterior superior iliac spine (ASIS) tract towards the anterior superior ⅓ of the iliotibial tract (ITB). For conditions involving the knee, measure a length of tape from the proximal tibia to the ASIS.

Tape application

The starting anchor is applied with zero tension on the anterior superior iliac spine. With the tissue in a lengthened position, the base of the tape is applied with 15–25% tension towards the iliotibial band. The final anchor is applied to the ITB with zero tension. For conditions involving the knee, complete the taping at the proximal lateral tibia with zero tract tension. Rub the tape to activate the glue.

Reassessment

Reassess the client for changes in strength, tonal changes, functional changes and symptoms.

8

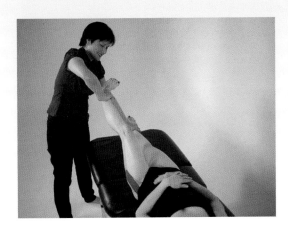

KINESIO TAPING
Tensor fasciae latae

LENGTH TAPING

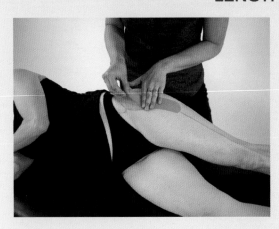

Client position

The client is in a sidelying position. The non-taped leg is below with the hip and knee flexed. This lower knee may be held by the client in order to assist with support. The hip to be taped is on top with the hip in extension, external rotation and hip adduction towards the floor over the edge of the bed.

Measurement of tape

A length of tape is measured from the anterior superior iliac spine towards the anterior superior ⅓ of the iliotibial tract. For conditions involving the knee, measure a length of tape from ASIS all the way to the proximal tibia.

Tape application

The starting anchor is applied with zero tension on the iliotibial band just distal to the insertion. With the tissue in the lengthened position, the base of the tape is applied with 15–25% tension towards the ASIS. The final anchor is applied to the ASIS with zero tension. For conditions involving the knee, place the starting anchor on the proximal lateral tibia. Rub the tape to activate the glue.

8

LENGTH TAPING

Reassessment

Reassess the client for changes in length, strength, tonal changes, functional changes and symptoms. If components of the testing were found to be significant on pre-testing, these should be reassessed for changes. For testing where strength was also in deficit, re-test for a normalisation of strength bias testing.

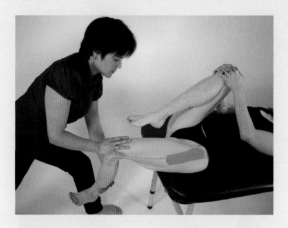

8

ANATOMY
Gluteus medius and gluteus minimus

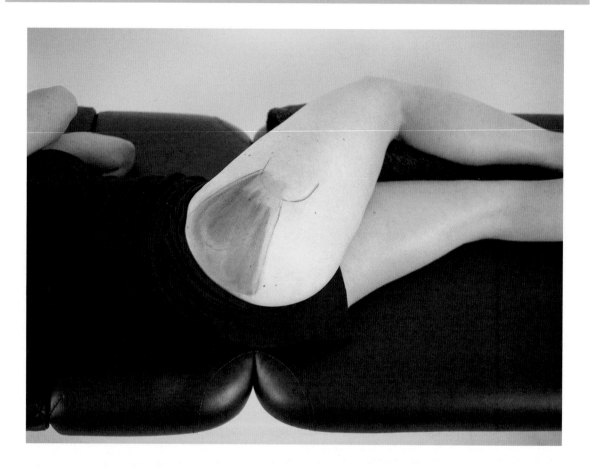

Gluteus medius

Origin:	External surface of the ilium between the iliac crest and the posterior gluteal line and anterior gluteal line; gluteal aponeurosis
Insertion:	Oblique ridge on the lateral surface of the greater trochanter for the femur
Nerve supply:	Nerve root: L4, 5, S1 Peripheral nerve: superior gluteal
Function:	Abducts the hip joint. Anterior fibres medially rotate and may assist in hip flexion. Posterior fibres laterally rotate and may assist in extension

Gluteus minimus

Origin:	External surface of the ilium between the anterior and inferior gluteal lines and margin of the greater sciatic notch
Insertion:	Anterior border of the greater trochanter of the femur and hip joint capsule
Nerve supply:	Nerve root: L4, 5, S1 Peripheral nerve: superior gluteal
Function:	Abducts, medially rotates and may assist in flexion of the hip joint

8

MUSCLE TESTING
Gluteus medius—posterior fibres

STRENGTH BIAS TESTING

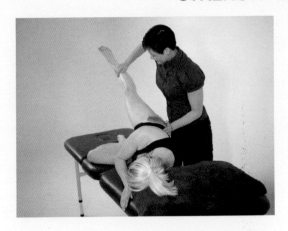

Client position
The client is in a sidelying position with the lower hip and knee flexed so that the feet are at the level of the calf of the leg being examined. This creates a more stable base of support for testing.

Instruction to client
The client is instructed to maintain the abducted hip position with the hip externally rotated whilst the examiner applies a downward force.

Examiner position and notes
The examiner stands behind the client and stabilises the pelvis. The examiner places the hip being tested into a position of full hip abduction which is neutral with regards to flexion/extension. The position of the client's foot may be a useful indicator for the rotatory elements in the lower limb.

An inability to achieve full external rotation may imply that the anterior tissue may be short or that the posterior fibres are compromised in their capacity to achieve the movement. If the client is not able to maintain full abduction range or the start position prior to the application of resistance force, this is a positive test and implies that taping may be appropriate.

Resistance
The examiner applies a force above the ankle in a direction of adduction towards the bed.

8

MUSCLE TESTING
Gluteus medius anterior fibres and gluteus minimus

STRENGTH BIAS TESTING

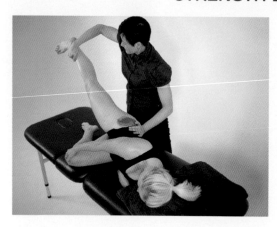

Client position

The client is in a sidelying position with the lower hip and knee flexed so that the feet are at the level of the calf of the leg being examined. This creates a more stable base of support for testing.

Instruction to client

The client is instructed to maintain the abducted hip position with internal rotation whilst the examiner applies a downward force.

Examiner position and notes

The examiner stands behind the client and stabilises the pelvis. The examiner places the hip being tested into a position of hip abduction which is neutral with regards to flexion/extension. The position of the client's foot may be a useful indicator for the rotatory elements in the lower limb.

If the client is unable to achieve full internal rotation of the hip (indicated by the foot) passively, this suggests a shortness of the external rotators, whereas an inability to maintain the range prior to resistance application suggests a weakness. If the client is not able to maintain full abduction range or the starting position prior to the application of resistance force, this may be indicative of a weakness. This test also implicates the tensor fasciae latae and so additional palpation and testing to ascertain which muscle is to be managed is appropriate.

Resistance

The examiner applies a force above the ankle in a direction of adduction towards the bed.

8

MUSCLE TESTING
Gluteus medius and gluteus minimus

LENGTH BIAS TESTING

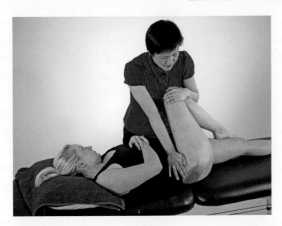

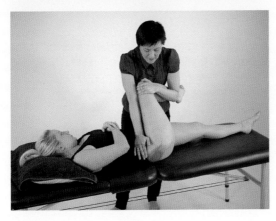

Client position
The client is lying supine with the contralateral leg in extension and the hip flexed to approximately 90 degrees and knee resting in a flexed position.

Instruction to client
The client is instructed to try to maintain the sacrum on the bed during testing.

Examiner position and notes
The examiner stands to the side of the client and assesses for range. Whilst stabilising the pelvis, the knee is taken in an arc to assess for specific restrictions in range. Once found, the direction and orientation of the tight fibres are assessed in order to determine the direction of tape placement. The range for which the hip is abducted across the body is noted with the appropriate angle for re-testing.

8

KINESIO TAPING
Gluteus medius and gluteus minimus

STRENGTH TAPING

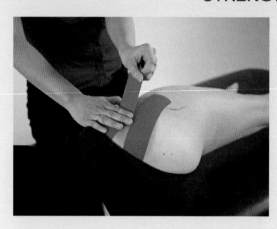

Client position

The client is in a sidelying position with the shaft of the femur angled to be in continuation of the fibres to be taped. For the posterior fibres, the hip is in some flexion with the leg adducted across the body and resting on the bed or towards the floor in front of the bed. For anterior fibres, the hip may be in a neutral position or in extension with hip adduction by allowing the leg to rest on or behind the bed.

Measurement of tape

For anterior fibres: A length of tape is measured from the anterior iliac spine towards the greater trochanter. This length of tape will assist with the anterior fibres of gluteus medius which have the same function as the gluteus minimus. The position of taping is similar to tensor fasciae latae taping.

For posterior fibres: A length of tape is measured from the posterior iliac crest to the greater trochanter.

Additional tape may be useful for larger clients or those requiring more stimulation. Conversely, smaller clients may have the tape cut into a Y-strip.

Tape application

The starting anchor is applied with zero tension on the iliac crest. With the tissue in a lengthened position, apply the base of the tape with 25–35% tension towards the greater trochanter. The final anchor is applied to the greater trochanter with zero tension. Reposition the client for additional fibres at the appropriate angles. Rub the tape to activate the glue.

8

STRENGTH TAPING

Reassessment
Reassess your client for changes in strength, tonal changes, functional changes and symptoms.

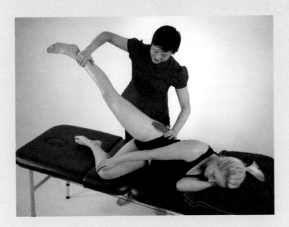

KINESIO TAPING
Gluteus medius and gluteus minimus

LENGTH TAPING

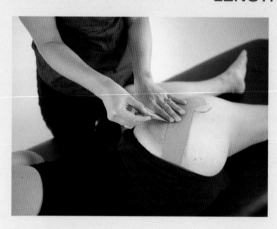

Client position

The client is in a sidelying position with the shaft of the femur angled to be in continuation of the fibres to be taped. For the posterior fibres, the hip is in some flexion with the leg adducted across the body and resting on the bed or towards the floor in front of the bed. For anterior fibres, the hip may be in a neutral position or in extension with hip adduction by allowing the leg to rest on or behind the bed.

Measurement of tape

For anterior fibres: A length of tape is measured from the anterior iliac spine towards the greater trochanter. This length of tape will assist with the anterior fibres of gluteus medius which have the same function as the gluteus minimus. The position of taping is similar to tensor fasciae latae taping.

For posterior fibres: A length of tape is measured from the posterior iliac crest to the greater trochanter.

Additional tape may be useful for larger clients or those requiring more stimulation by covering a larger surface area. Conversely, smaller clients may have the tape cut into a Y-strip.

Tape application

The starting anchor is applied with zero tension on the greater trochanter. With the tissue in a lengthened position, apply the base of the tape with 15–25% tension towards the iliac crest. The final anchor is applied to the iliac crest with zero tension. Reposition the client for additional fibres at the appropriate angles. Rub the tape to activate the glue or instruct the client to activate the glue.

8

LENGTH TAPING

Reassessment

Reassess your client for changes in length, strength, tonal changes, functional changes and symptoms.

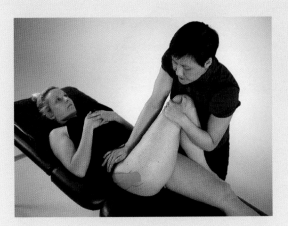

8

ANATOMY
Gluteus maximus

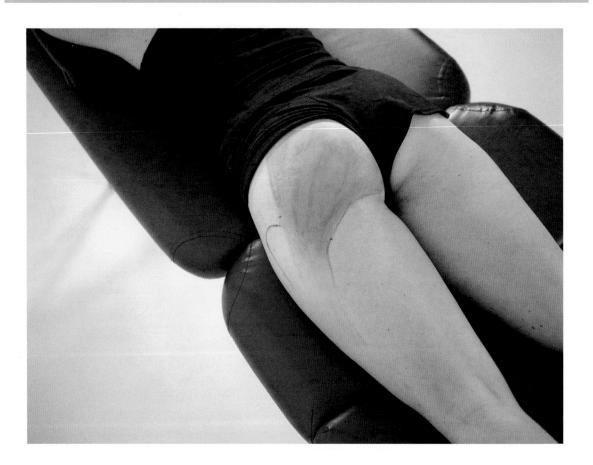

Gluteus maximus	
Origin:	Posterior gluteal line of the ilium, posterior surface of the lower sacrum, lateral coccyx, aponeurosis of the erector spinae, sacrotuberous ligament and gluteal aponeurosis
Insertion:	Superficial and proximal fibres into the iliotibial tract and fascia latae. Deep fibres at the distal portion to the gluteal tuberosity of the femur
Nerve supply:	L5, S1, S2, inferior gluteal
Function:	Extends and laterally rotates the hip joint. Lower fibres assist in adduction of the hip whilst the upper fibres assist in abduction. Via the insertion into the iliotibial tract, it may help to stabilise the knee in extension

8

MUSCLE TESTING
Gluteus maximus

STRENGTH BIAS TESTING

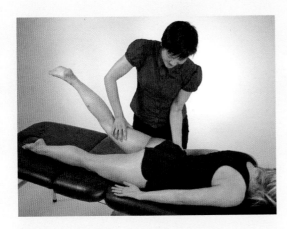

Client position
The client is prone with the knee at 90 degrees flexion (or more) to bias testing towards gluteus maximus as the hamstrings are in a shortened position. In the case of tight rectus femoris, the knee may be less flexed (as shown in the image above) during testing.

Instruction to client
The client is instructed to maintain the maximal passive hip extension achieved by the examiner (knee off the bed) whilst the examiner applies a downward force above the knee.

Examiner position and notes
The examiner is positioned to the side of the bed. The stabilising hand is placed around the ilium on the side being tested; an incorrect test has the ilium anteriorly rotating to achieve leg height. The examiner notes any compensations in movement which may indicate a weakness requiring an alternative strategy. An inability to maintain the maximal range achieved by the examiner prior to the application of resistance implicates a compromised strategy and is a positive test. The bias towards gluteus maximus testing is enhanced with greater knee flexion; however, this may be limited by rectus femoris tension. In the case where the knee is flexed beyond 90 degrees, the examiner will note a decreased range of hip extension due to restriction in range created by the rectus femoris.

Resistance
Resistance is applied proximal to the knee in a direction towards hip flexion.

8

MUSCLE TESTING
Gluteus maximus

LENGTH BIAS TESTING

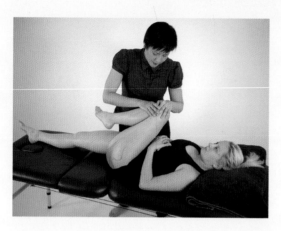

Client position

The client is lying supine with the contralateral leg extended.

Instruction to client

The client is instructed to maintain the sacrum on the bed as the examiner takes the ipsilateral knee to chest and across to midline. The end range is determined as soon as the pelvic position becomes compromised.

Examiner position and notes

The examiner stands to the side of the client and assesses for range. With a stable pelvis, the knee is taken cephalad (towards the chest) for end range resistance. The range for hip flexion is noted for reassessment. The testing assesses primarily posterior restrictions that limit hip flexion; further assessment and palpation to determine structure and angle of tension may be appropriate.

8

KINESIO TAPING
Gluteus maximus

STRENGTH TAPING

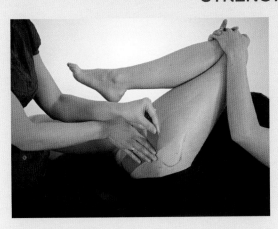

Client position
The client is lying supine. The non-taped leg is resting on the bed with the hip extended. The client holds the knee on the side to be taped towards the midline chest in full hip flexion with the knee relaxed in flexion.

Measurement of tape
A length of tape is measured from the sacrum to the posterior proximal iliotibial band (ITB).

Tape application
The starting anchor is applied with zero tension on the sacrum. With the tissue in the lengthened position, the base of the tape is applied with 15–25% tension towards the posterior aspect of the ITB. The final anchor is applied to the ITB band and lateral femur with zero tension. Rub the tape to activate the glue.

Reassessment
Reassess the client for changes in strength, tonal changes, functional changes and symptoms.

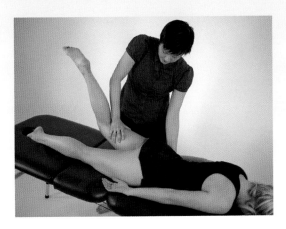

8

KINESIO TAPING
Gluteus maximus

LENGTH TAPING

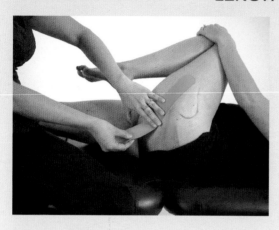

Client position

The client is lying supine. The non-taped leg is resting on the bed with the hip extended. The client holds the knee on the side to be taped towards the midline chest in full hip flexion with the knee relaxed in flexion.

Measurement of tape

A length of tape is measured from the sacrum to the posterior proximal iliotibial band.

Tape application

The starting anchor is applied with zero tension on the posterior iliotibial band. With the tissue in the lengthened position, the base of the tape is applied with 15–25% tension towards the sacrum. The final anchor is applied to the sacrum with zero tension. Rub the tape to activate the glue.

Reassessment

Reassess the client for changes in length, strength, tonal changes, functional changes and symptoms. For testing where strength was also in deficit, re-test for a normalisation of strength bias testing.

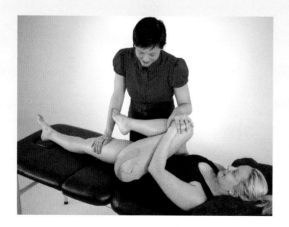

8

ANATOMY
Piriformis

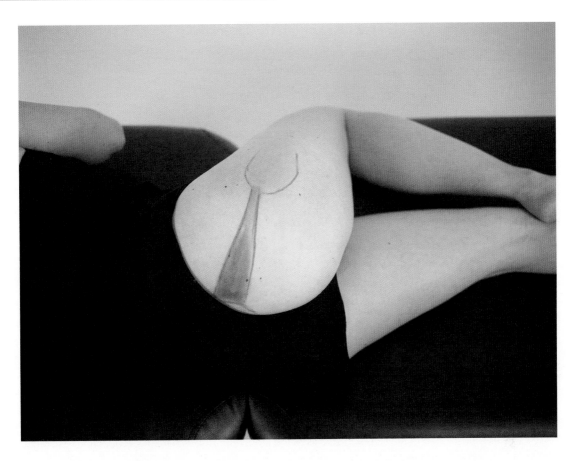

Piriformis

Origin:	Anterior surface of the sacrum and pelvic surface of the sacrotuberous ligament
Insertion:	Superior border of the greater trochanter for the femur
Nerve supply:	Nerve root: L5, S1, S2 Peripheral nerve: sacral plexus
Function:	Lateral rotator of the hip in its anatomical position. May assist in extension. May assist in abduction when the hip is flexed. Is a medial rotator of the hip when hip flexion range is greater than 60 degrees

8

MUSCLE TESTING
Piriformis

STRENGTH BIAS TESTING

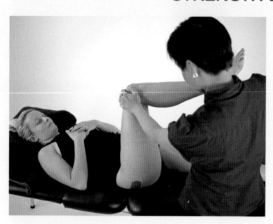

Client position

The client is lying supine with the hip and the knee flexed to 90 degrees. The contralateral leg is in extension.

Instruction to client

The client is instructed to maintain the position as the examiner applies a force to the outside of the lower leg. The client attempts to rotate the heel away from the midline whilst keeping the knee fixed in space. The piriformis is a medial rotator of the hip in this position and so the test is for medial rotation strength.

Examiner position and notes

The examiner is positioned to the side and stabilises the knee laterally, with the hand applying resistance placed at the lateral heel/ankle.

Resistance

Resistance is applied at the lateral ankle or heel to take the ankle towards the midline so that the client is required to engage the medial rotators to maintain the position.

8

MUSCLE TESTING
Piriformis

LENGTH BIAS TESTING

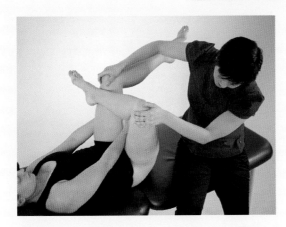

Client position
The client is lying supine with both hips in flexion and the feet resting on the bed.

Instruction to client
The client is instructed to rest the testing leg on the opposite thigh above the knee (shin resting on thigh in a figure 4 shape). Both hips are flexed as the client reaches to support the contralateral thigh with clasped hands. Whilst keeping the tailbone connected to the bed, the client flexes both hips. The movement is ceased once a restriction is felt or the pelvic position is lost.

Examiner position and notes
The examiner stands to the side of the client and can assist in hip flexion by supporting the contralateral leg. End range resistance can be assessed by placing some overpressure to either the hip flexion component or the hip lateral rotation component.

Placing the hip in lateral rotation with abduction, as shown, is appropriate to assess for the length of the piriformis when the hip has greater than 60 degrees of flexion.

8

KINESIO TAPING
Piriformis

STRENGTH TAPING

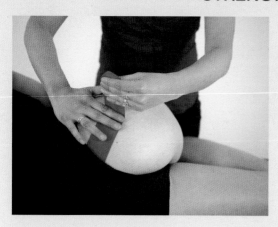

Client position

The client is in a sidelying position with the shaft of the femur angled to be in continuation of the fibres to be taped. The hip is in some flexion with the leg adducted across the body and resting on the bed.

Measurement of tape

A length of tape is measured from the sacrum to the greater trochanter.

Tape application

The starting anchor is applied with zero tension on the sacrum. With the tissue in the lengthened position, the base of the tape is applied with 25–35% tension towards the greater trochanter. The final anchor is applied to the trochanter with zero tension. Rub the tape to activate the glue.

Reassessment

Reassess the client for changes in strength, tonal changes, functional changes and symptoms.

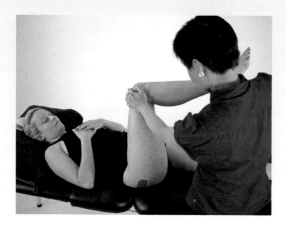

KINESIO TAPING
Piriformis

LENGTH TAPING

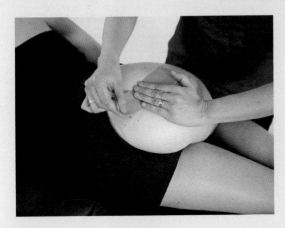

Client position
The client is in a sidelying position with the shaft of the femur angled to be in continuation of the fibres to be taped. The hip is in some flexion with the leg adducted across the body and resting on the bed.

Measurement of tape
A length of tape is measured from the sacrum to the greater trochanter.

Tape application
The starting anchor is applied with zero tension on the greater trochanter. With the tissue in the lengthened position, the base of the tape is applied with 15–25% tension towards the sacrum. The final anchor is applied to the sacrum with zero tension. Rub the tape to activate the glue.

Reassessment
Reassess the client for changes in length, strength, tonal changes, functional changes and symptoms. For testing where strength was also in deficit, re-test for a normalisation of strength bias testing.

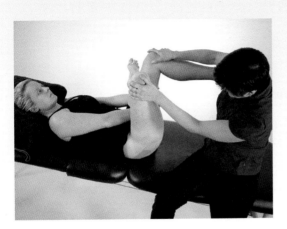

8

ANATOMY

Quadratus femoris and obturator externus

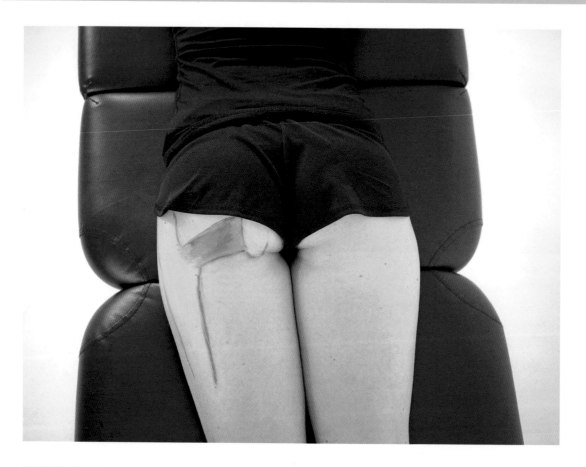

Quadratus femoris

Origin:	Proximal part of the lateral border of the ischial tuberosity
Insertion:	Distal to the intertrochanteric crest on the proximal part of the quadrate line of the femur
Nerve supply:	Nerve root: L5, S1, S2 Peripheral nerve: sacral plexus
Function:	Lateral rotator of the hip

Obturator externus

Origin:	Pubic and ischial rami and external surface of the obturator membrane
Insertion:	Trochanteric fossa of the femur
Nerve supply:	L3, 4 Peripheral nerve: obturator
Function:	Lateral rotator of the hip. May assist in adduction of the hip joint

8

MUSCLE TESTING
Quadratus femoris and obturator externus

STRENGTH BIAS TESTING

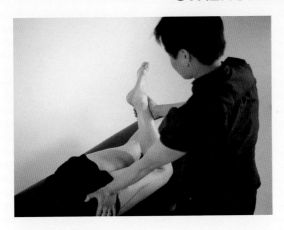

Client position

The client is lying prone on the bed with the hip in a neutral position and the knee flexed to 90 degrees. The contralateral leg is resting in neutral.

Instruction to client

The client is instructed to try to maintain the position as the examiner applies a force to the inside of the lower leg. The client attempts to take the ankle over to the contralateral side whilst keeping the knee on the bed in order to create lateral rotation of the hip.

Examiner position and notes

The examiner is positioned on the ipsilateral side and applies a force to the inside of the ankle to rotate the ankle away from the midline. The examiner places the stabilising hand over the ipsilateral hip and ensures that the thigh stays on the bed during the testing. The examiner should note any compensatory strategies such as flexing the hip or abduction. The examiner may assist with stabilising the pelvis or knee during testing.

Resistance

The examiner applies a force above the ankle in a direction away from the midline so that the client actively engages the lateral rotators to maintain the position.

MUSCLE TESTING
Quadratus femoris and obturator externus

LENGTH BIAS TESTING

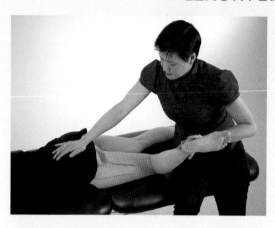

Client position

The client is lying prone on the bed with the hip in a neutral position and the knee flexed to 90 degrees. The contralateral leg is resting in neutral.

Instruction to client

Whilst keeping the knee fixed on the bed and the knee bent at 90 degrees, the client is instructed to allow the ankle to fall to the side and take this to the maximal available range.

Examiner position and notes

The examiner is positioned to stabilise the hip during the test. The examiner may test for passive range by further rotating the hip by taking the ankle away from the midline. An increase in passive range may indicate a motor control deficit on the internal rotator of the hip rather than a length issue of the external rotators. The examiner notes any asymmetries in movement upon comparing both sides.

8

KINESIO TAPING
Quadratus femoris and obturator externus

STRENGTH TAPING

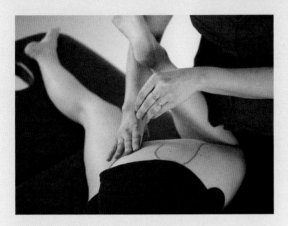

Client position
The client is in a sidelying position with the side being taped uppermost. The upper hip and knee are flexed with the knee resting on the bed in adduction and the ankle is resting on a pillow or against the practitioner to create internal rotation.

Measurement of tape
A length of tape is measured from the proximal ischium to the greater trochanter.

Tape application
The starting anchor is applied with zero tension on the ischial tuberosity. With the tissue in the lengthened position, the base of the tape is applied with 25–35% tension towards the greater trochanter. The final anchor is applied to the trochanter with zero tension. Rub the tape to activate the glue.

Reassessment
Reassess the client for changes in strength, tonal changes, functional changes and symptoms.

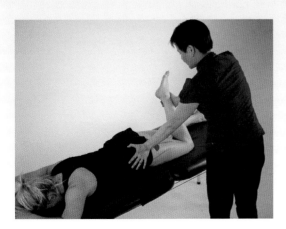

8

KINESIO TAPING
Quadratus femoris and obturator externus

LENGTH TAPING

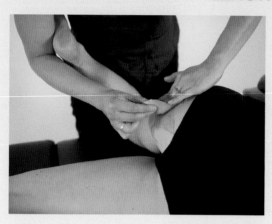

Client position

The client is in a sidelying position with the side being taped uppermost. The upper hip and knee are flexed with the knee resting on the bed in adduction and the ankle is resting on a pillow or against the practitioner to create internal rotation.

Measurement of tape

A length of tape is measured from the ischial tuberosity to the greater trochanter.

Tape application

The starting anchor is applied with zero tension on the greater trochanter. With the tissue in the lengthened position, the base of the tape is applied with 15–25% tension towards the ischial tuberosity. The final anchor is applied to the ischial tuberosity with zero tension. Rub the tape to activate the glue.

Reassessment

Reassess the client for changes in length, strength, tonal changes, functional changes and symptoms. For testing where strength was also in deficit, re-test for a normalisation of strength bias testing.

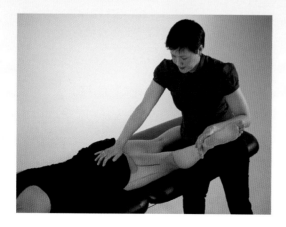

8

ANATOMY

Gemellus superior, gemellus inferior and obturator internus

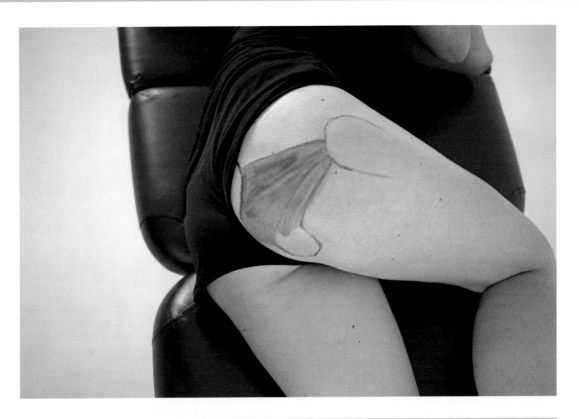

Gemellus superior

Origin:	External surface of the spine of the ischium
Insertion:	Medial surface of the greater trochanter of the femur proximal to the trochanteric fossa
Nerve supply:	Nerve root: L5, S1, S2 Peripheral nerve: sacral plexus
Function:	Lateral rotator of the hip. May assist in abduction of the hip joint when the hip is flexed

Gemellus inferior

Origin:	Proximal part of the ischial tuberosity
Insertion:	Medial surface of the greater trochanter of the femur proximal to the trochanteric fossa
Nerve supply:	Nerve root: L4, L5, S1, S2 Peripheral nerve: sacral plexus
Function:	Lateral rotator of the hip. May assist in abduction of the hip joint when the hip is flexed

Obturator internus

Origin:	Pelvic surface of the obturator membrane and margin of the obturator foramen as well as the ischial surface proximal to this; obturator fascia
Insertion:	Medial surface of the greater trochanter of the femur proximal to the trochanteric fossa
Nerve supply:	Nerve root: L5, S1, S2 Peripheral nerve: sacral plexus
Function:	Lateral rotator of the hip. May assist in abduction of the hip joint when the hip is flexed

8

MUSCLE TESTING
Gemellus superior, gemellus inferior and obturator internus

STRENGTH BIAS TESTING

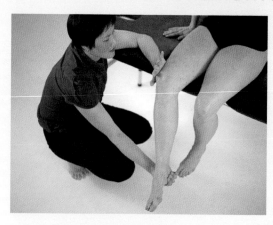

Client position

The client is seated with the pelvis in a neutral position and the hip and knee flexed to 90 degrees. The feet are unsupported. This test can also be done in a supine position with the hip and knee flexed to 90 degrees on the side to be tested.

Instruction to client

The client is instructed to maintain the position as the examiner applies a force to the medial ankle or heel.

Examiner position and notes

The examiner is positioned to the side. The examiner should note any compensatory strategies such as flexing the hip, knee or spine, or abducting the hip. The examiner stabilises the lateral knee during testing.

Resistance

The examiner applies a force at the ankle or heel in a direction away from the midline so that the client actively engages the lateral rotators to maintain the position.

8

MUSCLE TESTING
Gemellus superior, gemellus inferior and obturator internus

LENGTH BIAS TESTING

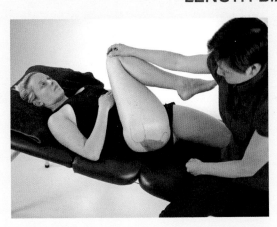

Client position

The client is lying supine with the contralateral leg resting on the bed and the tested hip held at the knee. Alternatively, this test may be done in sitting with the leg initially resting on the opposite thigh before the knee is taken to the chest.

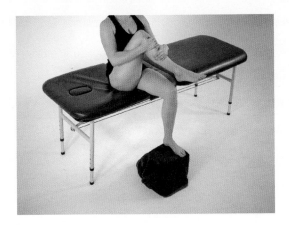

Instruction to client

The client is instructed to take the knee across the body towards the opposite shoulder without moving the pelvis, a cue to sink the sit bones into the bed or back in the seat is usually sufficient.

Examiner position and notes

The examiner is positioned to the side of the client and assesses for end range, and palpates for any particular restrictions or discomfort.

8

KINESIO TAPING
Gemellus superior, gemellus inferior and obturator internus

STRENGTH TAPING

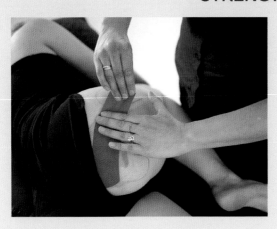

Client position

The client is in a sidelying position with the side being taped uppermost. The upper hip and knee are flexed so that the shaft of the femur is in line with the fibres to be taped (knee to chest). The knee is resting on the bed in adduction and the ankle can also be resting on a pillow to create internal rotation.

Measurement of tape

A length of tape is measured from the inferior lateral angle of the sacrum to the greater trochanter. This longer length of tape assists in maintaining the tape on the body for longer as it is typically held by the underwear and the edges are less likely to be caught with moving the underwear throughout the day.

Tape application

The starting anchor is applied with zero tension on the inferior lateral angle of the sacrum. With the tissue in the lengthened position, the base of the tape is applied with 25–35% tension towards the greater trochanter. The final anchor is applied to the trochanter with zero tension. Rub the tape to activate the glue.

Reassessment

Reassess the client for changes in strength, tonal changes, functional changes and symptoms.

8

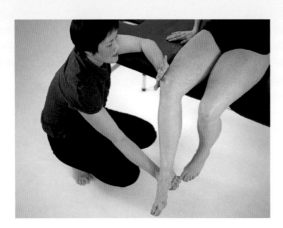

KINESIO TAPING
Gemellus superior, gemellus inferior and obturator internus

LENGTH TAPING

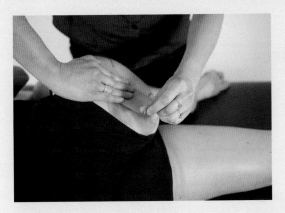

Client position

The client is in a sidelying position with the side being taped uppermost. The upper hip and knee are flexed so that the shaft of the femur is in line with the fibres to be taped (knee to chest). The knee is resting on the bed in adduction and the ankle can also be resting on a pillow to create internal rotation.

Measurement of tape

A length of tape is measured from the inferior lateral angle of the sacrum to the greater trochanter. This longer length of tape assists in maintaining the tape on the body for longer as it is typically held by the underwear and the edges are less likely to be caught with moving the underwear throughout the day.

Tape application

The starting anchor is applied with zero tension on the greater trochanter. The base of the tape is applied with 15–25% tension towards the inferior lateral angle of the sacrum. The final anchor is applied to the sacrum with zero tension. Rub the tape to activate the glue.

Reassessment

Reassess the client for changes in length, strength, tonal changes, functional changes and symptoms. For testing where strength was also in deficit, re-test for a normalisation of strength bias testing.

8

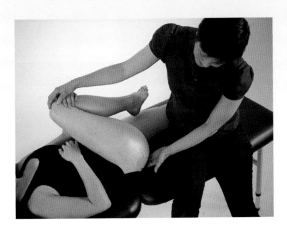

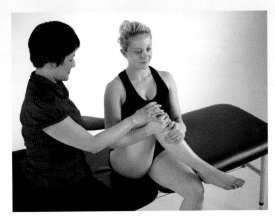

HIP ASSESSMENT SHEET

Clinic: .... Date: ....

Client name: ....

Functional review

Functional limitation	Pre-test measure	Post-test measure

Muscle testing

Tested priority	Muscle	Strength		Length		Comments
		Right	Left	Right	Left	
	Pectineus and adductor brevis					
	Adductor longus					
	Gracilis					
	Adductor magnus					
	Psoas major and minor					
	Iliacus					
	Tensor fasciae latae					
	Gluteus medius and gluteus minimus					
	Gluteus maximus					
	Piriformis					
	Quadratus femoris and obturator externus					
	Gemellus superior, gemellus inferior and obturator internus					

8

Treatment

Intervention	Re-test measures	Plan

Practitioner: .... Signature: ....

BIBLIOGRAPHY

Berryman Reese, N. M. (2012). *Muscle and sensory testing*. Missouri: Elsevier-Saunders.

Berryman Reese, N., & Bandy, W. D. (2010). *Joint range of motion and muscle length testing*. Missouri: Saunders Elsevier.

Calais-Germain, B. (1993). *Anatomy of movement* (12 ed.). Seattle: Eastland Press.

Comerford, M., & Mottram, S. (2012). *Kinetic control: the management of uncontrolled movement*. Sydney, Australia: Elsevier.

Kase, K., Hashimoto, T., & Okane, T. (1998). *Kinesio Taping perfect manual: amazing taping therapy to eliminate pain and muscle disorders*. Albuquerque: Kinesio Taping Association.

Kase, K., & Rock Stockheimer, K. (2006). *Kinesio Taping for lymphoedema and chronic swelling*. Albuquerque: Kinesio Taping Association.

Kase, K., Wallis, J., & Kase, T. (2003). *Clinical therapeutic applications of the Kinesio taping methods*. Albuquerque: Kinesio Taping Association.

Kendall, F. P., McCreary, E., Provance, P., Rodgers, M., & Romanic, W. (2005). *Muscles: testing and function with posture and pain*. Baltimore: Lippincott Williams Wilkins.

Standring, S., Borely, N., Collings, P., Crossman, A., Gatzoulis, M., Healy, J., … Wigley, C. (2008). *Gray's anatomy: the anatomical basis of clinical practice* (S. Susan Ed. 40 ed.). London, United Kingdom: Churchill Livingstone Elsevier.

8

Techniques for testing and taping the knee

Popliteus

Rectus femoris

Vastus lateralis

Vastus medialis

Sartorius

Semitendinosus and semimembranosus

Biceps femoris

Gracilis

ANATOMY
Popliteus

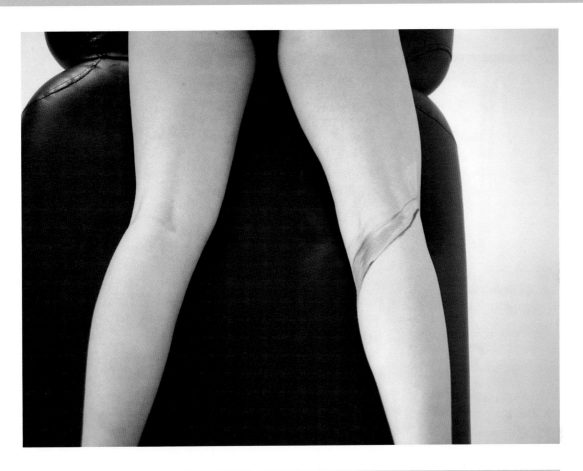

Popliteus

Origin:	Anterior part of the lateral femoral condyle and oblique popliteal ligament (and lateral meniscus) of the knee joint
Insertion:	Triangular area proximal to the soleal line on the posterior surface of the tibia and fascia
Nerve supply:	Peripheral nerve: Tibial Nerve root: L4, 5, S1
Function:	With origin fixed or non-weight-bearing; medially rotates the tibia on the femur and flexes the knee joint. In weight-bearing with the insertion fixed: laterally rotates the femur on the tibia and flexes the knee joint. It is a key muscle involved in unlocking the knee (yield) upon heel strike. Popliteus helps to reinforce the posterior ligaments of the knee drawing the meniscus posteriorly during knee flexion to prevent crushing of the meniscus

9

MUSCLE TESTING
Popliteus

STRENGTH BIAS TESTING

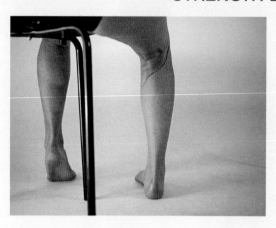

Client position
In sitting with the knee flexed at 90 degrees with the foot resting on the ground.

Instruction to client
Instruct the client to medially rotate the tibia on the femur by turning the foot inwards whilst maintaining heel contact with the floor.

Examiner position and notes
The examiner is not required to apply resistance in this test as it is used primarily to indicate whether the muscle is active.

Resistance
The examiner is not required to apply resistance in this test.

9

MUSCLE TESTING
Popliteus

LENGTH BIAS TESTING

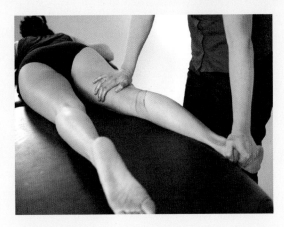

Client position
The client is prone with the knee extended and the foot just resting off the bed.

Instruction to client
The client is instructed to move the leg into lateral rotation of the tibia on the femur by rotating the foot out.

Examiner position and notes
The examiner stands to the side of the bed and applies additional force to rotate the lower tibia into external rotation whilst stabilising the thigh. With good joint integrity the examiner may use the leverage of the foot by cupping the calcaneus with the hand to create the rotary force.

The examiner assesses for range of the movement and quality of the movement. The examiner should note any symptoms that are reproduced during the testing for re-evaluation after the intervention. Range should be compared to the non-affected side for a baseline of normal range when available.

KINESIO TAPING
Popliteus

STRENGTH TAPING

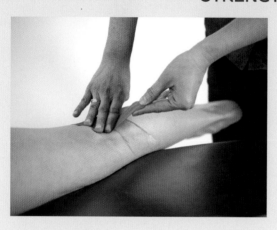

Client position

The client is lying prone with the hip abducted so that the knee is extended and the lower leg externally rotated on the bed.

Measurement of tape

Measure a length of tape from the lateral femoral condyle to the medial tibia.

Tape application

Apply the starting anchor on the lateral condyle with zero tension. With the tissue in a lengthened position, apply the base of the tape with 25–35% tension obliquely towards the medial proximal tibia. Apply the final anchor with zero tension on the medial tibia. Rub the tape to activate the glue.

Reassessment

Reassess your client for changes in strength, tonal changes, functional changes and symptoms.

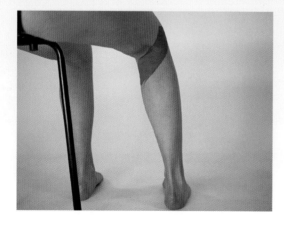

KINESIO TAPING
Popliteus

LENGTH TAPING

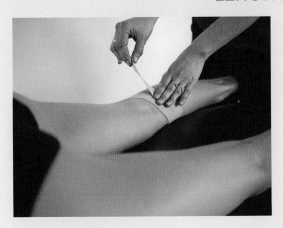

Client position

The client is lying prone with the hip abducted so that the knee is extended and the lower leg externally rotated on the bed.

Measurement of tape

Measure a length of tape from the lateral femoral condyle to the medial tibia.

Tape application

Apply the starting anchor on the medial proximal tibia with zero tension. With the tissue in a lengthened position, apply the base of the tape with 15–25% tension obliquely towards the lateral femoral condyle. Apply the final anchor with zero tension on the lateral femoral condyle. Rub the tape to activate the glue.

Reassessment

The client is reassessed for range of movement and symptoms, and palpated for changes in tone. A restoration of length may also yield strength improvements where a strength deficit was detected prior to the taping; in these circumstances, the strength should also be reassessed. Any functional deficits can also be reassessed for changes.

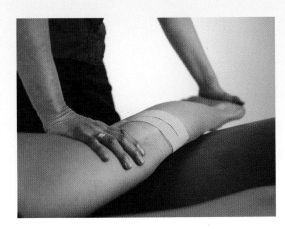

9

ANATOMY
Rectus femoris

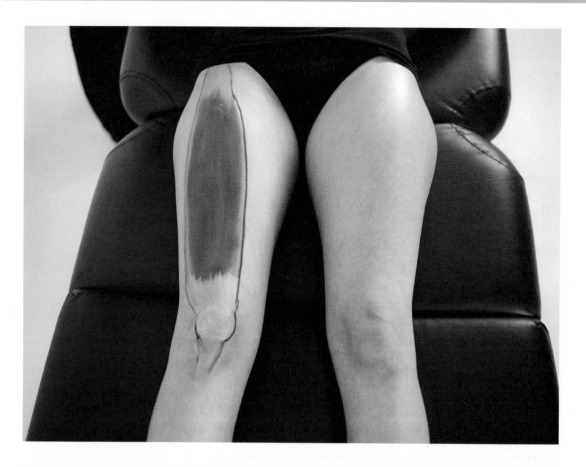

Rectus femoris

Origin:	Straight head: anterior inferior iliac spine Reflected head: from the groove above the rim of the acetabulum
Insertion:	Proximal border of the patella, and via the patellar ligament onto the tuberosity of the tibia
Nerve supply:	Peripheral nerve: femoral Nerve root: L2, 3, 4
Function:	Extends the knee joint and flexes the hip joint

9

MUSCLE TESTING
Rectus femoris

STRENGTH BIAS TESTING

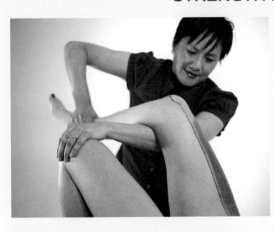

Client position
The client is lying supine with the hips and knees flexed so that the feet are resting on the bed.

Instruction to client
The client is instructed to extend the knee against the resistance applied by the examiner during the test.

Examiner position and notes
The examiner is positioned to the side of the bed. The proximal forearm slides under the tested knee so that the examiner's hand may rest on the contralateral knee. The examiner's proximal forearm thereby provides a fulcrum for movement of the knee during testing. The tested knee should then rest on the forearm with the foot resting off the bed. The examining hand is placed proximal to the ankle joint and the examiner's forearm should be angled down towards the bed in the same vector for which the resistance will be applied.

Resistance
The examiner applies a force in the direction of knee flexion towards the bed.

MUSCLE TESTING
Rectus femoris

LENGTH BIAS TESTING

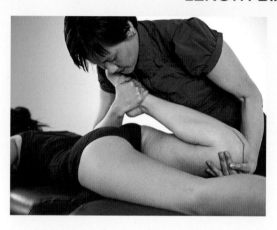

Client position
The client is lying prone.

Instruction to client
The client is instructed to take their heel to their bottom keeping the front of the hip connected to the bed. At the end of active range, the client may use their hands to achieve additional range. If the heel is able to touch the bottom, the client then attempts to lift the knee off the bed whilst maintaining the heel to the bottom and their hip on the bed.

Examiner position and notes
If the client is unable to perform the test independently the examiner may choose to do the test instead. The examiner is positioned in standing next to the bed and applies overpressure to the lower leg whilst stabilising the hip or assists in lifting the knee off the bed to assess for end range.

9

KINESIO TAPING
Rectus femoris

STRENGTH TAPING

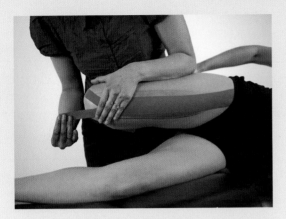

Client position

The client is positioned in sidelying with the leg to be taped uppermost. The client lengthens the tissue by holding the heel towards the bottom and with the hip in extension

Measurement of tape

Measure a length of tape from the proximal tibia to the anterior inferior iliac spine (AIIS). Cut one end into a Y-strip to place around the kneecap for management of symptoms around the kneecap. For conditions where symptoms exist under the patella or at the suprapatellar or infrapatellar bursa, the practitioner may choose to maintain a solid I-strip so as to ensure that the tape covers the bursa and patella to allow for symptomatic management rather than cut into a Y-strip.

Tape application

Apply the starting anchor on the AIIS with zero tension. Apply the base of the tape with 25–35% tension towards the patella. Complete the taping by applying the final anchor with zero tension on the tibia. Rub the tape to activate the glue.

Reassessment

Reassess your client for changes in strength, tonal changes, functional changes and symptoms.

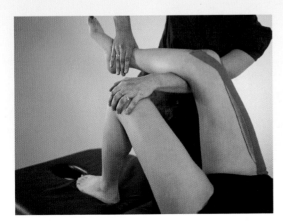

9

KINESIO TAPING
Rectus femoris

LENGTH TAPING

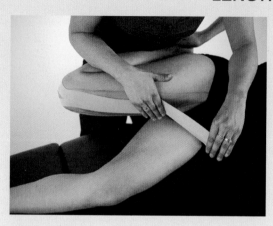

Client position

The client is positioned in sidelying with the leg to be taped uppermost. The client lengthens the tissue by holding the heel towards the bottom and with the hip in extension.

Measurement of tape

Measure a length of tape from the proximal tibia to the AIIS. Cut one end into a Y cut to place around the kneecap for management of symptoms around the kneecap. For conditions where symptoms exist under the patella or at the suprapatellar or infrapatellar bursa, the practitioner may choose to maintain a solid I-strip so as to ensure that the tape covers the bursa and patella to allow for symptomatic management rather than cut into a Y-strip.

Tape application

Tear the tape at the Y junction and apply each starting anchor with zero tension to the tibial plateau around the patella. With the tissue in the lengthened position, apply the base of the tape with 15–25% tension towards the AIIS. As the practitioner approaches the AIIS, the knee flexion component can be relaxed in order to achieve better hip extension and therefore tissue elongation for the taping. Complete the taping by applying the final anchor on the iliac spine with zero tension. Rub the tape to activate the glue.

9

LENGTH TAPING

Reassessment

Reassess your patient for changes in length, strength, tonal changes, functional changes and symptoms.

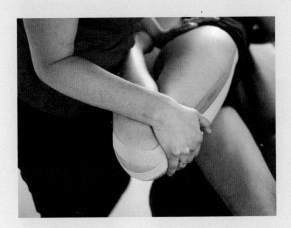

ANATOMY
Vastus lateralis

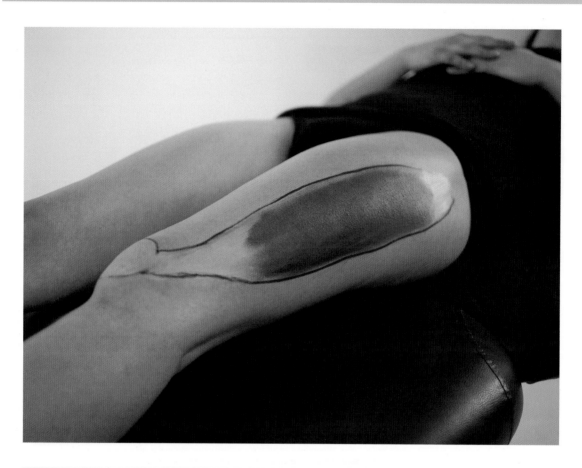

Vastus lateralis

Origin:	Proximal part of the intertrochanteric line, anterior and inferior borders of the greater trochanter, lateral lip of the linea aspera, and lateral intermuscular septum
Insertion:	Lateral and proximal border of the patella, and via the patellar ligament onto the tuberosity of the tibia
Nerve supply:	Nerve root: L2, 3, 4 Peripheral nerve: femoral
Function:	Extends the knee joint and provides lateral stability to the knee by assisting in patellar tracking and timing to balance with the forces produced by vastus medialis

9

MUSCLE TESTING
Vastus lateralis

STRENGTH BIAS TESTING

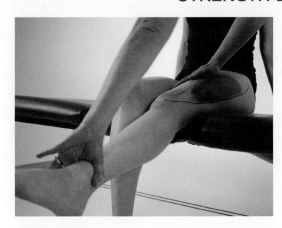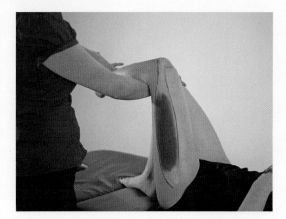

Client position

The client is seated with the thigh supported and the back of the knee just beyond the edge of the bed.

Alternatively, the client is in supine with the knees and hips flexed so that the feet are supported on the bed.

Instruction to client

The client is instructed to extend the knee against the resistance applied by the examiner during the test. The thigh is slightly internally rotated during the testing to bias the muscle into also working against gravity.

Examiner position and notes

Seated testing: The examiner is positioned to the side of the bed or seat. The proximal hand is placed over the thigh to stabilise the thigh in the slightly internally rotated position whilst the examining hand is place over the distal tibia.

Supine testing: The examiner is positioned to the side of the bed. The proximal forearm slides under the tested knee so that the hand may rest on the contralateral knee. The proximal forearm thereby provides a fulcrum for movement of the knee during testing. The tested knee should then rest on the forearm with the foot off the bed. The examining hand is placed proximal to the ankle joint and the examiner's forearm should be angled down towards the bed in the same vector for which the resistance will be applied.

Resistance

The examiner applies a force in the direction of knee flexion towards the bed.

9

MUSCLE TESTING
Vastus lateralis

LENGTH BIAS TESTING

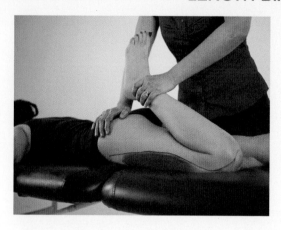

Client position
The client is lying prone.

Instruction to client
The client is instructed to take their heel to their bottom keeping the front of the hip connected to the bed. At the end of active range, the client may use their hands to achieve additional range. To add additional stress to the vastus lateralis muscles, the knee can be moved further towards or past midline. This creates adduction at the hip and may place the outer fibres of the quadriceps muscle group in a more lengthened position than the medial fibres.

Examiner position and notes
If the client is unable to perform the test independently the examiner may choose to do the test instead. The examiner is positioned in standing next to the bed and applies overpressure to the lower leg whilst stabilising the hip to assess for end range.

For additional testing, the knee may be adducted to midline to stress the vastus lateralis.

9

KINESIO TAPING
Vastus lateralis

STRENGTH TAPING

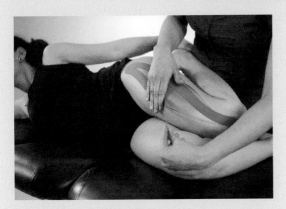

Client position

The client is positioned in sidelying with the leg to be taped uppermost. The client lengthens the tissue by holding the heel towards the bottom with the hip in extension. Additional adduction and/or internal rotation could be helpful in increasing tissue stretch when applying tape if the client's range permits.

Measurement of tape

Measure a length of tape from the anterior greater trochanter to the patella. Cut the tape down the centre into a Y-strip. For the management of local knee symptoms it may be useful to cut a longer tape to place around the kneecap and attach to the tibia.

Tape application

Apply the common starting anchor with zero tension at the proximal lateral thigh under the greater trochanter. With the tissue in the lengthened position, apply the base of each tail with 25–35% tension towards the proximal lateral patella. Complete the taping by applying the final anchor with zero tension. Rub the tape to activate the glue.

Reassessment

Reassess your client for changes in strength, tonal changes, functional changes and symptoms.

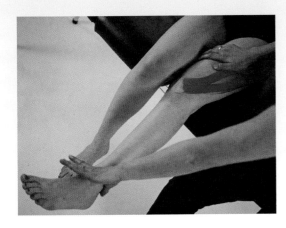
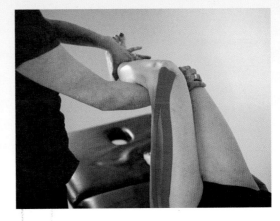

KINESIO TAPING
Vastus lateralis

LENGTH TAPING

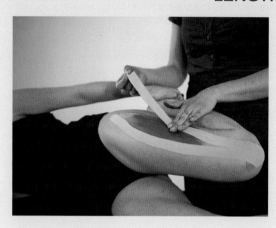

Client position

The client is positioned in sidelying with the leg to be taped uppermost. The client lengthens the tissue by holding the heel towards their bottom with the hip in extension. Additional adduction and/or internal rotation could be helpful in increasing tissue stretch when applying tape if the client's range permits.

Measurement of tape

Measure a length of tape from the anterior greater trochanter to the patella. Cut the tape down the centre into a Y-strip. For the management of local knee symptoms it may be useful to cut a longer tape to place around the kneecap and attach to the tibia.

Tape application

Apply the common starting anchor with zero tension to the patella. With the tissue in the lengthened position, apply the base of each tail of the tape with 15–25% tension towards the proximal anterior lateral thigh. Complete the taping by applying the final anchor adjacent to the greater trochanter with zero tension. Rub the tape to activate the glue.

9

LENGTH TAPING

Reassessment

The client is reassessed for range of movement and symptoms, and palpated for changes in tone. A restoration of length may also yield strength improvements where a strength deficit was detected prior to the taping; in these circumstances, the strength should also be reassessed. Any functional deficits can also be reassessed for changes.

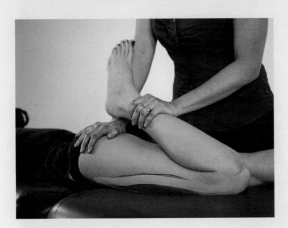

ANATOMY
Vastus medialis

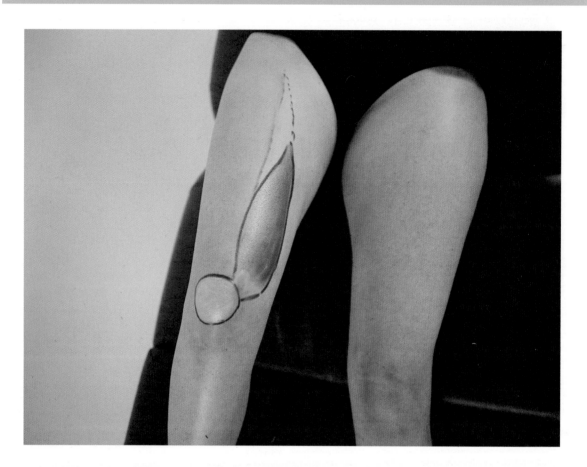

Vastus medialis

Origin:	Distal half of the intertrochanteric line, medial lip of the linea aspera, proximal part of the medial supracondylar line, tendons of adductor longus, and adductor magnus and medial intermuscular septum
Insertion:	Proximal and medial border of the patella, and via the patellar ligament onto the tuberosity of the tibia
Nerve supply:	Nerve root: L2, 3, 4 Peripheral nerve: femoral
Function:	Extends the knee joint and provides medial stability to the knee by assisting in patellar tracking and timing to balance with the forces produced by the vastus lateralis

9

MUSCLE TESTING
Vastus medialis

STRENGTH BIAS TESTING

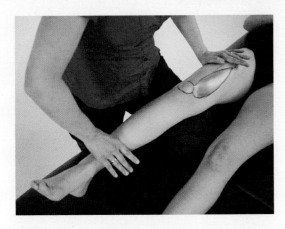

Client position

The client is lying supine with the knee to be tested resting on a bolster so that the knee is in some flexion approximately 15–20 degrees so as to test for terminal knee extension. Whilst the muscle is required throughout range, deficits may be better highlighted in their symptomatic range, in this case vastus medialis is tested for its role in terminal knee extension.

Instruction to client

The client is instructed to extend the knee against the resistance applied by the examiner during the test.

Examiner position and notes

The examiner is positioned to the side of the bed and stabilises the distal thigh. The examining hand is placed proximal to the ankle joint and the examiner's forearm should be angled down towards the bed in the same vector for which the resistance will be applied. To bias the test to implicate vastus medialis oblique (VMO), rotate the lower leg laterally so that the vastus medialis is placed to work against gravity.

Timing for VMO activation can be of more importance than direct strength to improving the client's function; the examiner may also test to compare vastus lateralis oblique (VLO) and VMO activation time to determine whether taping the VMO will be appropriate.

Resistance

The examiner applies a force in the direction of knee flexion towards the bed.

9

MUSCLE TESTING
Vastus medialis

LENGTH BIAS TESTING

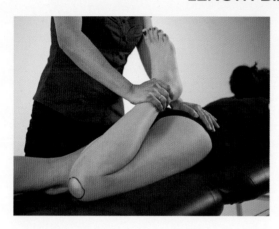

Client position
The client is lying prone.

Instruction to client
The client is instructed to take their heel to their bottom, keeping the front of the hip connected to the bed. At the end of active range, the client may use their hands to achieve additional range.

Examiner position and notes
If the client is unable to perform the test independently, the examiner may choose to do the test instead. The examiner stands next to the bed and applies overpressure to the lower leg whilst stabilising the hip to assess for end range.

For additional testing, the knee may be abducted from midline to stress the VMO.

9

KINESIO TAPING
Vastus medialis

STRENGTH TAPING

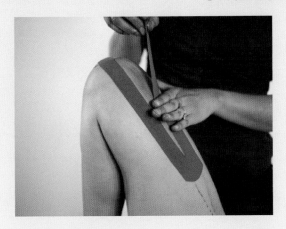

Client position
The client is lying supine with the knee in full flexion.

Measurement of tape
Measure a length of tape from the medial thigh where the VMO arises from between the border of sartorius and rectus femoris, to the patella. Cut the tape into a Y-strip. For the management of local knee symptoms it may be useful to cut a longer tape to place around the kneecap and wrap around the patella or attach to the tibia.

Tape application
Apply the common starting anchor with zero tension at the origin of the vastus medialis as it arises from the surrounding muscle in the middle of the medial thigh. Apply the base of each tail of tape with 25–35% tension on the vastus medialis oblique and vertical fibres respectively, towards the patella. Complete the tape by applying the final anchor to the patella with zero tension. Rub the tape to activate the glue.

Reassessment
Reassess your client for changes in strength, tonal changes, functional changes and symptoms.

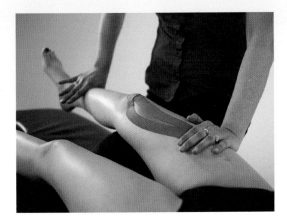

KINESIO TAPING
Vastus medialis

LENGTH TAPING

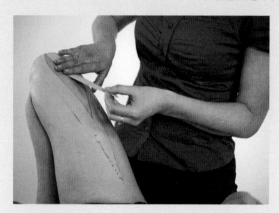

Client position

The client is lying supine with the knee in full flexion.

Measurement of tape

Measure a length of tape from the medial thigh where the vastus medialis oblique (VMO) arises from between the border of sartorius and rectus femoris, to the patella. Cut the tape into a Y-strip. For the management of local knee symptoms, it may be useful to cut a longer tape to place around the kneecap and wrap around the patella or attach to the tibia.

Tape application

Apply the common starting anchor with zero tension over the patella. Apply the base of each tape tail with 15–25% tension on the VMO and vertical fibres respectively. Complete the taping by applying the final anchor to the origin on the medial mid-thigh with zero tension. Rub the tape to activate the glue.

Reassessment

The client is reassessed for range of movement and symptoms, and palpated for changes in tone. A restoration of length may also yield strength improvements where a strength deficit was detected prior to the taping; in these circumstances, the strength should also be reassessed. Any functional deficits can also be reassessed for changes.

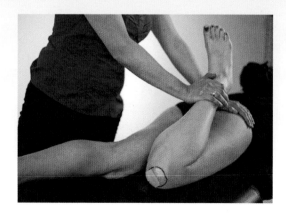

9

ANATOMY
Sartorius

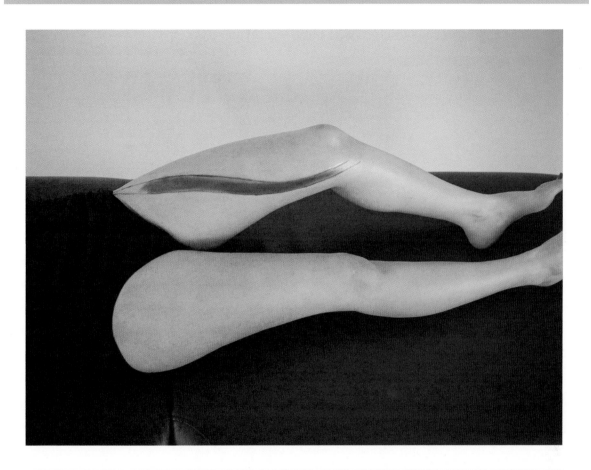

Sartorius	
Origin:	Anterior superior iliac spine and superior half of the notch just distal to the spine
Insertion:	Proximal part of the medial surface of the tibia near the anterior border
Nerve supply:	Nerve root: L2, 3, 4 Peripheral nerve: femoral nerve
Function:	Flexes, laterally rotates and abducts the hip joint. Flexes the knee and assists in medial rotation of the knee joint by working as part of the pes anserine muscle group in controlling tibial rotation

9

MUSCLE TESTING
Sartorius

STRENGTH BIAS TESTING

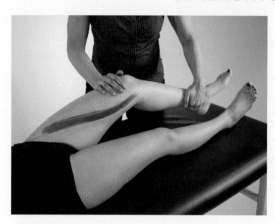

Client position
The client is lying supine with the legs extended.

Instruction to client
The client is to maintain the leg position that the examiner has placed them into for the testing, i.e. maintain hip flexion and knee flexion.

Examiner position and notes
The examiner stands to the side of the client and places the client into a position of hip flexion, external rotation and abduction of the hip, and knee flexion.

Resistance
The examiner places one hand lateral and above the knee joint to apply a force in the direction of hip extension, adduction and medial rotation. The other hand is placed against the posterior tibia above the ankle to apply a force in the direction of knee extension.

9

MUSCLE TESTING
Sartorius

LENGTH BIAS TESTING

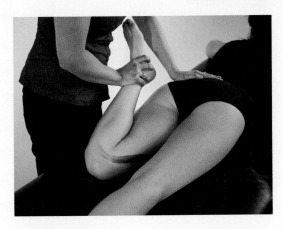

Client position

The client is lying prone.

Instruction to client

The client is instructed to take their heel to their bottom, keeping the front of the hip connected to the bed. At the end of active range, the client may use their hands to achieve additional range by taking the foot laterally and towards the bed adjacent to the pelvis. Alternatively, the examiner may perform the test.

Examiner position and notes

The examiner stands next to the bed and stabilises the hip with the proximal hand whilst taking the client's heel to bottom. At the completion of the knee flexion movement, the examiner takes the heel laterally and towards the floor. The examiner assesses for restriction and notes any reproduction of symptoms. This testing places significant pressure on the knee and hip and should be performed with caution.

KINESIO TAPING
Sartorius

STRENGTH TAPING

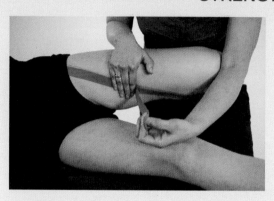

Client position

The client is in a sidelying position with the leg to be taped uppermost. The client lengthens the tissue in two stages, initially with the hip in extension for the proximal application of the tape and secondly with the knee in extension for the distal application of the tape. This assures maximal tissue stretch during the tape application for each joint that the muscle crosses and maintains a consistent tension on the tape relative to the client's maximal available range.

Measurement of tape

Measure a length of tape from the anterior superior iliac spine (ASIS) to the medial tibia. Depending on the width of the muscle, the tape may be cut into a 2.5 cm-wide strip.

Tape application

Apply the starting anchor with zero tension on the ASIS with the hip in extension and the knee flexed. Apply the base of the tape with 25–35% tension towards the middle of the thigh. Once the mid-thigh is reached, the knee is placed in extension with lateral rotation. Continue taping the muscle with 25–35% tension. Complete the taping by applying the final anchor over the medial tibia with zero tension. Rub the tape to activate the glue or instruct the client to activate the glue.

Reassessment

Reassess your client for changes in strength, tonal changes, functional changes and symptoms.

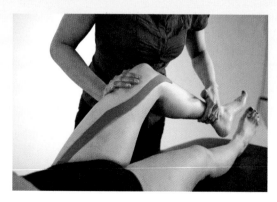

9

KINESIO TAPING
Sartorius

LENGTH TAPING

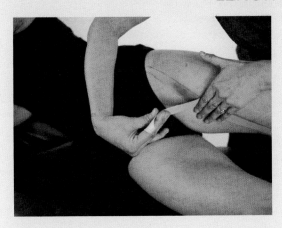

Client position

The client is in a sidelying position with the leg to be taped uppermost. The client lengthens the tissue in two stages, initially with the knee in extension for the distal application of the tape and secondly by placing the hip in extension as the proximal anchor is applied. This assures maximal tissue stretch during the tape application for each joint that the muscle crosses and maintains a consistent tension on the tape relative to the client's maximal available range.

Measurement of tape

Measure a length of tape from the anterior superior iliac spine (ASIS) to the medial tibia. Depending on the width of the muscle the tape may be cut into a 2.5 cm-wide strip.

Tape application

Apply the starting anchor with zero tension to the medial tibia with the knee in extension and lateral rotation of the lower leg. With the tissue in the lengthened position, apply the base of the tape with 15–25% tension towards the middle of the thigh. Once the mid-thigh is reached, the knee is flexed and the hip is placed in extension to maximise tissue stretch at the hip. Continue taping the muscle with 15–25% tension. Complete the taping by applying the final anchor on the ASIS with zero tension. Rub the tape to activate the glue.

9

LENGTH TAPING

Reassessment

The client is reassessed for range of movement and symptoms, and palpated for changes in tone. A restoration of length may also yield strength improvements where a strength deficit was detected prior to the taping; in these circumstances, the strength should also be reassessed. Any functional deficits can also be reassessed for changes.

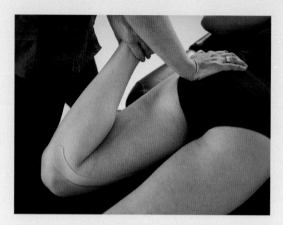

9

ANATOMY
Semitendinosus and semimembranosus

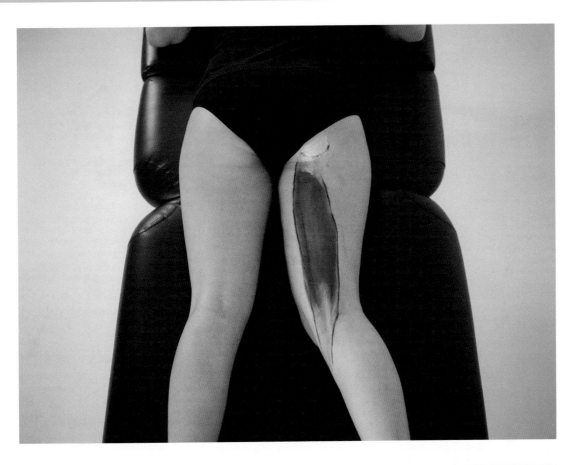

Semitendinosus

Origin:	Tuberosity of the ischium by the tendon common with the long head of the biceps femoris
Insertion:	Proximal part of the medial surface of the body of the tibia and deep fascia of the leg
Nerve supply:	Nerve root: L4, 5, S1, 2 Peripheral nerve: sciatic nerve tibial branch
Function:	Flexes and medially rotates the knee joint, extends and assists in medial rotation of the hip joint

Semimembranosus

Origin:	Tuberosity of the ischium, proximal and lateral to the biceps femoris and semitendinosus
Insertion:	Posterior medial aspect of the medial condyle of the tibia
Nerve supply:	Nerve root: L4, 5, S1, 2 Peripheral nerve: sciatic nerve tibial branch
Function:	Flexes and medially rotates the knee joint, extends and assists in medial rotation of the hip joint

9

MUSCLE TESTING
Semitendinosus and semimembranosus

STRENGTH BIAS TESTING

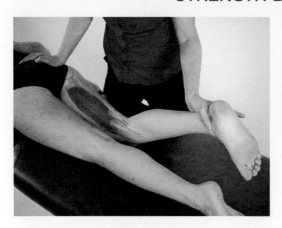 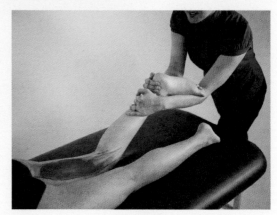

Client position

The client is lying prone with the knee flexed between 50 and 70 degrees. The tibia is then rotated medially and the rotated position is maintained during testing.

Instruction to client

The client is instructed to maintain knee flexion with medial rotation during the testing.

Examiner position and notes

The examiner stabilises the proximal hip and assesses for a hip flexion strategy. The examining hand is placed proximal to the ankle.

Alternatively, for stronger clients or smaller examiners, the examiner is positioned at the end of the bed and utilises their body weight to complete the test.

It is *not necessary* to apply resistance to the rotatory component of the test as this has been addressed with the starting testing position which the client is required to maintain. An inability to maintain the rotated position for testing indicates a positive test.

Resistance

The examiner applies a force proximal to the ankle in the direction of knee extension. This may be applied by leaning into the leg if standing to the side of the client or lunging back with body weight if standing at the end of the bed. It is unnecessary to apply resistance to the rotatory component of the test.

9

MUSCLE TESTING

Semitendinosus and semimembranosus

LENGTH BIAS TESTING

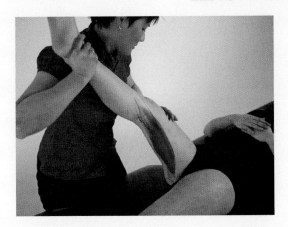 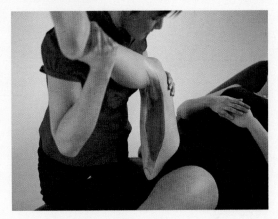

Client position

The client is lying supine with the back and pelvis in a neutral position.

Instruction to client

The client is instructed to raise the leg with the knee held in extension with slight external rotation of the tibia (foot turned out) to the maximum available range. The client is instructed to be aware of any compensatory movements and to stop when he or she is aware of utilising these. Compensatory movements are those not occurring at the joint being tested (the hip in this case); these can include, but are not limited to: lumbar flexion, external rotation of the contralateral leg, bracing through the upper body, knee flexion.

Alternatively, the hip is taken to 90 degrees of flexion by either the examiner or client. The knee is then extended and evaluated for knee extension range.

Examiner position and notes

The examiner maintains the knee extension whilst taking the leg into hip flexion range, noting for any compensatory strategies which would indicate when to stop testing, and the range available to the client before a compromise in strategy.

Alternative testing: The proximal thigh is stabilised by the examiner as the knee is taken into extension. The examiner assesses for restriction and compensation strategies which would indicate the available range had been reached without a compromise in technique.

9

KINESIO TAPING
Semitendinosus and semimembranosus

STRENGTH TAPING

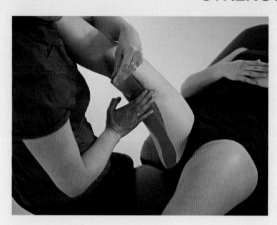

Client position

The client is lying supine for the tape application. For the proximal application, the hip is in full hip flexion and the knee relaxed. For the distal application of tape, the knee is taken to full extension with lateral tibial rotation and with the hip in a slightly flexed position. The two-stage tape application assures maximal tissue stretch during the tape application for each joint that the muscle crosses, and maintains a consistent tension on the tape relative to the client's maximal available range.

Measurement of tape

Measure a length of tape from the ischium to the medial tibia whilst in the length testing position.

Tape application

Apply the starting anchor at the ischium with zero tension. Place the tissue in a lengthened position by taking the knee to the chest with the knee flexed. Apply the tape with 25–35% tension over the proximal ½ of the posterior thigh. For the distal thigh, place the tissue in a lengthened position by allowing the knee to move away from the chest in order to achieve full knee extension with lateral rotation of the leg. Continue to apply the tape with 25–35% tension for the remaining distal ½ of the posterior thigh. Complete the taping by applying the final anchor with zero tension over the medial tibia. Rub the tape to activate the glue or instruct the client to activate the glue.

9

STRENGTH TAPING

Reassessment

Reassess your client for changes in strength, tonal changes, functional changes and symptoms.

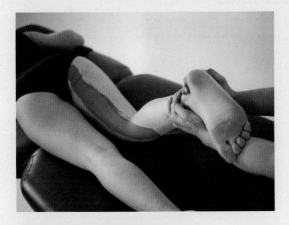

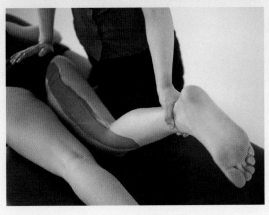

KINESIO TAPING
Semitendinosus and semimembranosus

LENGTH TAPING

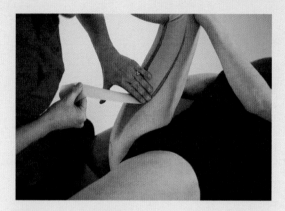

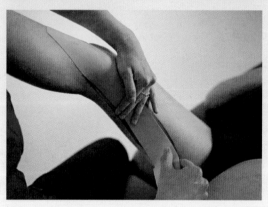

Client position

The client is lying supine for the tape application. For the proximal application, the hip is in full hip flexion and the knee relaxed. For the distal application of tape, the knee is taken to full extension with lateral tibial rotation and with the hip in a slightly flexed position. The two-stage tape application assures maximal tissue stretch during the tape application for each joint that the muscle crosses, and maintains a consistent tension on the tape relative to the client's maximal available range.

Measurement of tape

Measure a length of tape from the medial tibia to the ischium, taking care to measure the length component of the hip and the knee separately.

Tape application

Apply the starting anchor with zero tension on the medial tibia with the knee in extension and tibial lateral rotation. Apply the base of the tape with 15–25% tension over the belly of the muscle towards the posterior mid-thigh. Once the mid-thigh is reached, allow the knee to flex and then fully flex the hip. The client may assist this by holding the knee towards the chest. Continue applying the tape with 15–25% tension over the remaining proximal muscle Complete the taping by applying the final anchor over the ischium with zero tension. Rub the tape to activate the glue.

9

LENGTH TAPING

Reassessment

The client is reassessed for range of movement and symptoms, and palpated for changes in tone. A restoration of length may also yield strength improvements where a strength deficit was detected prior to the taping; in these circumstances, the strength should also be reassessed. Any functional deficits can also be reassessed for changes.

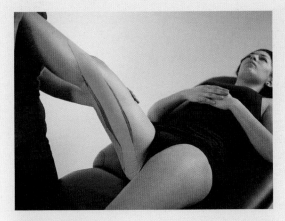

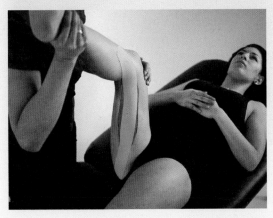

ANATOMY
Biceps femoris

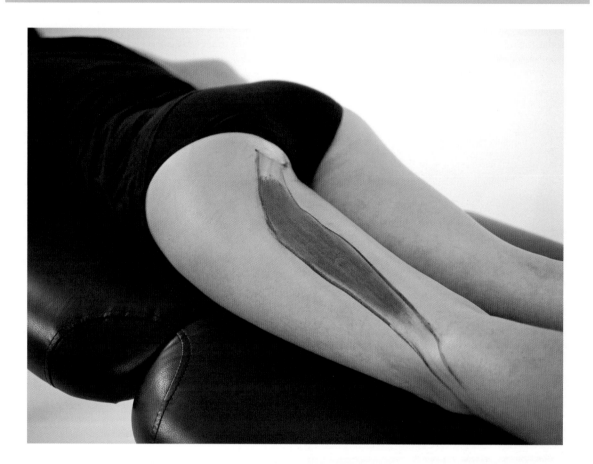

Biceps femoris

Origin:	Long head: distal part of the sacrotuberous ligament and posterior part of the ischial tuberosity Short head: lateral lip of the linea aspera, proximal ⅔ of the surpacondylar line and lateral intermuscular septum
Insertion:	Lateral side of the head of the fibula, lateral condyle of the tibia, deep fascia on the lateral side of the leg
Nerve supply:	**Long head** Nerve root: L5, S1, 2, 3 Peripheral nerve: sciatic nerve, tibial branch **Short head** Nerve root: L5, S1, 2 Peripheral nerve: sciatic nerve, peroneal branch
Function:	Both long and short heads flex and laterally rotate the knee joint. In addition, the long head extends and assists in lateral rotation of the hip joint

9

MUSCLE TESTING
Biceps femoris

STRENGTH BIAS TESTING

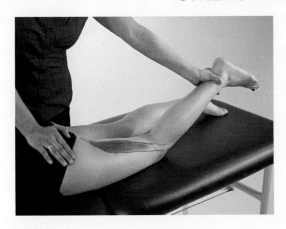 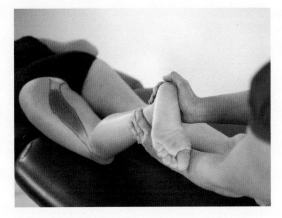

Client position
The client is lying prone with the knee flexed between 50 and 70 degrees, the tibia is then rotated laterally and the rotated position is maintained during testing.

Instruction to client
The client is instructed to maintain knee flexion with lateral rotation during the testing.

Examiner position and notes
The examiner stabilises the proximal hip and assesses for a hip flexion strategy. The examining hand is placed proximal to the ankle.

Alternatively, for stronger clients or smaller examiners, the examiner is positioned at the end of the bed and utilises their body weight to complete the test.

Resistance
The examiner applies a force proximal to the ankle in the direction of knee extension. This may be applied by leaning into the leg if standing to the side of the client or lunging back with body weight if standing at the end of the bed. It is unnecessary to apply resistance to the rotatory component of the test.

MUSCLE TESTING
Biceps femoris

LENGTH BIAS TESTING

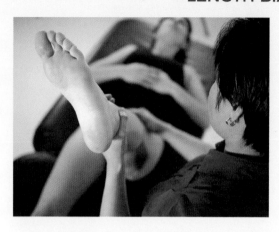 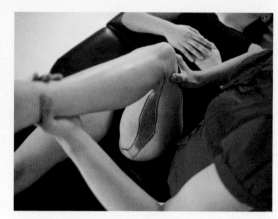

Client position

The client is lying supine with the back and pelvis in a neutral position.

Instruction to client

The client is instructed to raise the leg with the knee held in extension with slight internal rotation of the tibia (foot turned in) to the maximum available range. The client is instructed to be aware of any compensatory movements and to stop when he or she is aware of utilising these. Compensatory movements are those not occurring at the joint being tested (the hip in this case); these can include, but are not limited to: lumbar flexion, external rotation of the contralateral leg, bracing through the upper body, knee flexion.

Alternatively, the hip is taken to 90 degrees of flexion by either the examiner or client. The knee is then extended and evaluated for knee extension range.

Examiner position and notes

The examiner maintains the knee extension whilst taking the leg into hip flexion range, noting for any compensatory strategies which would indicate when to stop testing, and the range available to the client before a compromise in strategy.

Alternative testing: The proximal thigh is stabilised by the examiner as the knee is taken into extension. The examiner assesses for restriction and compensation strategies which would indicate the available range had been reached without a compromise in technique.

9

KINESIO TAPING
Biceps femoris

STRENGTH TAPING

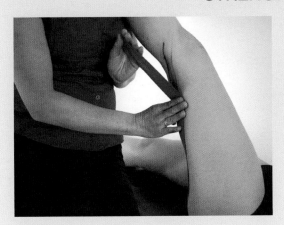

Client position

The client is lying supine for the tape application. For the proximal application, the hip is in full hip flexion and the knee relaxed. For the distal application of tape, the knee is taken to full extension with medial tibial rotation and with the hip in a slightly flexed position.

The two-stage tape application assures maximal tissue stretch during the tape application for each joint that the muscle crosses and maintains a consistent tension on the tape relative to the client's maximal available range.

Measurement of tape

Measure a length of tape from the ischium to the lateral tibia whilst in the length testing position.

Tape application

Apply the starting anchor at the ischium with zero tension. Place the tissue in a lengthened position by taking the knee to the chest with the knee flexed. Apply the tape with 25–35% tension over the proximal ½ of the posterior thigh. For the distal thigh, place the tissue in a lengthened position by allowing the knee to move away from the chest in order to achieve full knee extension with internal rotation of the lower limb. Continue to apply the tape with 25–35% tension for the remaining distal ½ of the posterior thigh. Complete the taping by applying the final anchor with zero tension over the lateral tibia. Rub the tape to activate the glue.

Reassessment

Reassess your client for changes in strength, tonal changes, functional changes and symptoms.

9

KINESIO TAPING
Biceps femoris

LENGTH TAPING

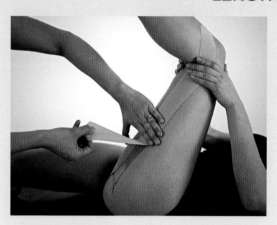

Client position

The client is lying supine for the tape application. For the proximal application, the hip is in full hip flexion and the knee relaxed. For the distal application of tape, the knee is taken to full extension with medial tibial rotation and with the hip in a slightly flexed position. The two-stage tape application assures maximal tissue stretch during the tape application for each joint that the muscle crosses and maintains a consistent tension on the tape relative to the client's maximal available range.

Measurement of tape

Measure a length of tape from the lateral tibia to the ischium, taking care to measure the length component of the hip and the knee separately.

Tape application

Apply the starting anchor at the lateral tibia with zero tension. Place the knee in the extended and internally rotated position to place the distal thigh tissue on stretch whilst the tape is applied with 15–25% tension over the distal ½ of the thigh. For tape placement higher than this, allow the knee to flex in order to take the hip into maximal hip flexion and apply the remaining base with 15–25% tension. Complete the taping by applying the final anchor with zero tension over the ischium. Rub the tape to activate the glue.

9

LENGTH TAPING

Reassessment

The client is reassessed for range of movement and symptoms, and palpated for changes in tone. A restoration of length may also yield strength improvements where a strength deficit was detected prior to the taping; in these circumstances, the strength should also be reassessed. Any functional deficits can also be reassessed for changes.

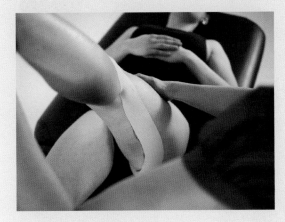
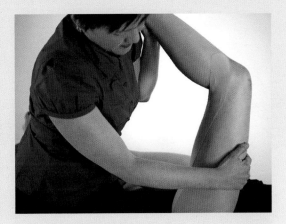

ANATOMY
Gracilis

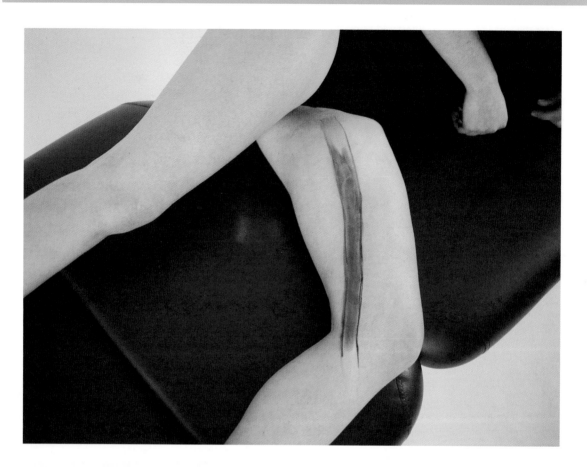

Gracilis	
Origin:	Ischiopubic ramus
Insertion:	Medial tibia distal to the condyle (pes anserinus)
Nerve supply:	Nerve root: L2, 3, 4 Peripheral nerve: anterior branch of obturator nerve
Function:	Adducts, flexes and medially rotates the knee; adducts the hip

9

MUSCLE TESTING
Gracilis

STRENGTH BIAS TESTING

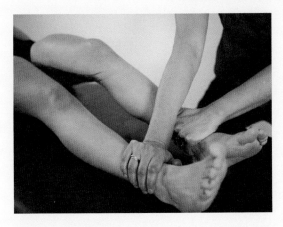

Client position
The client is lying supine with the leg to be tested in slight knee flexion and internal rotation of the tibia. The ankle is then taken towards the midline adjacent to the contralateral ankle.

Instruction to client
The client is instructed to keep the legs together whilst the examiner applies a force to attempt to separate the legs.

Examiner position and notes
The examiner stands to the side of the client and holds the legs above the ankle whilst standing in a stable lunge or squat position.

Resistance
The examiner applies a force at the ankle in the direction of abduction away from the opposite ankle.

9

MUSCLE TESTING
Gracilis

LENGTH BIAS TESTING

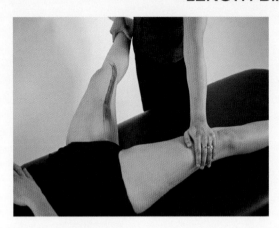

Client position

The client is lying supine with the hip and pelvis in a neutral position and the knee extended with lateral tibial rotation.

Instruction to client

The client is instructed to allow their leg to be taken out to the side as far as possible whilst keeping the knee extended and the pelvic position maintained.

Examiner position and notes

The examiner supports the leg in the horizontal plane and facilitates the abduction of the leg. The other hand may be used to stabilise the opposite lower limb. The leg is placed in lateral tibial rotation prior to the abduction. The examiner stops when a compensatory movement in the hip is noted or there is countermovement in the opposite leg.

9

KINESIO TAPING
Gracilis

STRENGTH TAPING

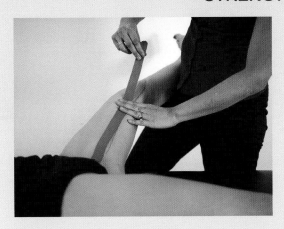

Client position

The client is lying supine with the hip in abduction, lateral rotation and flexion resting against a wall, the examiner's side or with the assistance of a belt around the foot.

Measurement of tape

Measure a length of tape from the ischiopubic ramus to the medial proximal tibia. Depending on the size of the muscle, the tape may be cut down its length to create a 2.5 cm-wide strip.

Tape application

Apply the starting anchor with zero tension as close to the ischiopubic ramus as possible. Apply the base of the tape with 25–35% tension towards the pes anserine on the proximal medial tibia. Complete the taping by applying the final anchor on the tibia with zero tension. Rub the tape to activate the glue or instruct the client to activate the glue.

Reassessment

Reassess your client for changes in strength, tonal changes, functional changes and symptoms.

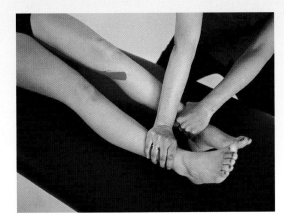

9

KINESIO TAPING
Gracilis

LENGTH TAPING

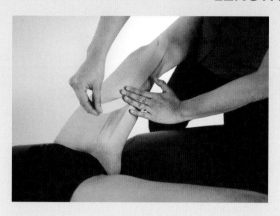

Client position

The client is lying supine with the hip in abduction, lateral rotation and flexion resting against a wall, the examiner's side or with the assistance of a belt around the foot.

Measurement of tape

Measure a length of tape from the ischiopubic ramus to the medial proximal tibia. Cut the tape into a 2.5 cm-wide strip if the client is smaller in size.

Tape application

Apply the starting anchor with zero tension over the pes anserine at the medial tibia. With the tissue in the lengthened position, apply the base of the tape with 15–25% tension towards the ischiopubic ramus. Complete the taping by applying the final anchor as close as possible to the ischiopubic ramus with zero tension. Rub the tape to activate the glue.

Reassessment

The client is reassessed for range of movement, symptoms and palpated for changes in tone. A restoration of length may also yield strength improvements where a strength deficit was detected prior to the taping; in these circumstances, the strength should also be reassessed. Any functional deficits can also be reassessed for changes.

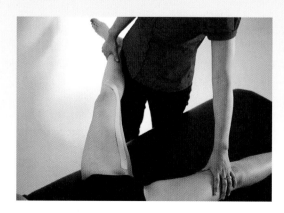

9

KNEE ASSESSMENT SHEET

Clinic: .... Date: ....

Client name: ....

Functional review

Functional limitation	Pre-test measure	Post-test measure

Muscle testing

Tested priority	Muscle	Strength		Length		Comments
		Right	Left	Right	Left	
	Popliteus					
	Rectus femoris					
	Vastus lateralis					
	Vastus medialis					
	Sartorius					
	Semitendinosus					
	Semimembranosus					
	Biceps femoris					
	Gracilis					

Treatment

Intervention	Re-test measures	Plan

Practitioner: .... Signature: ....

BIBLIOGRAPHY

Berryman Reese, N. M. (2012). *Muscle and sensory testing*. Missouri: Elsevier-Saunders.

Berryman Reese, N., & Bandy, W. D. (2010). *Joint range of motion and muscle length testing*. Missouri: Saunders Elsevier.

Calais-Germain, B. (1993). *Anatomy of movement* (12 ed.). Seattle: Eastland Press.

Comerford, M., & Mottram, S. (2012). *Kinetic control: the management of uncontrolled movement*. Sydney, Australia: Elsevier.

Kase, K., Hashimoto, T., & Okane, T. (1998). *Kinesio Taping perfect manual: amazing taping therapy to eliminate pain and muscle disorders*. Albuquerque: Kinesio Taping Association.

Kase, K., & Rock Stockheimer, K. (2006). *Kinesio Taping for lymphoedema and chronic swelling*. Albuquerque: Kinesio Taping Association.

Kase, K., Wallis, J., & Kase, T. (2003). *Clinical therapeutic applications of the Kinesio taping methods*. Albuquerque: Kinesio Taping Association.

Kendall, F. P., McCreary, E., Provance, P., Rodgers, M., & Romanic, W. (2005). *Muscles: testing and function with posture and pain*. Baltimore: Lippincott Williams Wilkins.

Standring, S., Borely, N., Collings, P., Crossman, A., Gatzoulis, M., Healy, J., ... Wigley, C. (2008). *Gray's anatomy: the anatomical basis of clinical practice* (S. Susan Ed. 40 ed.). London, United Kingdom: Churchill Livingstone Elsevier.

9

Techniques for testing and taping the ankle

Gastrocnemius

Soleus

Tibialis posterior

Tibialis anterior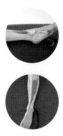

Extensor digitorum

Peroneus longus and peroneus brevis

ANATOMY
Gastrocnemius

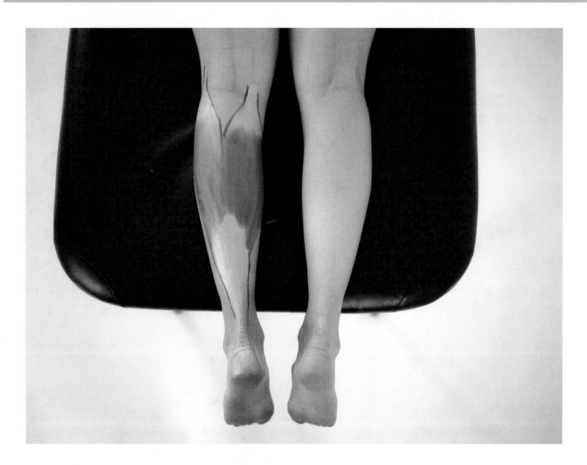

Gastrocnemius

Origin:	Medial condyle of the femur and adjacent popliteal surface Lateral condyle of the femur
Insertion:	Posterior surface of the calcaneus via the Achilles tendon
Nerve supply:	Nerve root: S1, S2 Peripheral nerve: tibial
Function:	Plantarflexion of the ankle and flexion of the knee

10

MUSCLE TESTING
Gastrocnemius

STRENGTH BIAS TESTING

Client position
The client is instructed to single-leg stand on the lower limb to be examined. The client may stand adjacent to a table or wall for balance if required, but be instructed not to use it for direct support.

Instruction to the client
The client is instructed to raise onto their toes with the knee fully extended. After the initial lift, testing can be based on repetitions or time to hold.

Examiner position and notes
The examiner is positioned to assess for height and quality of the movement. Whilst the testing is one of strength and not balance and proprioception, the Kinesio Taping intervention will aim to address the quality of movement control. The examiner should note the amount of effort and pain to produce the desired movement as well as the amount of completed repetitions or time to hold.

The client repeats the action until fatigued or until stopped by the examiner. A loss of height after a few repetitions when compared to the other side may indicate a positive test. The repetition required may be dependent on the load required by the client for function and training. Alternatively, a time-to-hold test may be appropriate for clients requiring endurance in the contracted position.

The client's history and symptoms may yield important information that may save on taping both medial and lateral heads. If the examiner is still unclear from the history and testing, both medial and lateral heads should be taped if the testing is positive.

Resistance
The client's body weight is used as a functional resistance. Repetitions of the task can provide a score for improvement or time held in the contracted position.

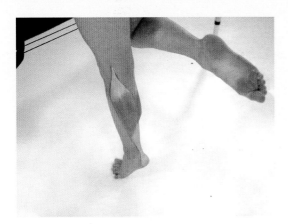

MUSCLE TESTING
Gastrocnemius

LENGTH BIAS TESTING A

Client position
The client is prone with the knee extended and the ankle when off the bed.

Instruction to client
The client is instructed to take their toes towards their head with the knee extended.

Examiner position and notes
The examiner may apply overpressure to the foot short of pain or discomfort and note the available range comparing both ankles. To bias the length testing towards the medial gastroc, the examiner may move the calcaneum into pronation. Alternatively to bias the testing to implicate a shortness of the lateral gastroc, the calcaneum can be moved into supination. Additional palpatory information can also be used to determine the best fibers for intervention.

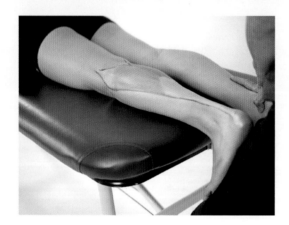

10

LENGTH BIAS TESTING B

Client position

The client stands in a lunge position with arms resting outstretched at the wall or a support and the torso vertical.

Instruction to client

The client is instructed to move the back foot back away from the wall whilst maintaining the heel on the floor, with the knee straight and the foot pointing forward.

Examiner position and notes

The ankle range being assessed is of the rear foot. This test uses the client's body weight as overpressure. A goniometer can be used to assess the angle achieved by the ankle.

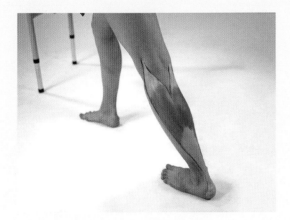

KINESIO TAPING
Gastrocnemius

STRENGTH TAPING

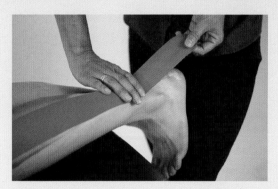

Client position

The client is lying in prone with the knee extended and the ankle and foot resting off the bed.

Measurement of tape

The client dorsiflexes the foot and a length of tape is measured from the sole of the foot under the calcaneus bone to the gastroc insertion onto the femoral condyle. The tape can be used as an I-strip to cover just the medial or lateral gastrocnemius (lateral shown).

When a practitioner is in doubt as to how long to make a piece of tape, it is recommended to err on the side of excess length as muscles operate in units and additional length of tape can provide beneficial stimulus to adjacent muscles.

Tape application

Apply the anchor on the medial OR lateral femoral condyle with zero tension. Dorsiflex the foot and apply the tape with 25–35% tension onto the target tissue. Complete the taping by placing the anchor onto the calcaneus with zero tension. Rub the tape to activate the glue.

Taping for the lateral gastrocnemius is shown. A second application over the medial head may also be appropriate if determined by the assessment.

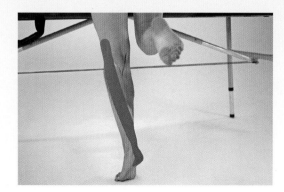

10

Reassessment

Reassess your client for changes in strength, tonal changes, functional changes and symptoms.

KINESIO TAPING
Gastrocnemius

LENGTH TAPING

Client position
The client is prone with the knee extended and the ankle and foot resting off the bed.

Measurement of tape
The client dorsiflexes the foot and a length of tape is measured from the sole of the foot under the calcaneus bone to the gastroc insertion onto the femoral condyle. The tape can be used as an I-strip to cover just the medial or lateral gastrocnemius (lateral shown) OR cut into a Y-strip to divide at the Achilles tendon so as to anchor on each condyle.

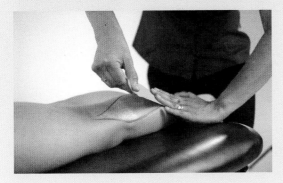

Tape application
Apply the anchor with zero tension on the calcaneus.

Apply dorsiflexion to the foot with the knee in extension and apply the tape with 15–25% tension over the gastrocnemius muscle. Pay close attention to covering areas with particularly tight bands of tissue that need to be relaxed. Complete the taping by placing the anchors with no tension onto the femoral condyle. Rub the tape to activate the glue.

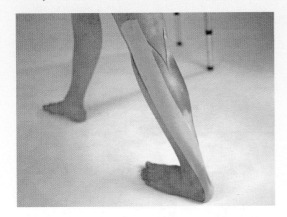

Reassessment
Reassess your client for changes in length, tonal change, function and reported symptoms.

Reassess your client for changes in strength.

ANATOMY
Soleus

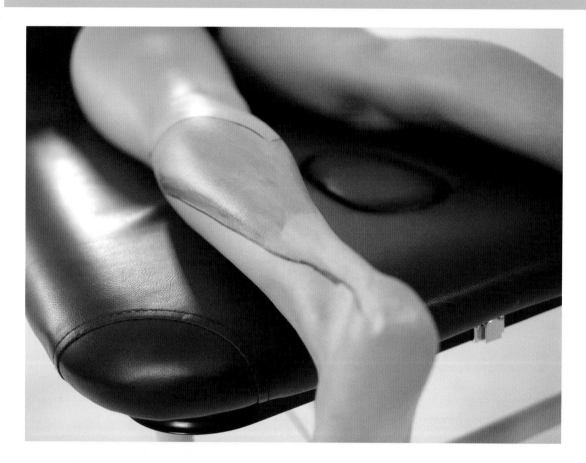

Soleus

Origin:	Posterior surface of the head of fibula, proximal ⅓ of the body of the fibula, soleal line and middle third of the medial border of the tibia
Insertion:	Posterior surface of the calcaneus via the Achilles tendon
Nerve supply:	Nerve root: S1, S2 Peripheral nerve: tibial
Function:	Plantarflexion of the ankle

10

MUSCLE TESTING
Soleus

STRENGTH BIAS TESTING

Client position

The client is in single-leg standing with the knee flexed maximally whilst still maintaining heel contact to the floor. The client may stand adjacent to a table or wall for balance if required, but be instructed not to use it for direct support.

Instruction to client

The client is instructed to raise onto their toes with the knee flexion maintained, to the full available range. After the initial lift, testing can be based on repetitions or time of hold.

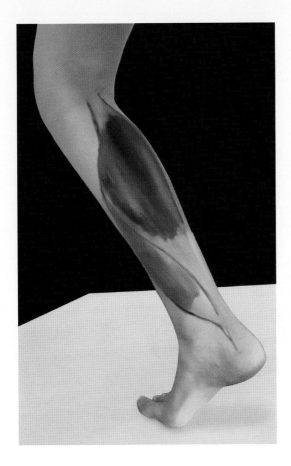

Examiner position and notes

The examiner is positioned to assess for height and quality of the movement. Whilst the testing is one of strength and not balance and proprioception, the Kinesio Taping intervention will aim to address the quality of movement control. The examiner should note the amount of effort and pain to produce the desired movement as well as the amount of completed repetitions or time of hold.

10

STRENGTH BIAS TESTING

The client repeats the action until fatigue or until stopped by the examiner. A loss of height after a few repetitions when compared to the other side may indicate a positive test. The repetition required may be dependent on the load required by the client for function and training. Alternatively, a time-of-hold test may be appropriate for clients requiring endurance in the contracted position.

The client's history and symptoms may yield important information that may save on taping both medial and lateral heads. If the examiner is still unclear from the history and testing, both medial and lateral heads should be taped if the testing is positive.

Resistance

The client's body weight is used as a functional resistance. Repetitions of the task can provide a score for improvement or time held in the contracted position.

10

MUSCLE TESTING
Soleus

LENGTH BIAS TESTING A

Client position
The client stands with the weight primarily on the lower limb to be examined with the knee flexed.

Instruction to client
With the knee maintained on the wall, the client is instructed to move the foot away from the wall whilst maintaining heel contact to the floor.

Examiner position and notes
A measuring tape can be used to measure the distance from the first toe to the wall. The greater the distance from the toe to the wall, the greater the flexibility/length of the tissue. This test uses the client's body weight as overpressure. A goniometer can also be used to assess the angle achieved by the ankle.

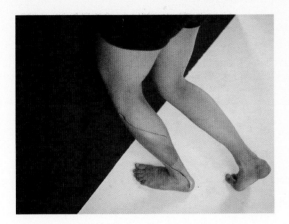

LENGTH BIAS TESTING B

Client position
The client is prone with the knee flexed to 90 degrees (see photo for Length Taping for client position).

Instruction to client
The client is instructed to turn the toes down towards the bed whilst keeping the knee flexed.

Examiner position and notes
The examiner applies overpressure in the direction of dorsiflexion and notes the ROM comparing both feet.

10

KINESIO TAPING
Soleus

STRENGTH TAPING

Client position

The client is lying prone with the foot resting over the edge of the bed. The practitioner flexes the client's knee and maintains the dorsiflexion position by applying force through the ball of the foot. The practitioner can use their thigh or torso to help maintain this position.

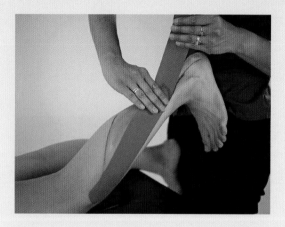

Measurement of tape

The client dorsiflexes the foot and a length of tape is measured from the sole of the foot under the calcaneus bone to the origin at the fibula (lateral) or tibia (medial).

When a practitioner is in doubt as to how long to make a piece of tape, it is recommended to err on the side of excess length as muscles operate in units and additional length of tape can provide beneficial stimulus to adjacent muscles.

Tape application

Apply the anchor on the origin at the fibula or tibia with zero tension (fibula origin is shown). Dorsiflex the foot and apply the tape with 25–35% tension onto the target tissue. Complete the taping by placing the anchor onto the calcaneus with zero tension. Rub the tape to activate the glue.

10

STRENGTH TAPING

Taping for the lateral soleus is shown. A second application over the medial head may also be appropriate if determined by the assessment.

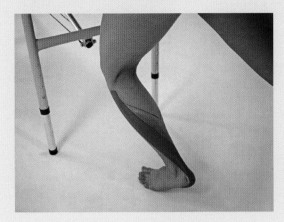

Reassessment

Reassess your client for changes in strength, tonal changes, functional changes and symptoms.

KINESIO TAPING
Soleus

LENGTH TAPING

Client position

The client is lying prone with the knee extended and the ankle and foot resting in dorsiflexion on the bed or against the practitioner's thigh or torso.

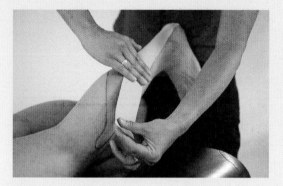

Measurement of tape

The client dorsiflexes the foot and a length of tape is measured from the sole of the foot under the calcaneus bone to the origin at the fibula (lateral) or tibia (medial). Alternatively, the tape can be cut into a Y-strip to divide at the Achilles so as to anchor on either side of the gastrocnemius belly.

Tape application

Apply the anchor with zero tension on the calcaneus. With the foot in dorsiflexion, apply the tape with 15–25% tension over the soleus muscle. Pay close attention to covering areas with particularly tight bands of tissue that need to be relaxed. Complete the taping by placing the anchors with zero tension onto the origin at the fibula or tibia. Rub the tape to activate the glue.

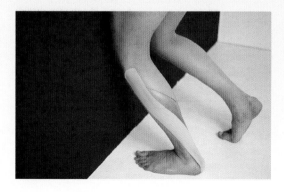

Reassessment

Reassess your client for changes in length, tonal change, function and reported symptoms.

Reassess your client for changes in strength.

10

ANANTOMY

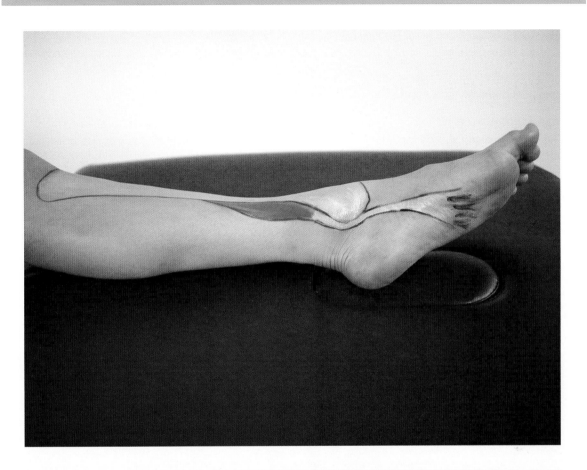

Tibialis posterior

Origin:	Posterior aspect of the interosseous membrane, posterior surface of the body of the tibia, proximal ⅔ of the medial surface of the fibula
Insertion:	Tuberosity of the navicular bone, cuboid bone, all three cuneiform bones, base of the metatarsals 2–4
Nerve supply:	Nerve root: L5, S1 Peripheral nerve: tibial branch
Function:	Inversion of the foot at the subtalar joint, plantarflexion of the foot at the ankle

MUSCLE TESTING
Tibialis posterior

STRENGTH BIAS TESTING

Client position

The client is in a sitting or supine position with the ankle resting beyond the edge of the bed.

Instruction to client

The client is instructed to plantarflex and invert the foot through the full available range of motion; pointing foot down and in.

Examiner position and notes

The examiner is positioned lateral to the ankle tested, in the opposite diagonal to the direction of the foot. They stabilise the ankle with their upper hand and using their lower hand to apply a resistance over the medial and dorsal foot in the direction of eversion and dorsiflexion. The examiner should stand in a lunge position and keep the testing arm outstretched.

Resistance

The examiner applies the resistance by dropping the body weight back onto the back leg. By keeping the arm outstretched, the examiner will be using their full body weight to test rather than just their arm muscles.

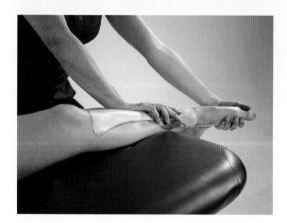

MUSCLE TESTING
Tibialis posterior

LENGTH BIAS TESTING

Client position
The client is in a sitting or supine position with the ankle resting beyond the edge of the bed.

Instruction to client
The client is instructed to dorsiflex and evert the foot to the maximum available range; pointing foot up and out.

Examiner position and notes
The examiner should note the amount of effort and whether there are symptoms provoked in order to produce the desired movement. The range and movement strategy should be compared to the non-affected limb. The examiner applies overpressure at the end of range to compare active to passive range as well as to assess for end feel.

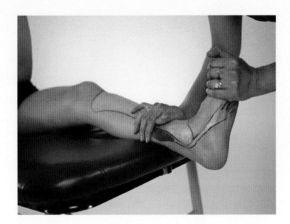

KINESIO TAPING
Tibialis posterior

STRENGTH TAPING

Client position

The client is in a sitting or supine position with the knee extended and the ankle and foot resting off the bed.

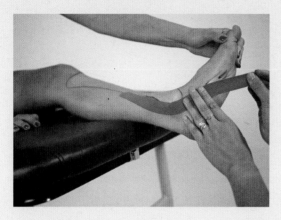

Measurement of tape

The client dorsiflexes and everts the foot. Measure a length of tape from the distal ⅓ of the medial tibia under the foot and onto the dorsal surface of the base of the fifth metatarsal.

Tape application

Apply the anchor with zero tension on the distal ⅓ to ½ of the tibia. Dorsiflex and evert the foot and apply the tape with 25–35% tension onto the target tissue. Complete the taping by placing the anchor onto the dorsal foot over the fifth metatarsal with zero tension. Rub the tape to activate the glue.

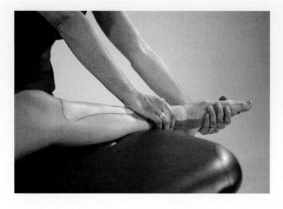

Reassessment

Reassess your client for changes in strength, tonal changes, functional changes and symptoms.

KINESIO TAPING
Tibialis posterior

LENGTH TAPING

Client position

The client is in a sitting or supine position with the knee extended and the ankle and foot resting off the bed.

Measurement of tape

The client dorsiflexes and everts the foot. Measure a length of tape from the lateral foot, under the foot and up to the medial tibia. The muscle is palpable in the distal ⅓ of the medial tibia before being covered by other muscles as it travels deep and posterior.

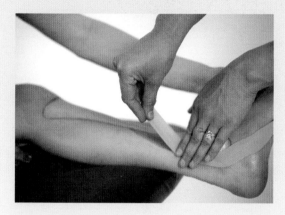

Tape application

Apply the anchor with zero tension on the dorsum of the fifth metatarsal. Apply dorsiflexion and eversion to the foot with the knee in extension and apply the tape with 15–25% tension over the tibialis posterior muscle. Complete the taping by placing the anchor with zero tension onto the tibia. Rub the tape to activate the glue.

Note: Whilst the muscle inserts onto the plantar surface of the foot, there is greater mechanical leverage when the tape is anchored around on to the lateral foot. Additionally, this assists with maintaining the tape on the foot for longer periods.

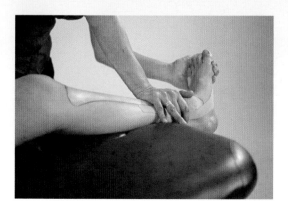

10

LENGTH TAPING

Reassessment

Reassess your client for changes in length, tonal change, function and reported symptoms.

Reassess your client for changes in strength.

ANATOMY
Tibialis anterior

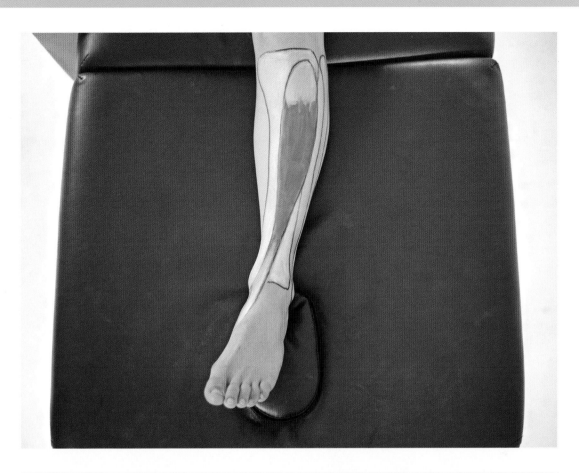

Tibialis anterior

Origin:	Lateral condyle and upper ⅔ of the lateral surface of the body of the tibia, interosseous membrane and deep crural fascia
Insertion:	Base of the first metatarsal, medial and plantar surfaces of the medial cuneiform bone
Nerve supply:	Nerve root: L4, L5, S1 Peripheral nerve: deep peroneal nerve
Function:	Dorsiflexion of the foot at the ankle, inversion of the foot at the subtalar and midtarsal joints

10

MUSCLE TESTING
Tibialis anterior

STRENGTH BIAS TESTING

Client position

The client is in a sitting or supine position with the ankle resting beyond the edge of the bed.

Instruction to client

The client is instructed to dorsiflex and invert the foot through the full available range of motion; pointing the foot up and in.

Examiner position and notes

The examiner is positioned lateral to the ankle tested, in the opposite diagonal to the direction of the foot. They stabilise the ankle with the upper hand and using the other hand apply a resistance over the medial and dorsal foot in the direction of plantarflexion and eversion. The examiner should stand in a lunge position and keep the testing arm outstretched. The examiner should attempt to shift their body weight backwards for the testing rather than strain through the upper limb.

Resistance

The examiner applies the resistance by dropping their body weight onto their back leg. By keeping their arm outstretched, the examiner will be using their full body weight to test rather than just their arm muscles

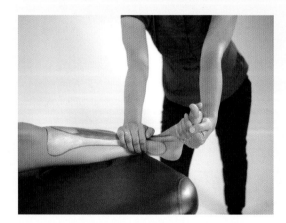

MUSCLE TESTING
Tibialis anterior

LENGTH BIAS TESTING

Client position
The client is in a sitting or supine position with the ankle resting beyond the edge of the bed.

Instruction to client
The client is instructed to plantarflex and evert the foot to the maximum available range; pointing the foot down and out.

Examiner position and notes
The examiner should note the amount of effort and whether there are symptoms provoked in order to produce the desired movement. The range and movement strategy should be compared to the non-affected limb. The examiner applies overpressure at the end of range to compare active to passive range as well as assess for end feel.

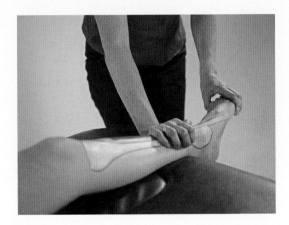

KINESIO TAPING
Tibialis anterior

STRENGTH TAPING

Client position

The client is in a supine position with the knee extended and the ankle and foot resting off the bed.

Measurement of tape

The client plantarflexes and everts the foot and a length of tape is measured from the first metatarsal up to the tibial condyle. Alternatively, the tape can be measured around the lateral foot, under the sole of the foot and up to the tibial condyle. The tape can last longer on the body with the longer anchor to the lateral foot.

When a practitioner is in doubt as to how long to make a piece of tape, it is recommended to err on the side of excess length as muscles operate in units and additional length of tape can provide beneficial stimulus to adjacent muscles.

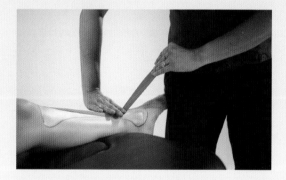

Tape application

Apply the anchor on the lateral tibial condyle with zero tension. Plantarflex and evert the foot, apply the tape with 25–35% tension onto the target tissue. Complete the taping by placing the anchor onto the first metatarsal or lateral foot with zero tension. Rub the tape to activate the glue.

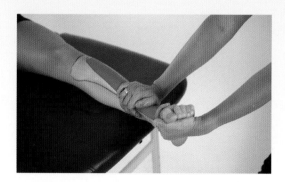

10

Reassessment

Reassess your client for change in strength, tonal changes, functional changes and symptoms.

KINESIO TAPING
Tibialis anterior

LENGTH TAPING

Client position
The client is in a supine position with the ankle and foot resting off the bed.

Measurement of tape
The client plantarflexes and everts the foot and the practitioner measures a length of tape from the first metatarsal to the tibial condyle.

Alternatively, the tape can be measured around the lateral foot, under the sole of the foot and up to the tibial condyle. The tape can last longer on the body by extending the anchor around to the lateral foot.

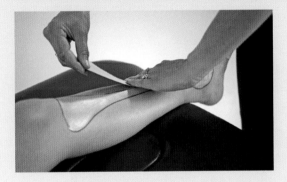

Tape application
Apply the anchor with no tension on the first metatarsal or the lateral border of the foot depending on your measurement. Apply plantarflexion and eversion to the foot with the knee in extension and apply the tape with 15–25% tension over the tibialis anterior muscle, paying close attention to covering areas with particularly tight bands of tissue that need to be relaxed. Complete the taping by placing the anchors with no tension onto the lateral tibial condyle. Rub the tape to activate the glue.

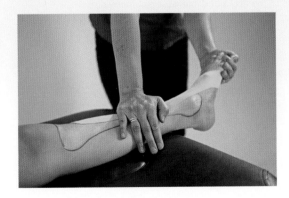

Reassessment
Reassess your client for changes in length, tonal change, function and reported symptoms.

Reassess your client for changes in strength.

10

ANATOMY
Extensor digitorum

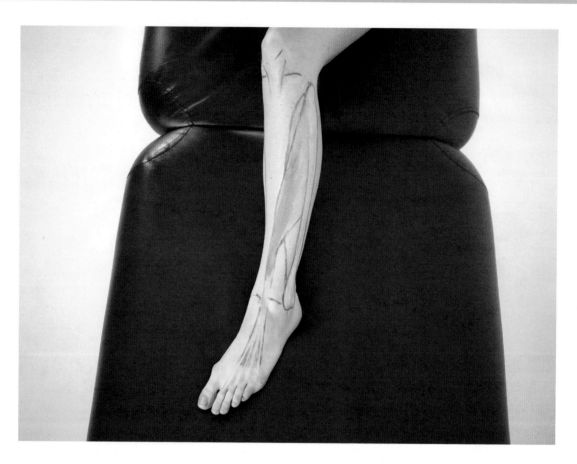

Extensor digitorum	
Origin:	Lateral tibial condyle, anterior surface of the fibula and interosseous membrane
Insertion:	Dorsum of the middle and distal phalanges
Nerve supply:	Nerve root: L4, L5, S1 Peripheral nerve: deep peroneal nerve
Function:	Extension at the metatarsal phalangeal joints of the lateral four toes

10

MUSCLE TESTING
Extensor digitorum

STRENGTH BIAS TESTING

Client position

The client is in a sitting or supine position with the ankle in dorsiflexion and eversion resting beyond the edge of the bed.

Instruction to client

The client is instructed to dorsiflex and evert the foot to the full available range of motion; pointing the foot up and out.

Examiner position and notes

The examiner is positioned in a lunge position standing medial to the ankle and in the opposite direction to the testing position of the foot. The examiner's upper hand should stabilise above the ankle whilst the lower hand applies resistance to the dorsal foot in the direction of plantarflexion and inversion.

Resistance

The examiner applies the resistance by dropping their body weight onto their back leg. By keeping their arm outstretched, the examiner will be using their full body weight to test rather than just their arm muscles.

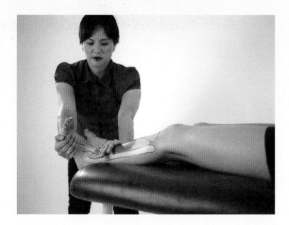

MUSCLE TESTING
Extensor digitorum

LENGTH BIAS TESTING

Client position
The client is in a sitting or supine position with the ankle resting beyond the edge of the bed.

Instruction to client
The client is instructed to plantarflex and invert the foot to the maximum available range; pointing the foot down and in.

Examiner position and notes
The examiner should note the amount of effort and whether there are symptoms provoked in order to produce the desired movement. The range and movement strategy should be compared to the non-affected limb. The examiner applies overpressure at the end of range to compare active to passive range as well as assess for end feel.

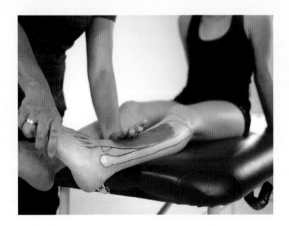

KINESIO TAPING
Extensor digitorum

STRENGTH TAPING

Client position

The client is in a sitting or supine position with the foot resting off the bed.

Measurement of tape

The client plantarflexes and inverts the foot and a length of tape is measured from the lateral tibial condyle to the dorsum of the foot. A fan cut to cover the various tendon attachments of the extensor digitorum may be beneficial in situations where foot conditions exist in addition to the positive ankle test.

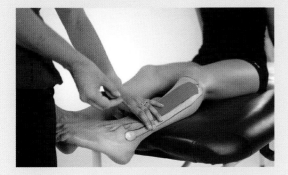

Tape application

Apply the anchor on the lateral tibial condyle with zero tension.

Plantarflex and invert the foot and apply the tape with 25–35% tension onto the target tissue.

Complete the taping by placing the anchor onto the dorsal foot with zero tension. Rub the tape to activate the glue.

When a practitioner is in doubt as to how long to make a piece of tape, it is recommended to err on the side of excess length as muscles operate in units and additional length of tape can provide beneficial stimulus to adjacent muscles.

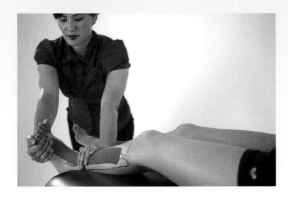

Reassessment

Reassess your client for changes in strength, tonal changes, functional changes and symptoms.

10

KINESIO TAPING
Extensor digitorum

LENGTH TAPING

Client position
The client is in a sitting or supine position with their foot resting off the bed.

Measurement of tape
The client plantarflexes and inverts the foot and a length of tape is measured from the dorsal foot to the tibial condyle.

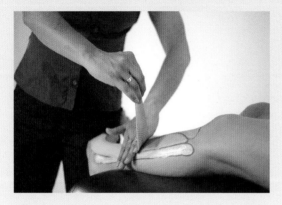

Tape application
Apply the starting anchor with zero tension on the dorsum of the foot. Apply plantarflexion and inversion to the foot with the knee in extension and apply the tape with 15-25% tension over the extensor digitorum muscle. Complete the taping by placing the anchor with zero tension onto the lateral tibial condyle. Rub the tape to activate the glue.

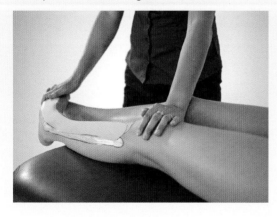

Reassessment
Reassess your client for changes in length, tonal change, function and reported symptoms.

Reassess your client for changes in strength.

10

ANATOMY
Peroneus longus and peroneus brevis

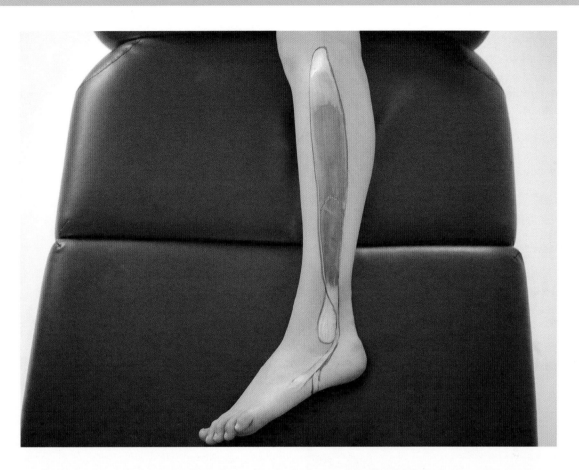

Peroneus longus

Origin:	Head and upper ⅔ of the lateral surface of the fibula
Insertion:	Base of the first metatarsal, lateral aspect of the medial cuneiform
Nerve supply:	Nerve root: L4, L5, S1 Peripheral nerve: superficial peroneal nerve
Function:	Eversion of the foot at the subtalar joint, weak plantarflexion of the foot at the ankle

Peroneus brevis

Origin:	Distal ⅓ of the lateral surface of the fibula
Insertion:	Tuberosity of the fifth metatarsal
Nerve supply:	Nerve root: L4, L5, S1 Peripheral nerve: superficial peroneal nerve
Function:	Eversion of the foot at the subtalar joint, weak plantarflexion of the foot at the ankle

10

MUSCLE TESTING
Peroneus longus and peroneus brevis

STRENGTH BIAS TESTING

Client position

The client is in a sitting or supine position with the ankle in plantarflexion and eversion resting beyond the edge of the bed.

Instruction to client

The client is instructed to plantarflex and evert the foot to the full available range of motion; pointing the foot down and out.

Examiner position and notes

The examiner is positioned in a lunge position standing on the opposite side of the bed to the foot being assessed. The examiner's upper hand should stabilise the tibia above the ankle whilst the lower hand applies resistance to the lateral and plantar surface of the foot in the direction of inversion and dorsiflexion.

Resistance

The examiner applies the resistance by dropping the body weight back onto the back leg. By keeping their arm outstretched, the examiner will be using their full body weight to test rather than just their arm muscles.

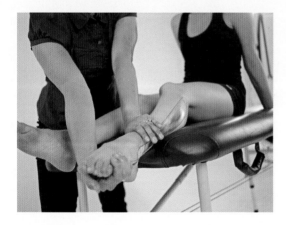

MUSCLE TESTING
Peroneus longus and peroneus brevis

LENGTH BIAS TESTING

Client position
The client is in a sitting or supine position with the ankle resting beyond the edge of the bed.

Instruction to client
The client is instructed to invert and dorsiflex the foot to the maximum available range; pointing the foot up and in.

Examiner position and notes
The examiner should note the amount of effort and whether there are symptoms provoked in order to produce the desired movement. The range and movement strategy should be compared to the non-affected limb. The examiner applies overpressure at the end of range to compare active to passive range as well as assess for end feel.

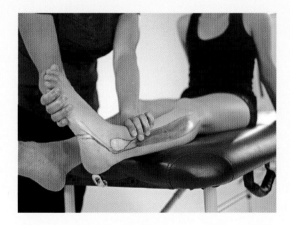

10

KINESIO TAPING
Peroneus longus and peroneus brevis

STRENGTH TAPING

Client position

The client is in a sitting or supine position with the ankle and foot resting off the bed. During the application the client may assist with maintaining the foot position by holding the foot with their hand.

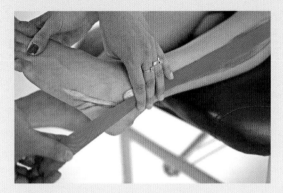

Measurement of tape

The client dorsiflexes and inverts the foot and the practitioner measures a length of tape from the head of the fibula, passing under the foot and onto the dorsal surface of the base of the first metatarsal.

Tape application

Apply the starting anchor on the head of the fibula with zero tension. Dorsiflex and invert the foot and apply the tape with 25–35% tension onto the target tissue. Complete the taping by placing the anchor onto the dorsal foot over the first metatarsal with zero tension. Rub the tape to activate the glue.

When a practitioner is in doubt as to how long to make a piece of tape, it is recommended to err on the side of excess length as muscles operate in units and additional length of tape can provide beneficial stimulus to adjacent muscles.

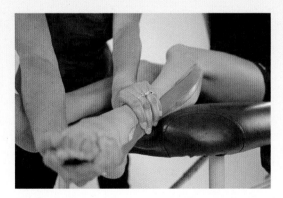

Reassessment

Reassess your client for changes in strength, tonal changes, functional changes and symptoms.

10

KINESIO TAPING
Peroneus longus and peroneus brevis

LENGTH TAPING

Client position
The client is in a sitting or supine position with the foot resting beyond the edge of the bed.

Measurement of tape
The client dorsiflexes and inverts the foot and a length of tape is measured from the first metatarsal under the foot and up to the head of the fibula.

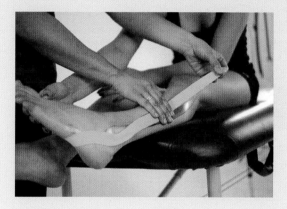

Tape application
Apply the starting anchor with zero tension on the base of the first metatarsal. Apply dorsiflexion and inversion to the foot with the knee in extension and apply the tape with 15–25% tension over the peroneus longus muscle. Complete the taping by placing the anchor with zero tension onto the fibular head. Rub the tape to activate the glue.

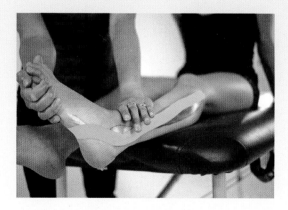

Reassessment
Reassess your client for changes in length, tonal change, function and reported symptoms.

Reassess your client for changes in strength.

10

ANKLE ASSESSMENT SHEET

Clinic: .... Date: ....

Client name: ....

Functional review

Functional limitation	Pre-test measure	Post-test measure

Muscle testing

Tested priority	Muscle	Strength		Length		Comments
		Right	Left	Right	Left	
	Gastrocnemius					
	Soleus					
	Tibialis posterior					
	Tibialis anterior					
	Extensor digitorum					
	Peroneus					

Treatment

Intervention	Re-test measures	Plan

Practitioner: .... Signature: ....

10

BIBLIOGRAPHY

Berryman Reese, N. M. (2012). *Muscle and sensory testing*. Missouri: Elsevier-Saunders.

Berryman Reese, N., & Bandy, W. D. (2010). *Joint range of motion and muscle length testing*. Missouri: Saunders Elsevier.

Calais-Germain, B. (1993). *Anatomy of movement* (12 ed.). Seattle: Eastland Press.

Comerford, M., & Mottram, S. (2012). *Kinetic control: the management of uncontrolled movement*. Sydney, Australia: Elsevier.

Kase, K., Hashimoto, T., & Okane, T. (1998). *Kinesio Taping perfect manual: amazing taping therapy to eliminate pain and muscle disorders*. Albuquerque: Kinesio Taping Association.

Kase, K., & Rock Stockheimer, K. (2006). *Kinesio Taping for lymphoedema and chronic swelling*. Albuquerque: Kinesio Taping Association.

Kase, K., Wallis, J., & Kase, T. (2003). *Clinical therapeutic applications of the Kinesio taping methods*. Albuquerque: Kinesio Taping Association.

Kendall, F. P., McCreary, E., Provance, P., Rodgers, M., & Romanic, W. (2005). *Muscles: testing and function with posture and pain*. Baltimore: Lippincott Williams Wilkins.

Standring, S., Borely, N., Collings, P., Crossman, A., Gatzoulis, M., Healy, J., … Wigley, C. (2008). *Gray's anatomy: the anatomical basis of clinical practice* (S. Susan ed. 40 ed.). London, United Kingdom: Churchill Livingstone Elsevier.

10

Index